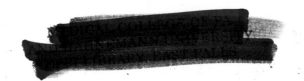
D1205993

Psychopharmacology

Psychopharmacology

An Introduction

Third Edition

RENÉ SPIEGEL

*Pharma Development, SANDOZ Pharma Ltd, Basel, Switzerland
and
Department of Clinical Psychology, University of Basel, Switzerland*

With contributions by R. Markstein and P. Baumann

Translated by Terry Weston

JOHN WILEY & SONS

Chichester · New York · Brisbane · Toronto · Singapore

QV
77
S755p
1996a

Other Wiley Editorial Offices

John Wiley & Sons, Inc., 605 Third Avenue,
New York, NY 10158-0012, USA

Jacaranda Wiley Ltd, 33 Park Road, Milton,
Queensland 4064, Australia

John Wiley & Sons (Canada) Ltd, 22 Worcester Road,
Rexdale, Ontario M9W 1L1, Canada

John Wiley & Sons (SEA) Pte Ltd, 37 Jalan Pemimpin #05-04,
Block B, Union Industrial Building, Singapore 2057

Library of Congress Cataloging-in-Publication Data

Spiegel, Rene
    [Einfuhrung in die Psychopharmakologie. English]
    Psychopharmacology : an introduction / Rene Spiegel ; with
contributions by R. Markstein and P. Baumann ; translated by Terry
Weston. — 3rd ed.
      p.   cm. — (A Wiley medical publication)
    Includes bibliographical references and index.
    ISBN 0 471 95729 1 (alk. paper)
    1. Psychopharmacology.   I. Markstein, R. (Rudolf)   II. Baumann,
P. (Pierre), 1944–   .   III. Title.   IV. Series.
    [DNLM: 1. Psychopharmacology.   QV 77 S755p 1996a]
RM315.S6513   1996
615'.78—dc20
DNLM/DLC
for Library of Congress   95–32202
                                                                    CIP

British Library Cataloging in Publication Data

A catalogue record for this book is available from the British Library

ISBN 0 471 95729 1

Typeset in 10/12pt Times by Dorwyn Ltd, Rowlands Castle, Hants
Printed and bound in Great Britain by Biddles Ltd, Guildford
This book is printed on acid-free paper responsibly manufactured from sustainable forestation,
for which at least two trees are planted for each one used for paper production.

Contents

Preface

Almost 14 years have passed since the first edition of this 'Introduction' was published by Kohlhammer-Verlag, and the second edition was published seven years ago by Hans Huber. The English version of the book was first published by John Wiley & Sons in 1983, who also brought out the second edition in 1989 and have now produced this third English edition.

This third edition essentially retains the structure of the second edition but its contents have been revised, with considerable changes in some parts. Thus, account is taken of the fact that a new generaton of antidepressants has been available for some years, that concepts of the mechanism of neuroleptic action have altered several times and have led to products with new mechanisms of action, and that therapeutic advances have even been recorded in a field which was only recently considered to be hopeless, namely Alzheimer's disease. New methodological developments, especially in the use of imaging techniques in psychiatry, and changes in opinions on the best possible use of psychopharmaceuticals and their duration of use in schizophrenia and depression have been suitably taken into account.

This book is aimed at doctors, psychologists and members of other professions dealing with patients and clients receiving short-term or continuous treatment with psychopharmaceuticals. It presents the desired actions and adverse effects of modern psychopharmaceuticals, their therapeutic uses and limitations, the history of psychopharmacology and research into potential new psychopharmaceuticals. The emphasis lies on the clinical and psychological aspects of psychopharmacology and psychopharmacotherapy, with only a basic consideration of the neurophysiological, molecular biological and neuroendocrinological aspects.

As in the previous editions, it was my aim to write a compact, interesting and easily read book, and to avoid specialist jargon and technical details as far as possible, but without losing sight of my own interests. I hope that the reader will profit from this effort. I thank Mrs A. R. Knecht, who, in addition to her other duties, advanced the production of this new edition through her great personal endeavours. My thanks also go to the management at Sandoz Pharma AG, who have consistently encouraged my activities as a lecturer and author, and the Clinical Psychology students of the Universities of Basel and

Fribourg, whose questions, comments and thoughts have contributed in many ways to the production of this book.

Please note that when referring to doctors, patients, students etc. I have used the pronoun 'he' as an abbreviation of the more politically correct form 'he/she'.

Basel, July 1995

Introduction

The prototypes of modern psychopharmaceuticals were discovered between 1952 and 1958. Since that time the successful treatment (critics of psychopharmacotherapy would say the suppression) of schizophrenic psychoses, depressions, states of tension and anxiety, and other mental disorders has become possible. Clinical psychiatry has changed greatly since 1952: fewer patients are hospitalized long term, care and treatment have largely shifted to outpatient departments, and in parallel with this there has been a tremendous swing to biologically orientated psychiatry.

It is desirable that as many persons as possible should be accurately informed about psychopharmaceuticals in use today: as doctors, psychologists, social workers and lawyers, but also as relatives or friends, we come into contact with patients, clients and neighbours who are being treated with these drugs, and at some time or other we may even find ourselves obliged to take psychopharmaceuticals. The reason and justification for this book are to be seen in that, although several pharmacotherapeutic compendia and excellent handbooks of psychopharmacology (Riederer *et al.*, 1992; Bloom and Kupfer, 1995) as well as specialized monographs and journals are available, there is no compact introduction to the subject readily available that puts the emphasis on psychological and general clinical aspects. This book is intended to close this gap and to help the reader gain a better insight into clinical psychopharmacology, its history, the major problems, the areas of intensive research and the research methods used. In addition, it should convey something of the fascination felt even after many years of personal involvement by the author and many of his colleagues in this dynamic, multidisciplinary field of work with its ever-changing focus.

The following comments apply to the design of our book:

Chapter 1 presents the psychopharmaceuticals known today. Their classification into therapeutic types is discussed together with the major indications (= therapeutic uses), typical actions and side effects of the individual classes of psychopharmaceuticals, and questions of nomenclature and dosage. The chapter contains tables and figures allowing rapid identification and allocation of medicaments on the basis of their names.

Chapter 2 summarizes the historical background of psychopharmacology. Psychopharmaceuticals in the modern sense have certainly existed only for about 40 years, but doctors, priests, medicine men, herbalists and others (witches!) have at all times been interested in chemical agents for the relief or cure of mental suffering. The history of psychiatry shows frequent swings between 'soft' methods of treatment (calming, protection, relief, understanding) and often very violent procedures (drill, intimidation, punishment) which reached their high point in the Europe of the so-called Enlightenment. The history of the discovery of modern psychopharmaceuticals is especially interesting as it illustrates two points: firstly, that drug therapies signify a real advance in psychiatric therapy, and secondly that the interaction of numerous individuals working in untiring research for years plus favourable circumstances were necessary to bring about this advance.

Chapter 3 should primarily be of interest to clinical and experimental psychologists since it deals with the effects of psychopharmaceuticals in healthy subjects. The emphasis is placed on methodological aspects of pharmacopsychology, for example the question of which test methods and mental functions are particularly sensitive to the effects of psychopharmaceuticals. Other topics discussed in this chapter concern the specificity of action of various psychopharmaceuticals in healthy subjects as well as the contribution which experiments in healthy subjects can make to the testing of new, unknown compounds in humans.

Chapter 4 continues the topic of Chapter 3 but is of a more specialized nature since some neurophysiological study methods applicable to humans and their application to psychopharmacology are discussed. Quantitative EEG studies, polygraphic sleep studies and evoked potential experiments are presented. This chapter, which is rather technical in parts, can be omitted by the non-specialist reader without detriment to an understanding of the following chapters.

In *Chapter 5*, which was written together with the biochemist Dr R. Markstein (Basel), we leave the descriptive level of drug effects and present some hypotheses or theories intended to explain the therapeutic effects of these medicaments. The chapter opens with a section on neurobiological terms and models, then deals with so-called mechanisms of action of substances exerting antipsychotic, antidepressant and anxiolytic effects. Among other things, this chapter shows clearly that we are still far from a complete understanding of the therapeutic actions of most psychopharmaceuticals.

On the basis of some examples, *Chapter 6* deals with questions of clinical research in psychopharmacology, i.e. with scientific studies carried out in sick persons. A review is first presented of the major ethical principles of clinical research that have to be taken into consideration today. A section written with the collaboration of PD Dr P. Baumann (Lausanne) discusses the relationships between drug concentrations in the patient's body and the observed clinical effects, and the following section considers the question of which features of a patient allow predictions of the result of treatment with given medicaments. This field, known by the name 'predictor research', has increased greatly in significance in recent years. The larger part of the chapter is devoted to the topic of testing new drugs in patients, with the emphasis on the partially contradictory demands that can arise from efforts to achieve scientifically faultless, relevant trials and out of the doctor's commitment to provide each individual patient with the best possible treatment.

Chapter 7 covers an area of psychopharmacology that has been developed intensively in recent years, namely the effects of drugs on human cognitive processes, especially memory performance. A summary is presented of experimental studies in healthy subjects and psychiatric patients regarding the question of whether certain psychopharmaceuticals administered short or long term can have beneficial or adverse effects on learning and memory functions. In view of the complexity of the topic and the corresponding experiments, it is not surprising to find that only a few of the questions asked can be answered unequivocally. The final sections of this chapter are devoted to attempts to use pharmacological remedies to alleviate dementias, i.e. the pathological changes in cognitive functions and behaviour which frequently occur with advancing age.

Chapter 8 deals with psychopharmacotherapy in the wider context of the treatment of mental disorders. Topics discussed include the necessary and useful duration of drug treatments, as well as the relationship between drug treatment and non-drug therapy. There are now results available from large-scale comparative studies which answer the question 'drug therapy and/or psychotherapy?' for various indications and which can therefore help therapists and their patients to reach rational decisions. Probably the most important lesson emerging from this chapter is the knowledge that there are several possible therapeutic approaches to many mental disorders and that pharmacotherapy and non-drug therapies are not mutually exclusive.

The *Epilogue* deals with some economic aspects of psychopharmacology and also contains thoughts on the topic of how far psychopharmacology has influenced modern psychiatry and psychology in theory and practice.

As the author of an 'Introduction' such as this book, one sees such an incredible flood of original studies and reviews in specialist journals, textbooks, handbooks and congress reports that the desire to write a topical and comprehensive book mainly as a solo effort seems almost presumptive. It has therefore been necessary to present a subjective and often perhaps arbitrary selection of references. Readers who wish to delve deeper into various topics in psychopharmacology are thus referred to the following two standard works:

Neuropsychopharmaka, a handbook of therapy issued in the German language by P. Riederer, G. Laux and W. Pöldinger, which appeared in six volumes in 1992 ff.;

Psychopharmacology: The Fourth Generation of Progress, edited by Floyd Bloom and David Kupfer (1995) in collaboration with the American College of Neuropsychopharmacology.

Both works contain dozens of chapters written in monograph form by leading scientists, and present the state of the art in all fields of psychopharmacology.

Works recommended for practical and therapeutic purposes include the continuously updated therapeutic guide *Psychiatrische Pharmakotherapie* by O. Benkert and H. Hippius (1980 ff.), and the book *Principles and Practice of Psychopharmacotherapy* by Janicak *et al.* (1993).

The most important journals are:

Psychopharmacology: Springer-Verlag (Berlin).
Pharmacopsychiatry: Thieme-Verlag (Stuttgart).
Journal of Psychopharmacology: British Association of Psychopharmacology.
Human Psychopharmacology: John Wiley (Chichester, UK).
Journal of Clinical Psychopharmacology: Williams & Wilkins (Baltimore, USA).
Progress in Neuro-Psychopharmacology and Biological Psychiatry: Pergamon Press (Oxford, UK).
Psychopharmacology Bulletin: NIMH, US Department of Health, Education and Welfare (Washington, DC).

Articles on topics of clinical psychopharmacology also appear in practically all known psychiatry journals (*Acta Psychiatrica Scandinavica, American Journal of Psychiatry, Archives of General Psychiatry, Biological Psychiatry, British Journal of Psychiatry, Nervenarzt, Psychiatry Research*, etc.).

CHAPTER 1

Modern psychopharmaceuticals

1.1 DEFINITION AND CLASSIFICATION

Psychopharmaceuticals are medicaments which can affect the behaviour and subjective state of man and are used therapeutically on account of these 'psychotropic' effects. Apart from psychopharmaceuticals, there are many other substances with psychotropic action, such as alcohol, nicotine, cocaine and heroin, which are characterized as social or addictive products and have no generally recognized therapeutic applications in Western medicine. Analgesics, antiepileptics and members of other drug classes also have direct or indirect actions on subjective state and behaviour but are not considered to be psychopharmaceuticals since they are not used primarily for their psychotropic effects.

Like other medicaments also, psychopharmaceuticals can be classified according to various principles: the chemist characterizes them by their chemical structure, the pharmacologist by their actions in representative biological test systems, the doctor by their therapeutic uses or indications. One such classification according to *clinical criteria* today covers the following classes of psychopharmaceuticals:

– *Neuroleptics* for the symptomatic treatment of schizophrenia and of states of agitation occurring in other psychiatric syndromes; these medicines are also occasionally called antipsychotics or, in English-speaking areas, major tranquillizers.
– *Antidepressants* for the treatment of depression; other names are thymoleptics (= mood stabilizers) or thymeretics (= mood activators) for a more stimulant group of antidepressants. *Lithium*, administered prophylactically, is also counted as a medicament with antidepressant action.
– *Tranquillizers* (synonym: anxiolytics) for the treatment of states of anxiety and tension of varied origins; in English-speaking areas they are also called minor tranquillizers. The sleep-inducing agents (hypnotics) most used today are chemically and pharmacologically closely related to tranquillizers.
– *Psychostimulants* are medicaments which can increase drive and performance. They are also called stimulants or, less commonly today, analeptics. *Nootropics* are meant substances which, especially in the elderly, may have a beneficial effect on cognitive functions without inducing general stimulation.

Table 1.1.   Classification of psychotropic substances

Position of psycho-recognized tropic effect	Medicaments having a therapeutic action	Substances having no recognized therapeutic action
Psychotropic effect = main effect, desired action	*Psychopharmaceuticals* Neuroleptics Antidepressants Tranquillizers, hypnotics Psychostimulants, nootropics	*'Social drugs'*, *'Drugs'* Alcohol Nicotine Cocaine, heroin, etc.
Psychotropic effect = side effect, undesired action	Analgesics Narcotics Antihistamines Antihypertensives Appetite suppressants	

Apart from psychopharmaceuticals there are many other substances that also affect subjective state and behaviour.

- *Analgesics* (pain-killers) and *narcotics*: some of these products not only have an analgesic and anaesthetic action but, especially in larger doses, also have euphoriant and, to some extent, hallucinogenic actions and can therefore be abused.
- Some *antiepileptics* or *anticonvulsants*, i.e., medicaments which prevent epileptic seizures, can have a beneficial effect on the patient's mood and behaviour.
- *Social* drugs such as alcohol and caffeine have little or no therapeutic applications in Western medicine but undoubtedly affect subjective state and behaviour, whilst the use of *'drugs'* such as marijuana, LSD, cocaine and heroin involves risks which, according to today's opinion, outweigh the possible benefits.

Other medicaments, which will not be discussed in the following chapters, have psychotropic actions that are considered to be side effects or adverse effects. Thus, some antihistamines (i.e., products used to counteract allergic reactions) induce fatigue and drowsiness, and the same applies to some myorelaxants. Antihypertensives (i.e., agents reducing blood pressure) such as alpha-methyldopa (Aldomet®) or clonidine (Catapres®) can cause fatigue and depression (Douglas, 1980; Bianchine, 1980; Blaschke and Melmon, 1980).

Many medicaments have indirect psychotropic effects in that they relieve pain and other complaints and so improve well-being. Analgesics, antipyretics and anti-inflammatory products are the best-known examples. They are not considered to be psychotropic substances since they have no direct action on behaviour and subjective state when given in therapeutic doses.

The following sections of this chapter concentrate on psychopharmaceuticals in the sense of Table 1.1, i.e. neuroleptics, antidepressants, tranquillizers and psychostimulants; attention will also be paid to hypnotics and so-called nootropics.

1.2   NEUROLEPTICS

1.2.1   Clinical actions and uses

Neuroleptics are calming medicaments used to counteract marked inner unrest, psychomotor agitation and severe insomnia. These states can arise within the following contexts:

- schizophrenic psychoses, especially catatonic and paranoid forms (ICD F20.0 and F20.2, also F20.9, 23.1, 23.2, etc.);
- mania (ICD F30.1–30.9; F31.1 and 31.2);
- psychotic syndromes as sequelae of organic brain disorders (e.g. old age paranoia, ICD F22.0);
- depressions, especially those with anxious, agitated symptoms (ICD F23.2, F33.3).

Patients treated with neuroleptics find that they have a pronounced calming effect which differs from that of other sedative medicaments (tranquillizers and hypnotics) in two major respects. Firstly, in contrast to most tranquillizers, neuroleptics are not myorelaxant and, unlike sleep inducers, are not narcotic even in high doses. Secondly, apart from their calming action they also act on some psychotic symptoms (hence the expression 'antipsychotics'). The antipsychotic effects of a neuroleptic generally develop only after several days or weeks of treatment. Delusions and ideas of persecution recede and partially or entirely lose their frightening character, while threatening and demanding voices become quieter or are totally silenced. The patient gives the outward impression of being able to cope with his surroundings in a more meaningful and comprehensible manner; his subjective state and behaviour are less 'psychotic'.

The therapeutic effect of neuroleptics consists of a 'calming action on psychomotor agitation, aggressive behaviour, affective tensions, psychotic illusions, psychotic delusions, catatonic behavioural disturbances, and schizophrenic ego-disturbances' (Benkert and Hippius, 1980, p. 86). This descriptive list also expresses the fact that neuroleptics have a primarily sedative action at the start of a treatment and, depending on the dose and product, may also act as sleep inducers. Delay and Deniker (1953), the discoverers of the first neuroleptic, chlorpromazine (see Chapter 2), described the gradual waning of the general calming effect and the appearance of the antipsychotic action during therapy as follows: 'Following a transient, somnolent phase, the patients seem calm, indifferent and distant (in French "lointains"), their bearing is affectively and emotionally neutral and passive, although the intellectual faculties do not appear to be impaired' (Delay and Deniker, 1953, p. 350).

On the basis of studies with healthy subjects and observations in psychotic patients, Degkwitz (1967, p. 108 ff.) distinguishes between **three phases of action** of neuroleptic drugs:

1st phase (duration about one week): the patient tends to doze and sleep, even during daytime, and his drive is clearly reduced; he has no initiative, appears lethargic and indifferent to his environment; there is a certain detachment from worries and anxieties also from those psychotic in nature – interpretative delusions, reference ideas, paranoid–hallucinatory experiences become less frequent.

2nd phase (duration about one week): the neuroleptic–sedative effect recedes whilst the 'antipsychotic' effect is retained; during this phase, despite a pronounced reduction in emotional tension, there is still a danger of undesirable emotional outbreaks and over-reactions.

3rd phase: the general loss of drive is only minor whereas emotional responsiveness is still reduced; the patient seems to be indifferent and shows little spontaneity; the antihallucinatory drug effect is retained and, in many cases, the patient's insight into his illness (and hence also the possibility for psycho- and sociotherapeutic measures) increases.

On the basis of a critical literature survey, Keck *et al.* (1989) came to the conclusion that the course of action of neuroleptics, particularly the onset of their specific antipsychotic action, has still not yet been studied accurately enough. Although there have been hundreds of open trials, such as those of Degkwitz (1967), there have been hardly any controlled studies in which clear distinction was made between the non-specific calming action and the antipsychotic effects of neuroleptics.

1.2.2 The best-known products

More than 40 neuroleptics are currently marketed in German-speaking countries (and a few less in English-speaking areas), the best known of which are presented in Table 1.2. The following explanations apply to this table and the others in this chapter.

Trade names (first column): they are chosen by the manufacturers and are protected as trade marks. They can vary from one country to another for the same compound. Medicaments are mostly designated by their trade names in everyday clinical use.

Non-proprietary or generic names (second column): these give, in abbreviated form, an indication of the chemical structure of a medicament and, since they are the same in all countries, promote international understanding (in publications, congresses, etc.) better than trade names. However, generic names are rarely used in everyday clinical speech.

Table 1.2. A selection of widely used neuroleptics (complete list given in Dietmaier and Laux, 1992)

Trade name	Generic name	Customary oral daily doses (mg)
Ciatyl®, Sordinol®	Clopenthixol	20–300
Dapotum®, Lyogen®, Omca®	Fluphenazine	3–20
Dipiperon®	Floropipamide	80–360
Dogmatil®	Sulpiride	100–600
Fluanxol®	Flupenthixol	1–10
Haldol®	Haloperidol	1–20
Largactil®, Megaphen®	Chlorpromazine	50–600
Leponex®, Clozaril®	Clozapine	12.5–600
Mellaril®	Thioridazine	75–700
Neuleptil®, Aolept®	Periciazine	20–150
Neurocil®, Nozinan®	Laevomepromazine	50–600
Orap®	Pimozide	3–10
Prazine®, Protactyl®	Promazine	50–1000
Risperdal®	Risperidone	4-8mg
Sedalande®	Fluanison	5–80
Truxal®, Taractan®	Chlorprothixene	50–600

Customary oral daily doses (third column): the smallest and largest recommended daily doses of the same medication may differ by a factor of 5–50. These wide dosage ranges are due to the fact that neuroleptics are used in various indications and that their efficacy and tolerability vary from patient to patient. Thus, elderly patients are given the smallest possible neuroleptic doses, whereas large doses may be required in young, acutely psychotic patients.

1.2.3 Differences between different products

In view of the extent of Table 1.2 and the aforementioned number of 40 commercially available neuroleptics, the obvious question is whether so many neuroleptics are actually needed or in what ways the various products differ in clinical use.

Two different aspects have to be considered in the answer: the economic and the scientific. An economical interest to have a variety of products in the market exists on the part of those pharmaceutical companies which have developed and marketed or are developing neuroleptics. As a result, their advertising places the emphasis on the special features and advantages of individual medicaments, even though the differences between many products are clinically not always very relevant. Nevertheless, the differences which actually exist between products with regard to their pharmacokinetic and pharmacodynamic properties are of scientific interest.

Pharmacokinetics (= study of the movements of a medicament): neuroleptics and other medicaments show differences in absorption, distribution, metabolism and excretion as a result of their different chemical structures and pharmaceutical preparations (capsule, tablet, injectable) and in relation to the conditions within the body (see Chapter 6). The transfer of a medicament from the blood into the brain tissue across the so-called brood–brain barrier and its binding to specific brain structures and thus its actions depend on the physicochemical properties of the molecule. The interplay of these and other factors explains why neuroleptics of different chemical structures are not equally effective milligram for milligram (Table 1.2: column 3) and why they differ with regard to onset and duration of action.

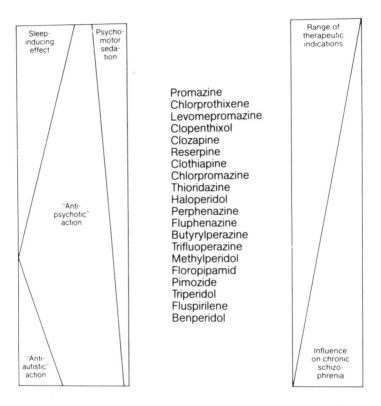

Figure 1.1.   Spectrum of action of neuroleptics. The diagram (after Pöldinger, 1975, reproduced by permission of Editiones 'Roche', Basel) shows the relative sleep-inducing, antipsychotic and anti-autistic potency of a number of neuroleptics. Preparations in the medium range have the most pronounced antipsychotic effect; medicaments in the upper range are above all sleep-inducing and have a sedative action on the psychomotor system. The width of the range of indications is inversely proportional to the therapeutic effect in chronic schizophrenics (right half). This somewhat out-dated diagram is only intended to provide a rough guide, since individual components of action can differ in intensity according to patient, phase of the illness and dose administered

Pharmacodynamics: neuroleptics also differ in their pharmacodynamics, i.e., their pharmacological and clinical profiles of action. Rough distinction is made between highly sedative, hypnotic neuroleptics (e.g. clopenthixol, levomepromazine) and other products with weaker initial sedative action (e.g. fluphenazine and haloperidol). Sedative neuroleptics are prescribed for states of major internal and external unrest, often combined with insomnia, whereas the less sedative neuroleptics are preferred for patients suffering from delusions and hallucinations but in whom heavy sedation is undesirable.

Some 20 years ago, Pöldinger (1975) sought to classify neuroleptics on the basis of their spectrum of clinical actions. His classification (Fig. 1.1) illustrates the fact that neuroleptics do not have a uniform type of action and are therefore not entirely interchangeable one with another.

All neuroleptics have a certain antipsychotic effect although this is not equally strong in all compounds of the group. The neuroleptics listed in the medium range of the Pöldinger diagram have the most pronounced effect on hallucinations, delusions and schizophrenic emotional disturbances. Certain preparations have, in addition, a so-called antiautistic action; i.e., they can exert a favourable drive-enhancing effect in patients with 'negative symptoms' who live a withdrawn, lethargic existence. In the case of these neuroleptics there is no sleep-inducing effect, not even in the initial phase, and their psychomotor sedative effect is of little importance.

Thanks to their different patterns of action, neuroleptics can be individually selected for use in patients displaying differing symptoms. In the case of disturbed, agitated patients representing a danger to themselves and to their surroundings, the doctor will generally choose a medicament having a pronounced sedative and initially sleep-inducing effect, whereas for withdrawn, chronic schizophrenics who cut themselves off from the outside world he will tend to select a preparation having an antiautistic effect. Despite the very varied supply, most doctors restrict themselves to using just a very few neuroleptics with which they had become familiar during their training and clinical activities. A polypragmatic approach constantly making different choices of medicaments from the vast selection is generally frowned upon.

1.2.4 Side effects ('adverse effects') of neuroleptics

The clinical choice of a neuroleptic is not only determined by the diagnosed illness and the prevailing symptoms, but also on the basis of what side effects the treating doctor regards as being acceptable in each individual case. Neuroleptics are not only strong acting with respect to their desired effects, but also with respect to their undesirable actions, known as side effects. Table 1.3 provides a summary of the commonest side effects of neuroleptics.

In general, the sedating, initially hypnotic neuroleptics, especially in larger doses, often induce vegetative side effects such as orthostatic hypotension, mostly accompanied by acceleration of pulse rate, modifications of myocardial activity that are revealed in the ECG (electrocardiogram), sweating, dry mouth and sometimes impaired sexual function, especially in men. In contrast, neuroleptics having a pronounced antipsychotic action often lead to extrapyramidal motor symptoms, namely dyskinesias (disturbed movements), iatrogenic (= treatment-induced) Parkinsonoid states and, after prolonged use, tardive dyskinesias (see Section 1.2.5). The 'atypical' neuroleptic clozapine is an exception to this rule since it exhibits marked antipsychotic activity associated with a spectrum of side effects more typical of a sedating, weakly antipsychotic neuroleptic (Baldessarini and Frankenberg, 1991). Irrespective of the type of action, neuroleptics may also trigger adverse hormonal shifts (elevation of prolactin levels) and often, as a result, amenorrhoea and (transient) sterility, breast enlargement (gynaecomastia) and lactation.

In view of the large number of potential adverse effects, the benefits and risks of neuroleptic treatment have to be carefully weighed against each other in each individual patient: the unrestricted prescription of these medicaments is just as unwarranted as total abstinence from medication. Questions of risks and benefits also apply to the discontinuation of neuroleptic therapy, which is desirable at the earliest possible opportunity (see Chapter 8, pp. 216–220).

1.2.5   Neuroleptics and tardive dyskinesias: unanswered questions

Tardive dyskinesias are motor disturbances which sometimes arise following long-term treatment with neuroleptics. The first symptoms to appear are generally rolling and gyratory movements of the tongue. These are followed by sucking and smacking movements of the lips and, finally, the trunk and extremities may also be affected. The dyskinesias disappear entirely during sleep and subside during wakefulness when the parts of the body involved are moved intentionally, e.g. during talking, eating or writing.

Opinions vary as to the incidence and causes of tardive dyskinesias and their precise connection with the use of neuroleptics. Estimates of their incidence extend from 0.5% to 56% of all chronically hospitalized psychiatric patients – a discrepancy which is attributed above all to the differences in criteria governing the selection of patients for various investigations and to heterogeneous assessment criteria (Kane and Smith, 1982). Tardive dyskinesias may arise during treatment with neuroleptics, but are also observed months or years after the medicament has been discontinued. Tardive dyskinesias are more commonly seen in older patients, although motor disturbances in varying forms are in any event more frequent in advanced age (Varga *et al.*, 1982). Moreover, older patients being treated with neuroleptics generally have a longer history of illness and drug therapy than do younger patients. Some authors take the view that the cumulative neuroleptic dose over a period of time (and not the duration of treatment) represents the decisive risk factor for the appearance of tardive dyskinesias. However, this

Table 1.3. Side effects of neuroleptics (see Hinterhuber and Haring, 1992)

Vegetative disorders[a] (particularly with sedative–hypnotic neuroleptics)
- Decrease in blood pressure, especially on standing up (= orthostatic hypotension)
- Acceleration of pulse rate
- Modification of myocardial activity (ECG changes)
- Sweating, dry mouth, constipation
- Impotence, ejaculation disorders, anorgasmia

Extrapyramidal motor disorders (particularly with neuroleptics having a pronounced antipsychotic action)

Early dyskinesia (uncontrolled movements which may arise at the commencement of therapy)
- Spasms of the tongue, visual spasms, pharyngospasms
- Grimacing, stiff neck, trismus
- Gyratory and rotatory movements of the upper extremities

Neuroleptic Parkinsonoid (after several weeks' treatment)
- Restriction of motor movement (akinesia)
- Loss of facial expression (hypomimia), festinating gait
- Increased muscle tension (rigor); trembling (tremor)

Acathisia (after prolonged treatment)
- Restlessness, inability to remain seated
- Urge to move continuously

Tardive dyskinesia (after prolonged treatment and particularly in older patients)
- Involuntary chewing, smacking of lips, swallowing and rolling movements of the tongue
- Gyratory and flailing movements of the extremities

---

[a] The *neuroleptic malignant syndrome* (NMS, see Shalev and Munitz, 1986), a rare but very hazardous complication of neuroleptic treatment, is also counted among the vegetative disorders but may also occur after the use of neuroleptics with pronounced antipsychotic action. This syndrome is characterized by immobility, rigidity, tremor, greatly elevated body temperature (= hyperthermia), accelerated pulse, bouts of sweating and white blood count shifts. Figures for the incidence of NMS vary from 0.4% to 1.4% of all patients treated with neuroleptics (Pope *et al.*, 1986); young men are affected relatively more frequently (Kellam, 1990).

view has also been contradicted on the basis of empirical studies (Bergen *et al.*, 1992).

It has been found repeatedly that those patients tending to suffer more from extrapyramidal side effects in the earlier stages of neuroleptic treatment, and thus requiring appropriate concomitant medication (anticholinergics), tend to exhibit more tardive dyskinesias in later years. It is as yet unclear whether this relationship is attributable to a long-term unfavourable effect of anticholinergics or to other factors. In discussing tardive dyskinesias it must also be considered that older authors (e.g. Bleuler, 1911) had found that movement disorders of all types can be part of the pathological spectrum of the disease itself in unmedicated chronic schizophrenics.

Furthermore, it has still to be established to what extent tardive dyskinesias can remit spontaneously and whether some neuroleptics tend to lead to dyskinetic symptoms more than others. Whilst some tardive dyskinesias may be suppressed by renewed administration of neuroleptics, or by increasing their dosage, this does not solve the problem, but merely postpones and possibly augments it. As yet there exist no effective therapy and/or safe prophylactic measures against what are, for many patients, very unpleasant late consequences of neuroleptic treatment (Jeste and Wyatt, 1982).

1.3 ANTIDEPRESSANTS

1.3.1 Clinical actions and uses

Antidepressants are medicaments used to treat depression, i.e., states of severe dejection lasting for weeks or months. The term 'depression' does not designate a single disease but a syndrome which needs to be characterized more precisely on the basis of the prevailing symptoms present and taking the patient's prior history into account. On the basis of the patient's clinical status, differentiation is made between inhibited and agitated forms of depression; states of depression that are almost exclusively expressed in the form of physical complaints and symptoms are termed vegetative, somatized or masked depressions.

Antidepressants are primarily prescribed for their mood-elevating action, which generally develops after several days of treatment and often only after some weeks. The expressions 'thymoleptic' (= mood-stabilizing medicament) and 'thymeretic' (= mood-activating medicament) designate two antidepressant groups that differ partially in their pharmacological and clinical actions. Neither thymoleptics nor thymeretics act to improve mood or produce euphoria in healthy, non-depressed subjects, so that in this respect their mood-lightening effect can be considered depression-specific.

A major indication for antidepressants is endogenous depression (Fig. 1.2) which, by definition, has its origin neither in a physical cause nor in a psychologically traceable development or cause. In the case of so-called psychogenic depression, on the other hand, antidepressants are of only secondary importance; in such cases therapy should primarily be based on psychotherapeutic procedures.

Combined pharmacotherapeutic and psychotherapeutic approaches are also successful in psychogenic depression (see Chapter 8). In the case of somatogenic depression, which by definition is based on a physical illness, causal therapy is wherever possible directed at the underlying physical ailment, antidepressants possibly being used to provide an additional symptomatic relief.

Thymoleptics and thymeretics are not 'happy pills', nor are they euphorics. In the case of endogenous depression there is a balancing out of pathological low mood, an effect which is normally obtained in two to three weeks or even longer in many cases. As is the case in patients suffering from psychogenic depression, the first effect to become apparent in endogenous depression is the calming one, with the result that anxiousness, unrest and sleep disturbances can be reduced quickly and hence the patient's confidence in the treatment increases. Drugs which may be stimulating or cause euphoria in healthy volunteers, such as amphetamine, alcohol or cocaine, are not suitable for use as antidepressants.

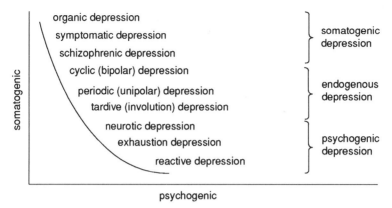

Figure 1.2. Nosological classification of depression. The scheme (Kiel-holz, 1979) differentiates depressive disorders according to their causes and not their clinical manifestations. For example, organic, periodic and reactive depressions may occur both as inhibited and as agitated forms. Depressions are characterized by mental and physical symptoms. The mental symptoms include profound sadness, anxiety, loss of drive (or inner unrest, agitation), suicidal thoughts, self-reproach and feelings of guilt, while the physical symptoms include insomnia, fatigue, loss of appetite, loss of sexual drive and somatic complaints of all types

If an antidepressant is discontinued too early in a patient whose depression has subsided under pharmacotherapy, rapid and serious relapse may result. This indicates that, whereas antidepressants may suppress a depressive phase, they cannot definitely end – and hence cure – it. The attenuation of depressive symptoms is thus not a sufficient criterion for withdrawing drug therapy (Chapter 8, p. 227 ff.). The decision as to when an antidepressant may be discontinued is thus often difficult – especially since the majority of preparations can have pronounced and very unpleasant side effects for the patient (see Section 1.3.4).

1.3.2   The best-known products

There are about 30 antidepressants marketed in most European countries at present (fewer in the USA), differing in their pharmacokinetic and pharmacodynamic properties. The best-known products are listed in Table 1.4. In clinical terms distinction is made between initially sedative, drive-neutral and activating antidepressants. Initially sedative antidepressants such as amitriptyline and doxepine are prescribed primarily for depressions with anxious-agitated symptoms, and act initially to calm and promote sleep; their mood-lightening effect develops later. Weakly sedative and drive-enhancing antidepressants (e.g. nortriptyline, desipramine, fluoxetine) are prescribed when sedation of the patient is not indicated or is undesirable (Fig. 1.3). Products that have been introduced in the last 10 years are generally characterized by better tolerability and greater safety.

Table 1.4. A selection of well-known antidepressants (for complete list, see Dietmaier and Laux, 1993)

Trade name (UK and US)	Generic name	Customary oral daily doses (mg)
Agedal®*	Noxiptiline	75–450
Anafranil®	Clomipramine	50–300
Manerix®	Moclobemide	150–600
Prozac®	Fluoxetine	10–60
Insidon®	Opipramol	150–300
Ludiomil®	Maprotiline	75–200
Aventyl®	Nortriptyline	30–100
Noveril®*	Dibenzepine	120–720
Pertofran®*	Desipramine	50–300
Seropram®	Citalopram	20–60
Seroxat®	Paroxetine	20–60
Sinequan®	Doxepin	75–300
Surmontil®	Trimipramine	50–400
Tofranil®	Imipramine	75–200
Tolvon®	Mianserin	10–60
Molipaxin® (UK), Desyrel® (US)	Trazodone	75–200
Tryptizol®, Amyline® (UK), Elaril®, Endep® (US)	Amitryptiline	75–300
Vivalan®*	Viloxazine	150–200

* Not currently marketed

Lithium is a substance with a prophylactic action against manic and depressive episodes occurring in the context of endogenous depressions. In contrast to the antidepressants described so far, lithium is not a complex synthetic compound, but a metal found in nature in the form of a number of salts. Lithium has an important place in the treatment of emotional psychoses since it can not only be used against manias and for secondary prophylaxis of some depressions, but can also suppress or at least attenuate the phasic occurrence of certain schizoaffective psychoses. Under lithium medication, the intervals between the individual episodes gradually become longer and the protection against relapse becomes all the more pronounced, the longer lithium is regularly taken. This effect is usually observed after a minimum of 6 months' treatment (for details, see Baldessarini, 1985, Chapter 3).

1.3.3 How effective are antidepressants?

It is not always easy to assess the success of antidepressant treatment accurately since depression very often tends to spontaneous healing or remission. Cyclic and periodic forms of endogenous depression follow a phasic pattern: the depressive episode lasting weeks or months, can, in the bipolar form, shift into mania or there is a gradual lightening of the depression, as may be observed in the unipolar forms. The depressions of middle and old age (involutional and late depressions) are also subject to spontaneous remission or healing even though the tendency to chronicity is intensified and the risk of recurrence of depression is greater (review by Jablensky, 1987). Psychogenic

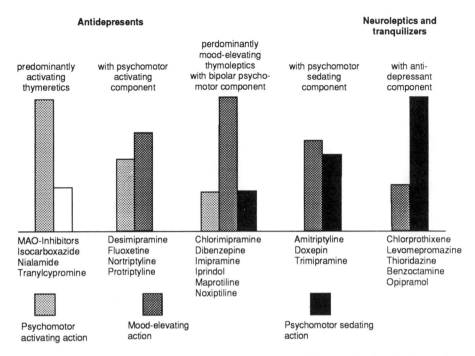

Figure 1.3. Spectra of action of antidepressants. The diagram (modified after Pöl-dinger, 1975, reproduced by permission of Editiones 'Roche', Basel) shows some typical medicaments which are used to treat depression. The drive-enhancing drugs on the left with little or no sedative action are mainly used in inhibited forms of depression. The neuroleptics and tranquillizers with some antidepressant properties on the right are used in patients with anxious–restless forms of depression. In the middle are the 'classic' antidepressants with, relatively speaking, the most pronounced mood-elevating effect

MAO inhibitors = monoamine oxidase inhibitors (see Chapter 5)

depression often subsides when the exterior (social, familial) or internal (psychodynamic) surroundings of the patient change, whereas somatic depression is generally also relieved when the physical cause is eliminated. In the individual case it is consequently often difficult to distinguish between a cure *post hoc* or *propter hoc*: has the antidepressant agent contributed to the shortening of the depressive phase, or would it have subsided spontaneously?

The difficulties associated with a precise assessment of the success of treatment in each individual case are also reflected to some extent in the published results of controlled clinical studies with antidepressants in larger groups of patients. Controlled trials, i.e., comparisons between an active product such as an antidepressants and placebo (a medicament containing no active ingredient), do not always produce the expected results (Table 1.5). According to an early review by Morris and Beck (1974), placebo was therapeutically equal to the studied antidepressant in 31 of 88 published comparative trials, i.e., in 35% of

Table 1.5. Efficacy of antidepressants (Controlled studies against placebo: results of 88 comparative trials, modified from Morris and Beck, 1974, Archives of General Psychiatry 30, 667–674. Copyright 1974, American Medical Association)

	Hospitalized patients		Outpatients		Mixed groups		Total	
	Better than placebo	Not better	Better than placebo	Not better	Better than placebo	Not better	Better than placebo	Not better
Imipramine	23	15	6	4	1	1	30	20
Desipramine	3	2	1	0	0	0	4	2
Amitriptyline	7	4	7	2	0	0	14	6
Nortriptyline	4	3	1	0	0	0	5	3
Protriptyline	1	0	2	0	0	0	3	0
Doxepin	1	0	0	0	0	0	1	0
Total	39	24	17	6	1	1	57	31

The figures correspond to the number of comparative, placebo-controlled clinical studies in which the superiority of the antidepressant in question over placebo was demonstrated or could not be demonstrated.

all studies. With these figures it also has to be considered that trials with a 'negative' outcome (no significant difference between active product and placebo) have a much smaller chance of being published than trials with a 'positive' outcome.

It is thus understandable why some authors previously doubted the efficacy of antidepressants in general (Welner *et al.*, 1980) or the advantages of newer antidepressants compared to 'classical' products (Song *et al.*, 1993). However, the great majority of doctors and scientific authors consider that the efficacy of first-generation antidepressants (imipramine, amitriptyline, nortriptyline) has been proved beyond a shadow of a doubt, and that efficacy has also been demonstrated for newer products such as trazodone or fluoxetine. Nevertheless, about one third of all depressed patients are considered refractory to therapy, i.e., do not respond to adequate doses of antidepressants within four weeks (Möller, 1991).

Methodological questions regarding the proof of efficacy of psychopharmaceuticals will be discussed in more detail in Chapter 6.

1.3.4 Side effects of antidepressants

The most common side effects of the older antidepressants, especially those of the sedative type, are vegetative and are mostly due to the anticholinergic action of these products: dry mouth, difficulties of visual accommodation, constipation, impotence in men as well as dizziness, increased sweating and palpitations. Of medical significance, especially in older patients, are decreases in blood pressure going as far as orthostatic collapse, delirium (state of confusion with disorientation in time and space) after overdosage, and heart function disorders (Table 1.6).

The side effects of antidepressants, sometimes very unpleasant, often lead patients to interrupt their treatment or to reduce the drug dose, which involves

Table 1.6.   The most common side effects of antidepressants

Mental symptoms
- Tiredness, pronounced daytime sedation; sleep disturbances
- Delirium (following overdosage, particularly in elderly patients)

Somatic symptoms
- Dry mouth, bad taste in the mouth, constipation
- Urinary retention, impotence
- Accommodation disorders (difficulty in near–far focusing of the eyes)
- Orthostatic hypotension, collapse (in elderly patients)
- Dizziness, headaches, palpitations
- Increased sweating

Complications
- Switch from depression to mania (in bipolar depressions)
- Attempted suicide (particularly with drive-enhancing antidepressants)

---

a great risk in view of the high relapse rate and danger of suicide in depression. The newer antidepressants such as trazodone, fluoxetine and other serotonin uptake inhibitors as well as moclobemide are characterized by better tolerability and lower toxicity, and are therefore preferred in the treatment of outpatients and elderly patients (Rudorfer and Potter, 1989). Nausea, headaches and weight loss are the most frequent side effects of these products.

Unfortunately *lithium* also is not devoid of undesired effects. A fine tremor often becomes apparent at the beginning of, and during therapy. In addition some patients complain of nausea, bloating and other gastrointestinal disorders (Schon, 1989). Thirst, polyuria (increased excretion of urine) and muscular weakness are not unusual and, although disturbances of thyroid and possibly kidney function are not common, they call for regular check-ups for the patient receiving lithium. Weight gain is another side effect of lithium; about 20% of all long-term patients gain 10 kg and more in weight. Since lithium has a narrow therapeutic range (i.e., the range between the therapeutically effective and the toxic dose) the concentration of the substance in the patient's blood has to be regularly monitored (Vestergaard *et al.*, 1988).

The antiepileptic agent carbamazepine (Tegretol®) has for many years been discussed as an alternative to lithium since it also has an antimanic effect and prophylactic activity against depression, with possibly better tolerability. However, carbamazepine has not yet been proven to be superior to lithium, and its precise indications have not been adequately defined (Prien and Gelenberg, 1989), so that it is mostly reserved for those patients who do not tolerate lithium or who do not respond to it.

1.4   TRANQUILLIZERS AND HYPNOTICS

1.4.1   Clinical actions and uses

Tranquillizers are medicaments with a calming action that are used in states of unrest, anxiety and tension of all types. The tranquillizers used today are almost all derived from the *benzodiazepine* group and have the advantage of lower toxicity and generally better tolerability than the older so-called sedatives of the barbiturate group.

Instead of 'tranquillizers' English-speaking authors also use the word 'anxiolytics' – i.e., anxiety-relieving medicaments. This has been criticized on account of the fact that anxiety states are part of differing psychopathological syndromes, may be qualitatively expressed in different ways, and thus necessitate specific forms of therapy. For this reason the term 'anxiolytic' is held to be too inexact. In respect of the expression 'minor tranquillizers', which also appears in English language literature, it has been said that this only makes a quantitative distinction against the 'major tranquillizers' (neuroleptics) – which corresponds to neither pharmacological nor clinical findings. In the present text we shall use the term 'tranquillizer' which, in its present-day connotation, relates to calming agents belonging to a few specific classes of substances, notably that of the benzodiazepines. Another group of anxiolytic compounds, the so-called beta-receptor blockers (Gastpar and Rimpel, 1993), which are not psychopharmaceuticals in the conventional sense, will be dealt with briefly in Chapter 8.

Whereas neuroleptics and antidepressants are used mainly in 'major psychiatry', i.e., in the treatment of schizophrenia and depression, tranquillizers are mostly used in general medicine for the treatment of neurotic, vegetative, psychosomatic and even purely physical conditions. This multiple usage is promoted by the fact that tranquillizers of the benzodiazepine type have an almost exclusively central action so that vegetative effects (dry mouth, sweating, visual disturbances, urine retention, constipation, fall in blood pressure) which can be unpleasant for patients or even hazardous are practically absent.

Most of the *hypnotics* used today are also benzodiazepines. They differ from tranquillizers mainly with regard to the timing of their action: hypnotics generally have a fast onset of action, but fading after a few hours so that there is no hangover in the form or tiredness and lack of alertness on the following morning. Compared with barbiturates, often used previously as sleeping pills, the modern hypnotics are characterized by greater safety; successful suicide attempts are rare with benzodiazepine derivatives alone.

1.4.2 The best-known products

About 20 benzodiazepines usable as tranquillizers or hypnotics are marketed at present; the best known of these are listed in Table 1.7. Here again there are striking differences between the doses of these products, which can be explained in the same way as for neuroleptics. The benzodiazepine derivatives show few qualitative differences even if the relevant advertising seeks to give a different impression. On the other hand, the time–effect features, i.e. the timing of onset of action and peak action as well as duration of action, mean that it is sensible to use different products for different purposes.

Table 1.7.   A selection of well-known tranquillizers and hypnotics

Trade name (UK and US)	Generic name	Dose (mg)	Use
Adumbran®, Seresta®* (UK), Serax® (US)	Oxazepam	20–150	Tranquillizer
Buspar®	Buspirone	15–30	Tranquillizer
Dalmane®	Flurazepam	15–30	Hypnotic
Euhynos®, Normison®, Tenox®	Temazepam	10–60	Hypnotic
Frisium®	Clobazam	20–60	Tranquillizer
Halcion®	Triazolam	0.25–1.0	Hypnotic
Lexotan®	Bromazepam	3–24	Tranquillizer
Librium® (UK), Limbritol® (US)	Chlordiazepoxide	5–150	Tranquillizer
Nitrados®, Somnite® (UK), Mogadon® (US)	Nitrazepam	5–15	Hypnotic
Restoril®	Temazepam	15–30	hypnotic
Noctamid®	Lormetazepam	0.5–2.0	Hypnotic
Rohypnol®	Flunitrazepam	2–6	Hypnotic
Ativan®	Lorazepam	2–10	Tranquillizer
Tranxene®	Clorazepate dipotassium	10–60	Tranquillizer
Valium®	Diazepam	5–60	Tranquillizer
Xanax®	Alprazolam	0.5–4	Tranquillizer

* Not currently marketed

1.4.3   Tranquillizers or psychotherapy?

What are the accepted indications for tranquillizers? Generally speaking, these medicaments are nowadays given when a patient suffers from anxiety states or symptoms to such an extent that his daily routine is considerably disrupted. It is quite clear from this formulation that the indications for tranquillizers can be less sharply defined than those of the neuroleptics and antidepressants: when can anxiety symptoms be said to so impair daily routine that one can speak of considerable disruption? And who is to determine whether a disruption is considerable or trivial: the patient, the doctor, the relatives?

Like almost all relevant authors, Lader and Petursson (1983) also advise against the long-term use of tranquillizers and emphasize that most anxiety states and phases of insomnia generally last for only a limited period of time; either the acute stress fades or the patient becomes used to the situation (or copes with it successfully), or a spontaneous remission occurs. In many cases the patient can be managed with advice and reassurance, and thus without medicaments.

Many patients with symptoms of anxiety and tension reject psychotherapy out of hand, often using extraneous and rather irrelevant grounds as a pretext. In addition, states of anxiety, tension and other forms of ego pain are frequently somatized; i.e., they manifest themselves in the form of physical complaints. Muscle tension, headaches, gastrointestinal disorders, sleep disturbances and other symptoms are often the physical equivalents of states

Table 1.8. Side effects of tranquillizers (somewhat similar to after-effects of benzo-diazepine hypnotics)

Sedation: feeling of fatigue, drowsiness, inattention
Deterioration of performance: decreased concentration and decreased physical
    capacity; anterograde amnesia (see Chapter 7)
Muscle relaxation, disturbed coordination, ataxia
States of disorientation: mostly in elderly patients
Paradoxical reactions: excitement, increased activity, aggressiveness
Euphoria, withdrawal symptoms, risk of dependency
So-called alcohol potentiation: the sedative action of tranquillizers is potentiated by
    alcohol. Relevant impairments are possible after the combined intake of
    tranquillizer doses and amounts of alcohol which, when taken alone, would
    produce no detectable actions (Mattila, 1984)

---

of psychic tension, and the worries and anxieties of patients are then directed at the physical symptoms, with the result that the original cause recedes into the background and is emotionally relieved. It thus becomes clear why there are broad and major fields of application for tranquillizers outside psychiatry, mainly in internal medicine, in rheumatology, gynaecology and paediatrics. Tranquillizers are therefore often referred to as panaceas, i.e., a cure for everything and everyone – a criticism that is only partly justified in the opinion of many doctors: should counseling or psychotherapeutic measures be ruled out in a patient for extraneous or pertinent inner reasons, then it would not be 'medically ethical' to refrain on reasons of principle from trying to treat the patient with a tranquillizer. It is, however, essential that therapy using medicaments be constantly monitored in order to avoid the development of habituation or dependence.

1.4.4 Side effects of tranquillizers

The normally excellent tolerability of these preparations has contributed greatly to the widespread use of tranquillizers. The commonest side effects (Table 1.8) are tiredness and muscle relaxation and these can generally be avoided by reducing the dose. Ataxia and paradoxical reactions such as irritability and increased activity occasionally arise in the elderly, but are rare in younger patients. Much attention has been focused on the negative effects of benzodiazepines on memory, but the clinical relevance of this amnestic drug action in everyday use is controversial (see Chapter 7).

1.4.5 Dependency on benzodiazepines

With their low toxicity, their action limited almost exclusively to the central nervous system and their other practical advantages (few pharmacokinetic interactions with other medicaments), tranquillizers and hypnotics of the benzodiazepine group apparently represent almost ideal medicaments. However, it is precisely the good tolerability and lack of subjectively unpleasant side effects, that can lead to problems: whereas hardly a single patient wants to take neuroleptics or antidepressants without a clinical need, there is a great risk of tranquillizer abuse. These medicaments have a relaxing and calming action, the world seems friendlier and more harmonious, real personal problems become less pressing. On the other hand, unrest, anxiety and distress reappear quickly and are often intensified after withdrawal of these medicaments, so that it is difficult to give up tranquillizers once the use of them has become a habit.

The problems of withdrawal of tranquillizers and hypnotics have been described in innumerable publications (reviews by Owen and Tyrer, 1983; Griffiths and Sannerud, 1987). Schöpf (1985) produced a compilation of the most common symptoms found after discontinuation of long-term benzodiazepine medication. According to him, the following symptoms arise 'frequently to regularly': dysphoria (ill humour), anxiety, insomnia, muscle pain and twitches, tremor, restlessness, nausea, loss of appetite and weight, headaches, sweating and blurred vision, i.e., to a large extent those symptoms against which the benzodiazepines were prescribed in the first place.

More striking are withdrawal phenomena having no connection with the original symptoms, namely disturbances of perception and sense of reality. These include hypersensitivity to noise, light and other sensory stimuli, as well as distorted perception in the visual, kinaesthetic and acoustic spheres. Disturbances affecting grasp of reality include transient depersonalization and derealization phenomena. Although these disturbances do not arise regularly but, according to Schöpf, 'only' in about 50% of cases, they are unpleasant for those affected, often causing anxiety and low spirits, especially since few doctors are aware of these symptoms and can suitably prepare their patients for tranquillizer withdrawal.

Many regimens intended to prevent the appearance of benzodiazepine dependency or to make the unavoidable withdrawal symptoms more tolerable have been devised and published (Marks, 1988; Sartory and Maurer, 1991). Trials have also been performed to compare abrupt and gradual withdrawal regimens and to assess the appearance of withdrawal symptoms after discontinuing benzodiazepines with long and short half-lives (Busto et al., 1986; Rickels et al., 1990; Schweizer et al., 1990). The results of these trials can be summarized as follows:

(1) Withdrawal symptoms are common after the discontinuation of benzodiazepines following prolonged use, and arise both with abrupt and with gradual withdrawal, and with products having short and long half-lives.

(2) After abrupt discontinuation, the withdrawal symptoms described by Schöpf (1985) are particularly severe and frequent during the first few days but then fade; with gradual discontinuation, the withdrawal symptoms are certainly less frequent but show hardly any decrease with the passage of time.

(3) The subjectively perceived severity of withdrawal symptoms and the readiness to withstand them without recourse to rescue medication vary greatly from one person to another.

(4) The discontinuation of benzodiazepines with a short half-life is particularly difficult and there is a great tendency to use rescue medication after both abrupt and gradual withdrawal.

It is continually being debated as to how far benzodiazepines form an epidemic that should be countered by more specific legislation. On the basis of a representative survey in more than 3000 adult Americans, Mellinger *et al.* (1984) came to the conclusion that only a small percentage of the population (1.6%) can be counted as 'long-term consumers' of these medicaments and that these patients are characterized by the following features: greater age, more women, more mental symptoms, more health problems. Since, according to the results of this survey, most long-term consumers maintain regular contact with their doctor and take their medicine as prescribed, Mellinger *et al.* saw no grounds for alarm or restrictive measures against benzodiazepines. In other respects the therapeutic utility of benzodiazepines is said to be sustained in most patients even during long-term medication so that there is no reason to prejudice patients against these useful medicaments by dramatic appeals or continual warnings (Uhlenhuth *et al.*, 1988). However, it is well known that not all authors share this view (see Allgulander, 1986; Chen and Lader, 1990).

1.4.6   Alternatives to benzodiazepines

In principle, all drugs with damping action on the central nervous system could be used as anxiolytics or hypnotics, but the pharmacological and/or pharmacokinetic properties of most compounds are not appropriate for their therapeutic use:

- As a substance known in almost all cultures, alcohol has only a non-specific sedating action, quickly creates dependency and is quite toxic.
- Opiates and the other natural products discussed in Chapter 2 are toxic and/or quickly create dependency.
- Barbiturates create dependency, have an unsuitable therapeutic safety margin and exhibit adverse interactions with other medicaments.
- Antihistamines which penetrate into the central nervous system have a non-specific sedative action, i.e. they can induce subjectively unpleasant side effects (see Table 1.6).

Since there is a great demand for anxiolytic and hypnotic substances and since the use of benzodiazepines should, in the opinion of many, be restricted, there is still great interest in obtaining effective, safe and non-habituating anxiolytics and hypnotics. The use of low doses of neuroleptics and (sedating) antidepressants has therefore been proposed in cases where a rapid onset of dependency is to be feared with benzodiazepines or where these products are contraindicated for other reasons, as in elderly patients at risk of stumbling and falling. According to the information summarized by Möller (1993a), the clinical results with some low-dose neuroleptics used as anxiolytics are very good, although the potential tardive sequelae of this type of treatment are still poorly known. Positive results have also been obtained with the sedating antidepressant trimipramine, which is used in low doses as a sleeping agent, primarily in elderly patients (Dietmaier and Laux, 1993).

The product buspirone represents another alternative, being an anxiolytic having a novel mechanism of action and which, unlike benzodiazepines, has no anticonvulsant or myorelaxant activities. Although buspirone has anxiolytic activity, it does not induce a spontaneous feeling of relaxation or of well-being and, insofar as clinical experience available allows this conclusion, has less potential to produce dependency than benzodiazepines. Buspirone also differs from benzodiazepines with regard to side effects: sedation, amnesia and ataxia practically do not occur, but the substance can lead to nausea, diarrhoea and, occasionally, headache. The disadvantages of buspirone are its low bioavailability (less than 10%), which can make dosage difficult, and the fact that its anxiolytic action develops only after several days of regular administration. Buspirone is therefore not indicated if rapid anxiolysis is required. On the other hand, it is particularly suitable when therapy is expected to last for a long time. Buspirone is not hypnotic.

1.5   PSYCHOSTIMULANTS AND SO-CALLED NOOTROPICS

1.5.1   Actions and uses of psychostimulants

Psychostimulants are psychically stimulating pharmaceuticals; synonyms are psychotonics, psychoanaleptics, psychic energizers. Using psychostimulants it is possible to prevent or suppress states of exhaustion and feelings of tiredness appearing after great exertion, during long and monotonous activity and following sleep deprivation. Alertness, concentration and enterprise are boosted through the use of psychostimulants and there may be pronounced well-being or even a state of euphoria, particularly after higher doses. The feeling of increased concentration and alertness is not merely subjective in nature; greater performance and improved consistency of performance may also be established objectively.

Despite these happy effects, psychostimulants do not enjoy a good reputation and are only rarely prescribed nowadays. The main reason for this is the potential for abuse of these medicaments in sport (doping) and among drug addicts (intravenously administered amphetamine products, 'speed', etc.). The uncontrolled use of stimulants in large doses can also lead to 'amphetamine psychoses', i.e., states of intense unrest and anxiety associated with delusions and (generally visual) hallucinations. Because of these risks, psychostimulants of the amphetamine type are available strictly on prescription only in almost all countries. Another drawback of known psychostimulants is tachyphylaxis: when used repeatedly, the products quickly lose their effect, so that long-term users are forced to increase the dose and, depending on the duration of use and dose, will go through a very unpleasant withdrawal syndrome in the form of insuperable drowsiness, lethargy or even depression if they want to stop the product temporarily or definitely.

Psychostimulants are used therapeutically in the hyperactive syndrome of children and in narcolepsy. *Hyperactive children* (ICD F90) are characterized by particular inattentiveness, motor unrest, learning disorders, impulsivity and affect incontinence. This severe conduct disorder (also known as hyper-motility and, in the USA, as attentional deficit hyperactivity disorder, ADHD) is often based on perinatal or postnatal brain damage. The preval-ence of ADHD is reported as 3–5% of all school-age children (in the USA); depending on the author, the syndrome is two to nine times more common in boys than in girls (Biedermann, 1991). Interestingly, stimulants do not cause a further increase in unrest in these children but lead to improved attentiveness, longer times spent on the same activity, increased self-control and thus im-proved adjustment to school and home life. This paradoxical effect of stim-ulants is explained by their action in regulating or stabilizing vigilance, and the success rates amount to about 65–75% of all treated children (Wilens and Biedermann, 1992). In the hyperactive syndrome, psychostimulants do not lose their efficacy even after prolonged use. Despite this, their use in central Europe is uncommon, contrary to the situation in the USA, where meth-ylphenidate is the most widely prescribed product, given to about 750 000 children in the 1980s (Barkley, 1990).

Narcolepsy (ICD G 47.4) and other types of hypersomnia are severe distur-bances of vigilance expressed as a sudden and irresistible requirement for sleep during the day, so-called sleep attacks (Aldrich, 1990). Apart from sleep attacks, the classical tetrad of narcolepsy includes cataplexy (sudden loss of muscular tone), sleep paralysis (waking from sleep with the feeling of not being able to move) and hypnagogic hallucinations (images or sequences of images of great apparent reality when falling asleep). Depending on the sever-ity of the illness, the patient drops off to sleep every few minutes or hours even when engaged in activities in which he had interest and joy. Narcoleptic syndromes are nowadays treated symptomatically with certain antidepres-sants and stimulants, often in combination.

1.5.2 The best-known psychostimulants

The best-known products come from the amphetamine group: Dexedrin® (generic name *d*-amphetamine) and Pervitin® (methamphetamine) were par-ticularly used in the 1950s and 1960s as stimulants and also as appetite sup-pressants, but today play hardly any role in medical practice. Ritaline® (methylphenidate) has some relevance: its psychostimulant action is weaker than that of amphetamines and it is apparently less abused than the latter. Since methylphenidate also possesses mild antidepressant activity, in some countries it is used to combat not only narcolepsy and hyperactive syndrome but also mild depressions without suicide risk (Satel and Nelson, 1989). Doctors in many European countries are, however, generally hesitant to prescribe methylphenidate.

1.5.3 Nootropics: medicaments acting on age-related disturbances of brain function

According to a definition by Coper and Kanowski (1983, p. 409), nootropics are 'centrally acting drugs intended to improve higher integrative noetic brain functions such as memory and the ability to learn, perceive, think and concentrate, but for which a specific, uniform mechanism of action is not known'. The expression 'nootropic' has not been adopted everywhere (Coper et al., 1987b) and in many works the old names 'geriatric agents' and 'brain metabolism enhancers' are still used. On the other hand, the older term 'cerebral vasodilators' has been dropped since it derived from an erroneous assumption concerning the mechanism of action of nootropics. The expression 'antidementia agents' is now being increasingly used (see Chapter 7).

What are nootropics and where are they used? Some slowing of sensory, cognitive and motor functions is seen as a normal sign of ageing, but if the deterioration in performance exceeds a certain (poorly defined) threshold, then depending on the school of thought adopted we speak of chronic organic brain syndrome (OBS) of the elderly or, according to more recent nomenclature, of incipient or advanced dementia. Most dementias are caused by cerebrovascular or neurodegenerative disorders, of which Alzheimer's disease is the most common and best known. At present there is no drug therapy available for treating advanced dementia, which is characterized by severe cognitive disorders, changes in behaviour and personality. In contrast, mild cognitive and affective symptoms of incipient senile dementia can be beneficially influenced by some nootropics (Orgogozo and Spiegel, 1987). The actions of these substances are of medical and social significance insofar as they contribute to keeping elderly patients independent for longer so that they can continue to live in their own homes. Particularly good tolerability is expected of nootropics since they have to be taken for months or years by elderly and frequently fragile patients who are often receiving other medical therapies also.

1.5.4 The best-known nootropics

Since the licensing requirements for medicines and thus for 'nootropics' are not equally strict in all countries, each country may have a large number or only a few of these medicaments on the market. In terms of chemical structures and pharmacological actions, the nootropics form a heterogeneous group of compounds whose therapeutic benefits have been a topic of discussion for years.

By converting the verbal assessments of efficacy expressed by the various authors into a score from 0 to 4, Table 1.9 quantitatively summarizes some of the major surveys of nootropic drug efficacy. From this compressed presentation it is first clear that different authors have applied criteria of variable strictness to the literature reviewed and particularly to the products evaluated. Thus, the mean efficacy score is lower for Goodnick and Gershon (1984) than for Wittenborn (1981); i.e., Goodnick and Gershon evaluated the practical benefits of nootropics more critically in general than Wittenborn. On the other hand, one product (Hydergine®, co-dergocrine mesylate) was scored highest throughout: the efficacy of Hydergine® in cognitive and affective disorders of the elderly has been demonstrated in more than 30 placebo-controlled clinical studies. Meanwhile, a summarizing analysis of efficacy has also been published for piracetam (Nootropil®), which indicates statistically confirmed activity as a nootropic agent (Fleischmann, 1990).

New approaches to pharmacotherapy in dementia are discussed in Chapter 7.

1.6 CONCLUDING COMMENTS ON CHAPTER 1

The foregoing sections apply a classification of psychopharmaceuticals based on the major therapeutic uses of these products. However, it should also be emphasized that the boundaries between the substance classes are often not as clear-cut as the terms used might suggest: thus, as already mentioned, low-dose neuroleptics may be used as anxiolytics or for the calming of agitated–depressed patients, and sedative antidepressants are often used in patients with chronic insomnia. In large doses or in combination with neuroleptics, tranquillizers of the benzodiazepine type can also be usefully applied in patients with acute schizophrenia (Lingjaerde, 1991; Wolkowitz and Pickar, 1991). The boundaries between the classes of psychopharmaceuticals are fluid and some of the newer medicaments cannot be clearly allocated to any of the prior categories. An example here is Dogmatil® (sulpiride), shown in Table 1.2: sulpiride is considered to be a weak neuroleptic but has no anticholinergic effects and thus does not induce the side effects typical for other weak neuroleptics (sedation, vegetative symptoms). In addition, sulpiride has a beneficial action on atypical depressions (see Langer and Schönbeck, 1983) and is also prescribed in internal medicine for so-called psychosomatic disorders.

Difficulties may arise when supposedly typical features of the actions of products in a given therapeutic category are blindly applied to new substances having the same indications. The history of the neuroleptic Leponex® (clozapine) illustrates this point: for years the empirical rule was that potent antipsychotic neuroleptics have marked extrapyramidal motor side effects, and many clinicians believed that a neuroleptic with vegetative and marked sedative effects could not be a very effective antipsychotic. When the clinical actions of clozapine were reported in the late sixties (marked antipsychotic efficacy combined with some anticholinergic side effects but no extrapyramidal symptoms), experts were very sceptical and it took several comparative studies between clozapine and other neuroleptics to eradicate the false general assumption that

Table 1.9. The efficacy of nootropics according to six major reviews

Trade name(s)	Generic name	Yesavage et al. (1979) 102, strict[a]	Reisberg et al. (1981) 96, n.d.[a]	Wittenborn (1981) 156, strict[a]	Branconnier (1983) 74, n.d.[a]	Goodnick and Gershon (1984) 140, n.d.[a]	Orgogozo and Spiegel (1987) 134, strict[a]
Cetal®	Vincamine	n.i.	n.i.	n.i.	1	0	n.i.
Cyclospasmol®	Cyclandelate	1–2	1–2	1–2	n.i.	0	1–2
Encephabal®	Pyritinol	1	n.i.	n.i.	1–2	n.i.	1
Pronestyl® (UK), Procainamide®, Durules® (US)	Procaine	n.i.	1	n.i.	n.i.	0–1	0
Helfergin®, Lucidril®	Meclophenoxate	n.i.	n.i.	0	1	1	n.i.
Hydergine®	Co-dergocrine mesylate	3	2–3	3–4	3	2	3
Nootrop®, Nootropil®	Piracetam	n.i.	1–2	1–2	1	1	1–2
Panergon®, Panervan® (UK), Rybarvin® (US)	Papaverine	1	1	1	n.i.	0	n.i.
Praxilene®, Dusodril®	Naftidrofuryl	2–3	2	1–2	1–2	0	1
Stugeron®	Cinnarizine	1–2	n.i.	n.i.	n.i.	0	n.i.
Duvadilan® (US)	Isoxsuprine	1	1–2	n.i.	n.i.	0	n.i.
Trental®	Pentoxyfylline	1	n.i.	n.i.	n.i.	n.i.	1

[a] Number of individual studies taken into consideration in the review in question and the strictness of the criteria applied to the evaluation of the individual studies (n.d. = criteria not defined in detail).
Key for evaluating the products (n.i. = no information on the product in question):
0 = No or no valid positive results.
1 = Few positive or only contradictory results.
2 = Positive results but of doubtful clinical relevance.
3 = Clinically relevant results reported.
4 = Clinically relevant *and* psychometrically objectivized results.

neuroleptics with strong antipsychotic effects must provoke extrapyramidal motor symptoms (Kane *et al.*, 1988; McKenna and Bailey, 1993).

Stereotyped assumptions of this type have a particularly invidious action in drug research since they can lead to sterile replication of existing patterns of pharmacological activity: the continued development of more and more antidepressants with 'amine-potentiating' and anticholinergic actions in the 1970s and 1980s provides an example of this. On the other hand, stereotyped assumptions may also prevent new developments: although the therapeutic potential of stimulant compounds is by no means exhausted (Chiarello and Cole, 1987), the search for novel performance-enhancing medicaments is overshadowed by the fear that all stimulants will bring the risks known for amphetamine derivatives (abuse, tachyphylaxis, risk of addiction). The history of psychopharmacology, which will be discussed in the next chapter, shows clearly that therapeutic advances can occasionally be made precisely where least expected and that false hypotheses can, by roundabout and wrong routes, lead to the correct answers and new, useful medicaments.

CHAPTER 2

The history of psychopharmacology

2.1 INTRODUCTION

When was psychopharmacology born? Is it, in fact, possible to pinpoint the date of its birth? Reference to some historical accounts yields a variety of replies: Hordern (1968) begins his history of psychopharmacology with Emil Kraepelin who, in 1882, embarked on a series of trials on various psychoactive substances in the laboratory of Wilhelm Wundt in Leipzig and who is looked upon as the founder of pharmacopsychology (see Chapter 3). Caldwell (1978) dates the birth of psychopharmacology as being 1951, with 'the utilization of drugs in restoring or maintaining mental health and for exploring the mind'. This year saw the discovery of the effect of chlorpromazine. In the opinion of Sack and De Fraites (1977) the modern era of psychopharmacology begins with the observation by J. Cade of the antimanic effect of lithium at the end of the 1940s.

We do not know when, and in what context, the term 'psychopharmaceutical' (psychopharmakon) was first used. In the transitional period between the Middle Ages and modern times – in 1548 to be precise – a collection of prayers of consolation and prayers for the dead was published under the title *Psychopharmakon, hoc est: medicina animae*. This was written by Reinhardus Lorichius of Hadamar, a member of the landed gentry of the German 'Land' of Hesse. Here the term 'psychopharmakon' relates to a spiritual medicine, which is to be used in miserable and hopeless situations of life.

Apart from psychopharmaceuticals in the spiritual sense, at all times and in most cultures psychotropic plant drugs have played a role in religious practices, magic rituals and healing. The substances best known in Europe and the Mediterranean area are *opium*, *hashish* and *hellebore*; in the medicine of India and other southeast Asian countries, *rauwolfia* has traditionally been of great significance (Wittern, 1983).

2.2 PSYCHOPHARMACOLOGY IN THE ANCIENT WORLD AND MIDDLE AGES

2.2.1 The most important substances

Opium is the solidified juice of the opium poppy (*Papaver somniferum*), which was cultivated even in prehistoric times: poppy residues have been found in Stone Age lake dwellings in northern Italy and Switzerland. The Sumerians living in the Tigris–Euphrates area 3000 years BC planted poppies and obtained its juice, which they called 'lucky' or 'happy', an indication that they well knew the mood-lightening, euphoriant action of opium. Finds from the second millennium BC in Asia Minor, Cyprus, Mycenae and Egypt show opium as a smoking material and healing agent; depending on the context, the opium poppy also stands as a symbol of fertility, sleep, death or immortality.

The sleep-inducing and analgesic actions of opium are described in the best-known medical writings from ancient times, the *Corpus Hippocraticum* and Galen's *Opus*. There is no mention of the risk of addiction, although Galen warns against overdosage and advises that the action of opium be attenuated by the addition of other substances; opium (under the name of *laudanum*) was almost always contained in the many variants of *theriak*, a compounded panacea known best in the Middle Ages.

Paracelsus, writing in the first half of the sixteenth century, called opium the philosopher's stone of immortality. In European medicine of the sixteenth and seventeenth centuries it found wide use as an analgesic and sedative, although opium abuse had become known from journeys of discovery to the Near and Far East. In the early nineteenth century a German pharmacist, Friedrich Sertürner, isolated the particularly active morphine from natural opium and this became widely used in military medicine as an analgesic and anaesthetic in the latter half of that century.

The resin of hemp (*Cannabis sativa*) is known as *hashish*; in general, the term marihuana covers the dried flowers, bracts and upper leaves of the female hemp plant. The intoxicating action of hashish was known to some peoples of ancient times but, except for its use against ear diseases, cannabis was never used in medicine. Hashish was very widely consumed in the Islamic world of the Middle Ages and even in Europe this intoxicant repeatedly appeared, although sporadically and often as a modish fad. However, hashish never played a recognized role in medicine and thus does not count as a psychopharmaceutical agent.

Hellebore root has been the psychopharmaceutical agent *par excellence* at various times. It is a plant of the Ranunculaceae family, the roots of which, as we now know, contain several glycosides, some of them rather toxic. White hellebore was traditionally used as an emetic (Vomitivum) and black helle-bore as a laxative (Purgativum); in both cases the guiding principle was that a mental illness has a physical cause that can be treated by physical effects, preferably by the removal of pathogenic substances from the body. Hellebore was so well known that it was mentioned in classical comedies: Aristophanes (Wasps, 1489) uses 'go drink hellebore' to mean 'you're crazy', and Plautus (Pseudolus, 1185) also means much the same when he says that some people should drink hellebore, i.e., should see a psychiatrist.

Hellebore found a very wide range of use: mania, melancholy, inflammation of the brain and mental retardation were included among the indications just as much as epilepsy, hydrophobia, violent temper and crazy ideas (Wittern,

1983, p. 14 ff.). White and black hellebore could also be combined and there is no difficulty in believing the ancient authors when they state that the simultaneous emetic and laxative treatment has a good calming effect! The use of hellebore declined in the nineteenth century since the product is difficult to dose and can induce seizures in large doses.

Decoctions of *Rauwolfia serpentina* (snakeroot) roots were traditionally used by Indians as a remedy for snake bites and also as a calming agent in some mental illnesses. The plant and its properties were known in Europe in the sixteenth and seventeenth centuries, so that rauwolfia made a successful career as a remedy for almost everything, but without finding a preferential position in psychiatry. Only in the early 1950s, after the active constituents of rauwolfia were discovered and produced in pure form, did the highly sedative and hypotensive alkaloid reserpine find transient use as an agent to control schizophrenic psychoses (Frankenburg, 1994).

2.2.2 Psychopharmaceuticals and the history of psychiatry

The precursors of modern psychopharmaceuticals, i.e., opium, hellebore and rauwolfia, cannot be considered in isolation but only by reference to their contemporary healing arts. Mental illnesses and their possible treatment have confronted people with the same questions at all times: where do the irrational ideas and impulses of the insane come from – their moods, notions, anxiety and illogical behaviour? Have these people sinned so that God has now cast an evil spirit into them as a punishment? What is this evil spirit: a spirit of nature, the ghost of an ancestor, a devil? Or is it the patient's body that produces the delusions without an outside agent – an unknown disease, a poison from within?

In the history of psychiatry, sketched here in just a few paragraphs, the different views held of man at different times are reflected in the constant swings between naturalistic and spiritualistic concepts of disease and the corresponding therapeutic approaches (see Kirchhoff, 1912; Heiberg, 1927; Ackerknecht, 1967).

In *Egypt* at the time of the Pharaohs, mental illnesses were a result of the wrath of gods, or even an expression of possession by demons. In agreement with this concept, the treatment given by the priest–doctor comprised: punishment or penance to appease the gods; exorcism and other means of driving out the demons; or the patient was isolated or banished to protect others from the frightening state. There is no record of the way in which opium, known in ancient Egypt, was part of the therapeutic procedures.

The *Old Testament* contains the impressive story about the first king of Israel, Saul, who was anointed by the prophet Samuel, whereupon 'the spirit of God came over him'; i.e., Saul had superhuman powers that even others could perceive. After the battle against the Amalek arch enemy, in which Saul did not follow God's instructions, the spirit of God left him and 'an evil spirit sent from God tormented him' (1 Samuel, 16: 14); Saul became depressed, suspicious, and subject to outbursts of anger. David, the later son-in-law and eventual successor, could initially soothe the king with singing and harping, but Saul's state subsequently deteriorated and he broke down after a serious military reverse in Gilboa. His illness seemed to be a dark fate sent by God; Saul became increasingly entangled in guilt from which he found no way out, and even David's singing and all efforts to restore his mental balance remained ineffective.

The start of a scientific approach to mental health is generally attributed to the ancient Greeks. In the sixth century BC, Alkmaeon of Croton carried out systematic autopsies and discovered the pathways connecting the eye and ears with the brain. As a result, the brain was seen as the seat of reason and the soul. Around 400 BC, Hippocrates and his school placed natural, i.e., physical, causes of mental illnesses in the foreground: they are expressions or results of an imbalance between the body fluids (humours) which are normally present in harmonious proportions. The *humoral theory of Hippocrates*, certainly one of the most influential concepts in the history of psychology and psychiatry, counted on four basic fluids corresponding to four temperaments or character types and, in the case of pathological predominance of one component, to four mental illnesses:

Humour	*Temperament: affectivity*	*Mental illness*
Blood	Sanguine: lively and weak	Mania, insanity
Phlegm	Phlegmatic: slow and weak	Calm insanity
Black bile	Melancholic: slow and strong	Melancholy
Choler	Choleric: lively and strong	Hysteria, especially in women

Since mental illnesses are due to an imbalance between the body fluids, treatment must seek to restore the balance. Methods directed to the body were recommended, such as diet, bathing and showering, blood-letting and laxatives (hellebore).

The writings of Hippocrates and his school have not been handed down to us. They reached Alexandria around 300 BC and were summarized by Celsus in the first century AD. The need for individual adaptation of each therapy was stressed here: frightened patients are to be reassured in a friendly manner, manic patients should be chained and perhaps starved; music and poetry lift the melancholy, the mad should be shunned or brought to other thoughts by sudden noises and, finally, adequate sleep should be ensured for all patients. Poppy (opium) and henbane were available for this, but rippling fountains could also have a calming and soporific action.

The major authority for medicine in the Middle Ages was *Galen* of Pergamon, who worked in Rome in the second century AD. Galen adopted the humoral theory of Hippocrates, including the classification of mental illnesses, and his therapeutic recommendations were also based on the tradition of the Hippocratic school: diet, vomiting, blood-letting and the administration of soporifics were the most important measures.

The *Middle Ages* are not a high spot in the history of psychiatry. This was the time of possession by the devil and demons, of mass movements with a clearly pathological nature (flagellants, children's crusade), witch-burning and gruesome exorcism of spirits. Science and medicine did not develop further in Christian Europe since 'the little that the Greeks knew was lost and an awful regression to earlier cultural stages occurred' (Ackerknecht, 1967, p. 18). However, this statement does not apply to the Islamic world: the Hippocratic–Galenic tradition was propagated further by Arabic doctors, and hospitals with separate departments for the mentally ill were available in Baghdad around AD 750 and in Cairo from AD 873. Treatment was based in the experience of the ancient world, so that measures directed to the body were predominantly used to overcome mental illnesses.

In the early Christian Middle Ages, however, a tradition arose that had a beneficial impact on the mentally ill, despite the fanaticism and incitement of later centuries: the tradition of *mercy*. Prayers were said for the possessed and the Church initially saw itself as a haven for the insane and epileptics also. Only in the eleventh century were some madmen considered to be envoys of the devil to be combated by all available means; in the fourteenth century there was a change to isolating the insane from the healthy population in lunatic asylums and madhouses. Therapeutic measures for those isolated in this way were superfluous at that time, especially since those who knew about herbs and poisons were often themselves suspected of being witches (Duerr, 1979).

Between the Middle Ages and modern times stand physicians such as Paracelsus (1491–1541), J. Weyer (1515–1588) and F. Platter (1536–1614), who turned more or less clearly against the concepts of witches and spirits which prevailed at that time, and restored natural causes to the centre-stage of mental illnesses. They had no new treatments to offer and, true to the Galenic tradition, prescribed blood-letting and purging to clean the body fluids, baths and massages for relaxation and to strengthen the body, soporifics and sedatives to stabilize excited minds.

2.3   THE MODERN AGE: PSYCHOPHARMACOLOGY BEFORE CHLORPROMAZINE

In the Age of Enlightenment and absolutism, psychiatry developed in different directions in the different European countries depending on local political and social circumstances (see Schrenk, 1973; Dörner, 1975; Foucault, 1978). The essential features of this development, which occurred in all countries sooner or later, are:

(1) The *spatial segregation of the insane* in houses that often lay outside the cities and towns, sometimes in one-time leper colonies.
(2) The gradual rediscovery of the *medical model* of mental illnesses, associated with research into pathological anatomical causes.

Table 2.1. Materia Medica (after P.J. Schneider, 1824)

Antagonists (For use in cases of excessive nervous sensitivity and insufficient physical sensitivity)	*Antiphlogistics* (Temperature-reducing measures)	*Narcotic agents* (Calming agents)	*Excitants, analeptics* (Nerve-invigorating agents)
A. Remedies promoting nausea and vomiting: Internal: Various emetics External: Revolving machine, revolving chair, swing, red-hot iron, whips with nettles, cupping glasses; suppurating head wounds, gentle rubbing of the skin Enemas, mustard plasters, blistering plasters, ants, scabies Cold baths, snow baths, sudden immersion, ice bags, tepid baths B. Cathartics (laxatives): Psychic disturbances are often located in the abdomen Medicaments, some of which are still in use today	Medical Surgical (e.g. bleeding, cupping)	A. Narcotics: saffron, thorn apple, henbane, tobacco. alraun, prussic acid, opium B. Strong narcotics: belladonna, hemlock, foxglove, verbena C. External agents: sack, cupboard, hollow wheel, strait-jacket, strait-cradle	A. Internal remedies: Camphor, sage, rosemary, lavender, balm mint, filix, valerian, green tea, arnica, cinnamon oil, juniper oil, cumin, fennel, aniseed, peppermint and terpentine oil Musk, castoreum, Spanish fly Many spices Naphthalene, old wines B. External remedies: Hot compresses on the head Sneezing powder, intake of irritants Electricity, galvanism, magnetism

(3) Attempts to return the insane (= social outcasts) to a normal life by means of work, useful tasks and a regulated daily routine, and to support them as *members of society*.

It is clear that these trends are contradictory to some extent. A spatially segregated patient cannot lead a normal life in society. The medical model of mental illnesses, with its objective of detecting and, where applicable, correcting anatomical or functional disorders in the patient's body, contradicts a socially orientated concept of the illness underpinning treatment by educational methods. Modern psychiatry has grown up with these contradictions and still lives with them today (Rosen, 1969).

Psychopharmacology emerged very gradually in modern times. One of the earliest compendia of psychopharmacology to appear in German was written by P.J. Schneider (1824), and describes in some 600 pages methods of psychiatric therapy used at the beginning of the nineteenth century. The description lacks discrimination in several respects and includes many measures which to us seem to be cruel or naive, insufficiently tested, and often contradictory. Some 400 pages are devoted to 'Materia Medica' and it is here that the majority of medicinal recommendations are to be found. However, many practices described in these Materia Medica are reminiscent of a torture chamber rather than of a hospital (Table 2.1) – and yet the author assures us that some of these measures were therapeutically effective in well-documented cases.

Psychotropic agents, in today's sense of the term, are classified by Schneider into the classes 'narcotic agents' and 'excitants, analeptics'. The list of allegedly useful substances, plants and extracts is comprehensive and colourful. An evaluation of the recommended active agents is hampered by the fact that the author provides no proof of efficacy according to present-day standards and that the reports of their effect are based on psychiatric terminology which is nowadays virtually incomprehensible. What does emerge clearly from this account is that Schneider numbered amongst the most effective medicaments the thorn apple (*Datura stramonium*), alraun, prussic acid, opium and belladonna. Alraun (*Mandragora*), henbane (*Hyoscyamus niger*) and belladonna (*Atropa belladonna*) are some of the traditional ingredients of witches' ointments and potions, to which was added the thorn apple at the beginning of the modern era (see Caldwell, 1978; Duerr, 1979).

Psychiatry made considerable advances in England and France in the early nineteenth century. A classification of mental illnesses based on precise clinical observations and statistical comparison was developed by Ph. Pinel (1745–1826) and J.E. Esquirol (1772–1840), and the cruellest of the treatment methods, including chaining the insane, had already been discontinued by the turn of the century. In 1818, Esquirol drew up an expert report on madhouses in France at the request of the French Home Office, and this shattering report led to a thorough reform of psychiatry. In his textbook of 1838, Esquirol spoke of 'maladie mentale' ('mental illness') instead of the previously used term 'alienation', and thus announced the victory of the medical model over spiritualistic concepts of psychiatric diseases. With Wilhelm Griesinger (1817–1868), the German school of psychiatry then underwent a similar transformation and, under Emil Kraepelin (1856–1926), a psychiatric classification was created, essential features of which still remain valid today.

Griesinger's textbook of psychiatry (1861) gives extensive information on only a very few centrally acting medicaments: particularly recommended are opium, ether and chloroform narcoses, as well as prussic acid. Opium was observed in appropriate cases to 'calm the sick, reduce hallucinations, dispel feelings of anxiety as well as delusions related thereto and occasionally to bring about their complete cure' (p. 488). Above all, younger patients whose ailment had not yet become chronic could, in Griesinger's experience, benefit from opium treatment – and interestingly enough no mention is made of the development of addiction.

Following narcoses, induced using either ether or chloroform, there was 'often (but by no means consistently) a temporary remission of the melancholia and mania . . . now and then even a complete *lucidum intervallum* . . . but the earlier clinical picture soon reappeared' (p. 489). According to Griesinger's observations, repeated use of ether and chloroform leads to the remissions becoming briefer and soon disappearing completely. The hope that had been laid on the medical treatment of mental disorders with synthetic substances was thus not fulfilled. Prussic acid is a secondary remedy listed by Griesinger and was said to be capable of calming moderate exaltation, melancholic anxiety and similar states. The author made no further remarks concerning other remedies (datura, belladonna, quinine and hashish) listed in his book.

Whilst Griesinger devotes only little space to the use of medicaments in the treatment of mental illness, Kraepelin's textbook of psychiatry (1899) made various references to the use of pharmaceuticals in the treatment of the mentally ill. Some of these are preparations having a certain tradition in psychiatry, whereas others were substances that had been discovered in the intervening period (Table 2.2). And yet, comparison of this list with Griesinger's recommendations shows how little progress had been made in the 40 or so years which had elapsed: although the number of hypnotics had grown somewhat, no fundamentally new types of activity had been found.

A similar stagnation is also apparent when one compares the first eight editions of the *Lehrbuch der Psychiatrie* (*Textbook of Psychiatry*) by Eugen Bleuler, which appeared between 1916 and 1949. Whilst the heading 'Hypnotics' already appears in the index of the first edition, the concept 'Treatment with medicaments' only appears in 1949, in the eighth edition. All in all, Bleuler used pharmaceuticals much more restrictively than Griesinger and Kraepelin: he regards opium as risky remedy that should be avoided in view of the danger of habituation. He also rejects alcohol – which was still

Table 2.2.   Psychopharmaceuticals listed by E. Kraepelin (1899)

1. *Narcotics: medicaments with calming action*
Opium: Excitation, anxiety states and pain-induced unrest respond to it; also pro-
   longed manic states
Morphine: Similar to opium, but simpler to dose. Risk of toxic effects and/or morphi-
   nism. Codeine, another opiate, offers no advantages
Hyoscine (scopolamine): A useful medicament, induces deep sleep rapidly. Especially
   for manic patients
Hashish: Hypnotic with unreliable action

2. *Hypnotics*
Chloral hydrate: Induces longer sleep, sometimes with drowsiness in the morning.
   Mordant, unpleasant taste. Paraldehyde: similar but more of a soporific
Sulfonal, trional: Pleasant to take, but often give rise to tiredness and feeling of
   weakness on the following day. Accumulation during prolonged use
Alcohol: Mild hypnotic, recommended dose 40–60 g (corresponds to > 100 ml co-
   gnac, whisky, etc.!); used in hysterical and neurasthenic, insomniac patients, and
   for insomnia in the elderly
Chloroform: For very severe states of excitation refractory to all other agents; the
   calming action does not last beyond the anaesthesia

3. *Bromine salts*
Give valuable service in epilepsy and neurasthenia, eliminate inner tension and insomnia. Risks during prolonged use: motor disorders, apathy

recommended by Kraepelin in 1899 – owing to the risk of alcoholism and, in
its place, recommends hyoscine (scopolamine) in states of pronounced agitation. As regards hypnotics proper, he advises against their prolonged use and
suggests that the remedies be changed from time to time in order to prevent
any habituation (Table 2.3). This reserved approach towards drug-based
therapy remained unchanged throughout the following editions of his textbook and, as already stated, hardly any additions were made to Bleuler's list
of recommended preparations between 1916 and 1949.

Apart from the slow progress in psychiatric pharmacotherapy it is striking
that, whereas Griesinger, Kraepelin, and Bleuler cited a large number of
sedatives and hypnotics, their recommendation included no stimulating
medicaments of any kind. While several preparations were available which
could be used to sedate raging, anxious, restless or sleep-disturbed patients,
the psychiatrists of the time were virtually powerless in the face of depressive
and stuporous states, if one discounts the not generally accepted use of opium.
Here a certain degree of progress was attained with the shock therapies:
insulin-induced coma, cardiazole-induced shock and, in particular, electroshock. Amphetamine was synthesized in 1927 and, thanks to its stimulating
properties, was used to a growing extent in the 1930s against narcolepsy and
similar disorders. However, it never acquired any great importance in psychiatric pharmacotherapy since it only displayed a modest effect in states of
exhaustion and slight depression, whilst remaining virtually ineffective in endogenous depression.

Table 2.3. Psychopharmaceuticals recommended by E. Bleuler (1916)

Hypnotics: Sulfonal, trional, chloral hydrate, veronal, paraldehyde. Whilst alcohol used as an hypnotic is pleasant for the patient, the risk of habituation makes it dangerous and ineffective

Bromine: In nervous agitation, less severe depression

Opiates: Can have a calming, sleep-inducing action. Less effective than expected in psychoses. Can be dispensed with, to be avoided because of the risk of addiction

Hyoscine (scopolamine): Useful in acute states of agitation, also in combination with morphine (Moscop)

2.4 THE DISCOVERY OF MODERN PSYCHOPHARMACEUTICALS

2.4.1 Chlorpromazine

A detailed account of the discovery of the antipsychotic effect of chlorpromazine has been given by two authors (Caldwell, 1970; Swazey, 1974); an abridged version is also to be found in Caldwell (1978). It emerges clearly from all three descriptions that this discovery was not the work of a single scientist or research group. Nor did it emerge as the result of a planned research project aimed at finding a pharmacological therapy for schizophrenia. What in fact happened was that several initially unrelated developmental trends converged at the end of the 1940s in the most fortuitous fashion and, thanks to precise clinical observations on the part of several doctors, led to the most significant advance in psychiatric therapy for many years. Swazey (1974) regards the following factors as critical:

- The efforts made by the French surgeon Laborit to find a safer anaesthetic technique and to prevent surgical shock.
- A pharmacological development programme embarked on by the firm Rhône–Poulenc in Paris to screen for medicaments having an antihistamine action.
- The readiness to experiment displayed by several biologically interested psychiatrists trying out pharmacological remedies to more effective psychiatric therapy.

Of special interest is the contribution made by H. Laborit, who had worked as an army surgeon during the Second World War and who, under the influence of his war experiences, devoted himself in subsequent years above all to the problem of shock.

The term shock when used in medicine relates to an acute state of weakness and the restriction of many vital functions: patients in shock are generally apathetic, their face is sunken, their expression full of anxiety. Their skin is moist, cold and grey, the pulse rapid and faint, blood pressure is normally low, musculature lax, superficial blood vessels empty. Respiration is superficial, basal metabolism reduced and urine formation considerably slower. Shock may be triggered by a variety of causes: by severe physical injury with excessive loss of blood, during surgery or severe psychic trauma; in predisposed persons it may also arise as a reaction to exogenous substances such as antibiotics or bee poison.

In the 1940s there were – and still are today – various current hypotheses as to the question of the biological or biochemical mechanisms of shock. In many years of research Laborit arrived at the view that endogenous substances having a transmitter function (adrenaline, acetylcholine and histamine, see Chapter 5) are involved in the triggering and full-scale development of shock. In his view, shock is a consequence of excessively strong biological emergency reactions no longer adapted to the situation, and can be combated by blocking the effects of the transmitters using appropriate pharmacological agents, if possible at several points simultaneously. In the light of this hypothesis, Laborit experimented with various substances known to have an inhibitory effect on adrenaline, acetylcholine and histamine. These included such medicaments as procaine, curare, atropine and – the class that was to decide future events – synthetic antihistamines.

This is where Laborit's interests coincided with those of the firm Rhône–Poulenc, which had already embarked on a chemical and pharmacological programme to develop antihistamine compounds several years before. An important point was reached when promethazine, an antihistamine with pronounced sedative and analgesic properties, was examined clinically by Laborit and other doctors. Not only was this medicament suitable, in combination with other substances, in preventing surgical shock, but Laborit observed that patients under promethazine were quieter and more relaxed and – even after major surgery – were in relatively good spirits.

Impressed by this success, Rhône–Poulenc decided in 1950 to look for more antihistamines in the same chemical class as promethazine having an even more pronounced central effect. This decision was by no means an obvious one, since the sedative effect of promethazine could barely be characterized using the contemporary methods of animal experiments. Furthermore, the sedating and sleep-inducing effect of promethazine was a distinct disadvantage in some therapeutic applications (hay fever, other allergies). In October 1950, disregarding these difficulties, P. Koetschet, one of the Rhône–Poulenc heads of research, suggested embarking on a well-directed search for promethazine analogues with a greater effect on the central nervous system. Although it was not possible to foresee what therapeutic applications these substances would have, Koetschet envisaged their exploratory use in anaesthesiology, in Parkinsonism, in psychiatry, and possibly also in epileptic patients. As early as March 1951 a substance, given the number 4560 RP, was available which was chemically related to promethazine whilst revealing a considerably more pronounced central effect in pharmacological tests in animals. In April 1951 human trials of 4560 RP commenced and the first applications confirmed that the compound augmented the sleep-inducing action of the barbiturates and also acted as a sedative when used on its own.

Laborit obtained 4560 RP in June 1951 and soon recognized the advantages of the new substance: it lessened the anxiety felt by patients prior to surgery, diminished surgical stress and made it possible to simplify the mixture of medicaments used by Laborit – the so-called lytic cocktails. Furthermore the compound had a low toxicity and could in consequence be used in a broader dosage rather than, for example, curare.

Under the effect of chlorpromazine, as 4560 RP was later to be named, patients did not lose consciousness, but merely became sleepy and uninterested in everything going on around them and being done to them (Laborit *et al.*, 1952). Laborit and his co-workers postulated that this strange central action suggested the use of chlorpromazine in psychiatry, for example in sleep therapy, where it was hoped to attain an improved effect and greater safety in comparison to hitherto known agents.

Laborit was not the only doctor conducting clinical trials on chlorpromazine at the instigation of Rhône–Poulenc: it emerged from reports given by other clinics that the substance produced a form of sedation which had previously been unknown. Based on these observations, Rhône–Poulenc decided, at the end of 1951, to extend the research programme to include the mentally ill and to use chlorpromazine, in combination with barbiturates, experimentally in sleep therapy and in the treatment of manic episodes. Independently of this, Laborit tried to encourage a few psychiatrists personally known to him to embark on clinical trials using chlorpromazine in restless patients. Eventually a group of doctors in a psychiatric military hospital decided to conduct an initial trial on a manic patient. After some three weeks of treatment with chlorpromazine in combination with other sedatives, the patient's condition improved to such an extent that he could be discharged and sent home. In a paper presented before the Société Médico-Psychologique, Hamon *et al.* reported on 25 February 1952 on their initial experiences with chlorpromazine, which they held to be interesting. However, since they did not consider the sedative effect of the new substance to be strong enough, they preferred the then customary electroshock therapy.

At about this time one of the best-known French psychiatrists of the day, J. Delay, commenced his own studies with chlorpromazine in conjunction with a colleague, P. Deniker. Deniker had learnt by private communications of Laborit's experiments with chlorpromazine in anaesthesiology, which were referred to as *hibernation artificielle*. He asked Rhône–Poulenc for drug samples and received them in February 1952. Unlike Laborit, who always used chlorpromazine in combination with other medicaments, Delay and Deniker decided to administer chlorpromazine without additional substances to manically agitated patients. Their first findings were so beneficial that they presented an initial report to the Société Médico-Psychologique after three months, a report which soon after appeared in written form (Delay *et al.*, 1952). During the following months the same authors published a number of reports in rapid succession on the effect of chlorpromazine in various psychiatric syndromes and thus helped to make the new medicament known in France and, in part, also abroad.

One of the first clinics outside France to show an interest in chlorpromazine was the Basel University Psychiatric Hospital. A young member of the clinic's staff (F. Labhardt) had been in Paris for postgraduate training from summer 1951 to spring 1952 and had heard there of the application of the new substance 4560 RP in anaesthesiology and psychiatry. An initial therapeutic trial commenced in Basel in January 1953 and was so successful that a rapid succession of patients with quite varied diagnoses underwent chlorpromazine cures. The first publication from the Basel clinic appeared in June 1953 (Staehelin and Kielholz, 1953): Largactil®, as the medicament was now named, was recommended in 'all severe psychic disturbances in which pronounced vegetative syndromes could be demonstrated', particularly in:

– emotional psychoses and other psychotic reactions;
– detoxification cures for addicts;
– severe neuroses, especially those with symptoms of anxiety and compulsion;
– symptomatic psychoses tinged with anxiety;
– certain forms of schizophrenia and manic-depressive psychosis.

This list shows clearly the extent to which the fields of indication of chlorpromazine had broadened in barely one and a half years. Of special importance was its use in schizophrenia which Labhardt presented shortly afterwards in a comprehensive lecture given at the First Largactil Symposium, which was held in Basel on 28 November 1953. According to data presented by Staehelin, the then head of the Basel clinic, of the approximately 500 patients in the clinic, some 200 were on Largactil® and over 130 discharged patients were continuing to take the medicament. Figures cited by Staehelin's colleagues in their lectures were equally impressive: Kielholz reported on results of treatment in 52 depressive patients, 16 drug addicts in withdrawal as well as more than 20 senile patients with nocturnal unrest. Labhardt presented data on the treatment of over 200 schizophrenic patients with chlorpromazine. To all this were added reports on therapeutic studies undertaken in other psychiatric hospitals in Switzerland and covering over 850 patients.

Particularly important consequences arose out of the findings presented by Labhardt (1954) on the treatment of schizophrenics: excellent results were obtained, not only in recently afflicted patients, but also in those who had been hospitalized for several years. In the case of chronic patients in whom the illness went back over five years or more, significant improvements were observed in almost 60% of the cases, and some of the patients who had previously had an almost hopeless prognosis according to prevailing opinions could be discharged from hospital.

Spectacular findings were not only being recorded with chlorpromazine in Paris and Basel; other centres also achieved favourable results. Thanks to chlorpromazine, the character of psychiatric hospitals and of psychiatric care in general underwent a radical change. Lunatic asylums became peaceful hospitals; many patients who had previously had to be institutionalized on account of the danger which they presented to their surroundings and to themselves could be discharged and partially rehabilitated. There was a marked reduction in the average stay in psychiatric hospitals. Thanks to chlorpromazine it was recognized that not only is schizophrenia an illness which can be treated, at least symptomatically by chemical means, but that it is in many cases an illness which can be cured – and the following years were to see a marked upswing in biologically orientated psychiatry (Chapter 5).

2.4.2 Antidepressants

The history of the first antidepressant, the monoamine oxidase (MAO) inhibitor iproniazid, is a complicated one for a number of reasons (Kline, 1970). Iproniazid was originally developed by the drug company Hoffmann-La Roche as a medicament for the treatment of tuberculosis, and attracted attention in 1951/52 during clinical trials on account of its stimulating and euphoriant effects: nervousness and sleep disorders occurred frequently and yet tubercular patients on iproniazid became cheerful and exuberant – moods strangely out of keeping with their condition. Initial applications in psychiatry, some in agitated, some in chronically apathetic schizophrenics, failed to lead to interpretable results, whereas the use of iproniazid against tuberculosis was increasingly being regarded as risky, mainly as a consequence of the stimulating effect of the preparation.

A more systematic clinical investigation of the antidepressant effect of iproniazid was only commenced in 1956 after animal experiments had suggested that the compound possessed an activity in this area. Pretreatment of animals with iproniazid prevented the so-called reserpine syndrome (Chapter 5) in mice and rats. Instead of being calm and tame, as is normally the case after reserpine alone, animals pretreated with iproniazid became hyperactive and, in some cases, aggressive, under the influence of reserpine. Initial clinical application in depressive patients revealed that iproniazid had a stimulating and mood-elevating effect in at least some of the patients. On the other hand, reports kept coming in of side effects caused by the preparation and these impeded its broader use. The manufacturers ultimately withdrew the preparation in the USA and in some other countries whilst it remained on sale in further markets – a confusing situation that went on for years (Kline, 1970). Some subsequently introduced MAO inhibitors such as isocarboxacid and tranylcypromine were also withdrawn after a short time on account of various types of side effects.

Another, by no means always straightforward, path was followed by the discovery of the so-called *thymoleptics*, which are today more important as antidepressants than are the MAO inhibitors. As in the case of Rhône–Poulenc, the firm Geigy in Basel had worked during the 1940s on antihistamine substances which were chemically similar to chlorpromazine and promethazine. In animal experiments one of these substances, preparation number G 22150, had an antihistamine as well as a sedative action and was tested in 1950 by the Swiss psychiatrist R. Kuhn in restless patients in view of its potential use as a sedative and hypnotic. As Kuhn wrote in 1957 the 'expected action was in most cases not found to be present . . . in the doses of 0.02–0.06 g used at that time. However, the preparation seemed to us to exert a pronounced calming effect in schizophrenics suffering from agitation, delusions and hallucinations'. However, 'this effect was assessed too much merely from the one-sided point of view of tranquillizing activity and hence the special interest of such substances was overlooked' (Kuhn, 1957, p. 1135).

In 1952 the first favourable results were obtained in psychiatry with chlorpromazine and Kuhn was amongst those to carry out trials with the newly discovered neuroleptic. And yet, as Kuhn wrote in 1970, chlorpromazine was too expensive to be used in his hospital in large quantities. He therefore approached Geigy in February 1954, pointing out the similarity between the effect observed with G 22150 and that of chlorpromazine. Further trial samples of G 22150 were supplied, but it became obvious that the Geigy preparation was inferior to chlorpromazine as an antipsychotic and, in addition, produced disturbing side effects. As a result, a further Geigy compound was selected for clinical trials: G 22355, which was chemically even closer to chlorpromazine than was G 22150. This substance was tested for about a year on some 300 patients with various mental illnesses and in spring 1956 Kuhn, to conclude his test series, also treated a few patients suffering from endogenous depression. It was discovered with surprise that the substance, later to be called *imipramine*, had a marked antidepressant effect which Kuhn (1957) described as follows:

– The patients' facial expression relaxes and regains its expressivity. The patients become livelier, friendlier, more sociable. They talk more and louder.
– The moaning, crying, and complaining stops, remarks relating to physical complaints decrease.
– The patients get up in the morning of their own accord, undertake activities under their own initiative; the lethargic pace of living returns to normal.
– The patients realize their improvement; feelings of heaviness, weakness and oppression decrease, feelings of guilt and depressive delusions disappear.
– Suicidal ideas and tendencies recede.
– Sleep disturbances and oppressive dreams become rarer. Daily mood swings with morning lows, lack of appetite and constipation cease.

According to Kuhn's observations, the effect of imipramine became apparent in some cases after a few days; in other cases several weeks passed before any therapeutic effect could be seen. He estimated his failure rate at 20–25%, but regarded his sample as too small for any reliable estimate to be made. If the medicament was discontinued too soon, there was said to be a danger of relapse. It was also not possible to ascertain from his observations whether imipramine shortened the natural duration of the depressive phase. The best therapeutic successes were recorded in 'endogenous depression and in cases of depression which first appeared at the menopause, in cases where vital symptoms were clearly in the foreground'. Kuhn also provided a comprehensive list of side effects of imipramine, which nevertheless in his view did not appreciably restrict use of the medicament. (None of the claims regarding the clinical pattern of action of imipramine made by Kuhn on the basis of open studies on 300 patients, 40 of whom suffered from endogenous depression, had later to be withdrawn or significantly modified.)

In contrast to iproniazid and imipramine, which were only synthesized in the early 1950s and then tested in man, *lithium* had been known to medicine for almost 100 years before J. Cade became aware of its specific antimanic action (see Cade, 1970). The starting point of this Australian psychiatrist's investigations was a hypothesis regarding the aetiology of manic-depressive illness, according to which mania was based on poisoning due to a surplus of an endogenous substance, whereas the depression was due to a deficiency of the same substance. In order to test this hypothesis, Cade injected the urine of manic patients into guinea-pigs and found this urine to display greater toxicity than that of healthy subjects. He then began his search for substances which would protect the guinea-pigs from the effects of the manic patients' urine. Via a few intermediate steps he came across lithium salts which had the desired effect. In addition it was noticeable that, with the administration of lithium, the animals became lethargic and showed virtually no reaction to stimuli, although they did not lapse into a state of sleep. As Cade wrote later: 'It may seem a long way from lethargy in guinea pigs to the control of manic excitement, but as these investigations had commenced in an attempt to demonstrate some possibly excreted toxin in the urine of manic patients, the association of ideas is explicable' (1970, p. 223). In any event, Cade conducted his first trials with lithium in manic patients in 1948 and reported in a publication on very good therapeutic findings in 10 out of 10 patients.

Despite this favourable result, lithium was hardly considered as a psychopharmaceutical for many years. There were a variety of reasons for this. Firstly, mania is not a very common psychosis and there is spontaneous remission in many cases. There were thus not so many occasions where lithium treatment was indicated. Secondly, lithium was considered to be toxic since it had for some time been given in excessive doses to patients with heart failure and had, in this way, led to a number of fatalities (Cade, 1970). Thirdly, a few years after Cade's first publication psychiatrists' attention had been claimed by chlorpromazine and the subsequent neuroleptics and antidepressants, thus explaining why lithium almost fell into oblivion. It was only in the 1960s that it once more attracted some interest, after a Danish psychiatrist, M. Schou, had shown that lithium salts were not only useful in the manic phase of manic-depressive illness, but could, in patients suffering from bipolar psychoses, also prevent the depressive phase.

2.4.3   Tranquillizers

Although the consumption of tranquillizers is more widespread than the use of neuroleptics and antidepressants (see Chapter 9), the discoveries of chlorpromazine and of imipramine are generally regarded as greater scientific advances than that of the tranquillizers. In making the public aware of the fact that mental disturbances can be treated with chemical agents, tranquillizers – owing to their widespread use – must, however, play as important a role as neuroleptics and antidepressants. For this reason, and in view of the economic significance of the consumption of tranquillizers, it is in order to set out briefly the history of the discovery of these medicaments.

As already mentioned in Chapter 1, sedatives – above all low dosages of sleep-inducing agents – were the historic precursors of the tranquillizers. The use of these medicaments was, however, severely restricted by their serious disadvantages: the narrow therapeutic range and the risk of habituation and addiction. A first link in the chain leading to present-day tranquillizers was forged by the compound *mephenesine*, which produced muscle relaxation, calm and a sleep-like state in animal experiments. Mephenesine was part of a chemical development programme which had been started shortly after the Second World War in an English pharmaceutical company (British Drug Houses), aimed at finding compounds active against penicillin-resistant bacteria. The pronounced muscle-relaxing action of mephenesine became apparent during toxicological testing (Berger, 1970) as a result of which clinical trials commenced to examine the muscle-relaxant properties of this substance. It soon became evident that mephenesine was not only muscle-relaxing, but anxiety-relieving and psychically relaxing too, whilst leaving the patient's mind clear and free of any mental impairment.

Mephenesine is rapidly broken down in the organism and therefore its effect is only of short duration. At an early stage, therefore, chemists directed their efforts at finding longer-acting, i.e., more slowly metabolized, analogues of mephenesine. Many preparations were synthesized and some were even marketed (see Ban, 1969, p. 313f.) but *meprobamate* was the first to display the desired profile of action since it had pronounced muscle-relaxing and anxiolytic effects, adequate therapeutic safety margin and long duration of action. Whilst the pharmacological profile of meprobamate was known as early as 1954, the substance was only accepted clinically as a tranquillizer in 1957. In the ensuing years, the practical application of meprobamate expanded to cover neurotic tension and complaints of all kinds and the compound enjoyed great commercial success, only to be halted with the advent of the benzodiazepines.

The history of the *benzodiazepines* has been set down by their inventor, the Polish–American chemist L. Sternbach (1978). He tells how in the mid-1950s Hoffman-La Roche, in the light of the success of the first psychopharmaceuticals, decided to investigate this field also. Of the possible approaches to chemical research – modification of already known and active molecules, synthetic work based on a specific biochemical hypothesis, synthesis of substances belonging to new chemical classes and their pharmacological screening in known experimental models – the firm chose the third. Sternbach based his chemical synthetic work on a class of substances which he had already examined earlier when working at the University of Cracow. Decisive in this choice was the fact that few scientists had concentrated on this class of chemicals and Hoffmann-La Roche could consequently expect to achieve a large number of patentable compounds. Furthermore, this class of substances was, as Sternbach emphasized, interesting for the chemist for scientific and technical reasons.

Regardless of these advantages, the newly synthesized compounds proved to be pharmacologically uninteresting and the programme was consequently already halted in 1957. Sternbach himself assumed new duties and was in the process of clearing the laboratory for new work when he came across two substances which had already been synthesized earlier, but had not yet been subjected to pharmacological tests. Without any great hopes, one of these substances was sent for pharmacological testing. Contrary to expectation it proved to be effective in the series of tests designed to indicate a tranquillizing effect. In mice it was muscle-relaxing, sedating, anticonvulsant and antiaggressive, and these effects were also confirmed in other species of animals. The compound, later to be called chlordiazepoxide (Librium®), was more effective in all the pharmacological tests than the reference substance meprobamate. It was not hypnotic even at high doses, had no vegetative effects and its toxicity was very low. A taming effect was observed in rhesus monkeys, which can be very vicious in captivity.

Initial clinical trials were conducted in geriatric patients in spring 1958: whilst the substance clearly displayed the expected sedative properties, it led in these patients to severe ataxia and to speech disturbances (Cohen, 1970), for which reason clinical trials were interrupted for some months. A member of the Hoffmann-La Roche clinical research department then had the idea of having lower doses of the preparation tested by practising psychiatrists in outpatients suffering from neurotic disorders. The results of these additional studies were encouraging: chlordiazepoxide led to a reduction in tension and states of anxiety, without causing any significant side effects such as disturbed wakefulness and impaired mental functioning. The preparation had a broad therapeutic range and no toxic effects were observed in man. 'This added up to an easily manipulated drug having a wide range of clinical application and minimal toxicity' (Cohen, 1970, p. 134). In view of these positive results, clinical trials were stepped up and as early as autumn 1959 a symposium was held at which reports were presented on experiences with chlordiazepoxide in several thousand patients. The American health authorities, the Food and Drug Administration (FDA), approved the medicament Librium® in February 1960, two years after commencement of clinical trials.

2.5   DISCUSSION: HOW WERE MODERN PSYCHOPHARMACEUTICALS DISCOVERED?

All prototypes of modern psychopharmaceuticals (lithium, chlorpromazine, meprobamate, imipramine and chlordiazepoxide) were discovered in a period of about 10 years (Fig. 2.1). Neither before nor since has such a series of therapeutic advances been made in psychiatry. Several authors dealing with the history of modern psychopharmacology have thus raised the question of which factors made a decisive contribution to the discovery of modern psychopharmaceuticals within such a short time. Two partial negative answers can certainly be given: (1) the discoveries followed no common pattern; (2) neither in the case of lithium nor in the case of chlorpromazine or imipramine can one speak of developments directed at a particular target, whereby a substance was developed with a specific therapeutic indication in view on the basis of pathophysiological knowledge and a given pharmacological hypothesis. To recapitulate the sequence of events once more:

- Chlorpromazine emerged from a series of compounds which aroused interest mainly on account of their antihistamine, and partly because of their anticholinergic, effects.
- Imipramine also came from a class of substances having antihistamine properties, and was earmarked and tested clinically as a possible competitor to chlorpromazine.
- Meprobamate was a further development based on a medicament (mephenesine), the muscle-relaxant effects of which had attracted attention as a side effect during toxicological trials and were then remodelled into a therapeutic application.

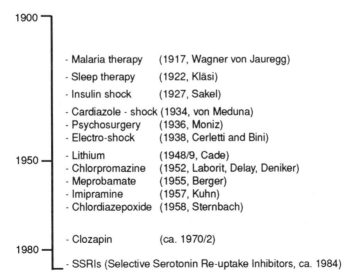

Figure 2.1.   The discovery of psychiatric somatotherapies

– In the case of MAO inhibitors also, a side effect that had been observed in conjunction with the use in another indication (tuberculosis) was converted into the therapeutic effect in a different group of patients.

Only in the case of chlordiazepoxide can one speak in terms of goal-directed development: here the intention was to find tranquillizing compounds in a new and patentable class of substances. In no case was there, however, a biochemical hypothesis concerning the illness or symptoms to be treated which would have led to the rational synthesis and development of appropriate pharmaceuticals.

2.5.1 Chance discovery

Is it then that the major discoveries in psychopharmacology are based on *coincidence* and, if so, what is meant by coincidence? A stroke of luck, whereby some psychiatrist, somewhere, experimenting with some kind of substance, unexpectedly hits on a major discovery, can certainly be ruled out in the case of chlorpromazine. For years Laborit had considered pharmacological ways of preventing shock, during which time he had systematically looked for suitable compounds and combinations of substances. In Delay's clinic efforts to alleviate psychoses by pharmacological means had had a long tradition; the experiments with chlorpromazine had been preceded by trials using other sympathicolytic and anticholinergic substances. The same also holds true for the Basel clinic, where the therapeutic indications of chlorpromazine were systematically expanded. An example to the contrary is given by Laborit's colleagues Hamon and his co-workers, who were able to test chlorpromazine even before Delay and Deniker had used it clinically, but did not recognize its potential.

How are the discoveries of imipramine, meprobamate, chlordiazepoxide and lithium to be assessed in this context? According to their inventors, luck was always involved, albeit in quite different ways. In Cade's own version of the story the choice of lithium as a medicament against mania was made on the basis of unrelated factors: in his experiments on the toxic effect of the urine of manic patients he was looking for a water-soluble form of uric acid and, in so doing, came across lithium urate. This molecule quite unexpectedly reduced the toxicity of the uric acid. Instead of lithium urate Cade consequently used lithium carbonate, which also protected his guinea pigs from the toxic effects of uric acid and this was the background against which the history of lithium as a psychopharmaceutical developed, as described in Section 2.4.2. Had it not been for Cade's systematic method of working, the chance discovery of lithium might in this case never have been made.

Looking back on it today, it would seem to us that chance played a smaller role in the discovery of the antidepressant effect of imipramine. The anti-manic effect of lithium was already known – although lithium was only being used in a few clinics – and the recently discovered antipsychotic effect of chlorpromazine suggested that psychoses could be symptomatically treated with pharmacological agents. Clinical trials in psychiatry with the chlorpromazine-like substances synthesized by Geigy were therefore a logical step; the critical contribution here was the persistent way in which R. Kuhn conducted his clinical studies, not simply confining himself to a single indication. Kuhn's personal conviction – a sort of magical belief that depression could be cured with pharmacological means – also played its part (Kuhn, 1970) and, taken together with the high price of chlorpromazine and the tight budget of a (non-university) psychiatric hospital in the mid-1950s, was probably decisive.

According to Sternbach's account of the discovery of chlordiazepoxide, chance was also at work in the laboratories of Hoffmann-La Roche, although in a negative way: of the series of substances which Sternbach had synthesized, why should it have been chlordiazepoxide, of all others, that had been left behind untested in the chemist's laboratory? Rather than stressing this chance occurrence, the well-conducted clinical trial of the experimental preparation should instead be emphasized. This was not restricted to a single indication or dosage range, but was extended – in the face of initial unfavourable results – into those indications within which the then standard preparation meprobamate achieved its best results (Cohen, 1970).

2.5.2 Serendipity and spirit of the age (Zeitgeist)

English-language literature, when referring to the discovery of the first psychopharmaceuticals, often states that '*serendipity*' was involved. This word, which comes from a Persian fairy tale, refers to the ability of a research worker to make a fortuitous and unexpected discovery, whilst leaving open upon what this ability is based. Jeste *et al.* (1979) have set out the etymology of the word and at the same time spoken against over-emphasis of the element of chance in the history of psychopharmacology. In their view, several impulses were needed to allow the development of the most important biological (pharmacological and other) methods of modern therapy in psychiatry:

- a strong individual motivation on the part of the research workers involved and the conviction that mental illnesses could be treated by physical methods;
- the ability to make precise observations and the persistence to follow up even unexpected results, and at the same time also the courage to extend laboratory observations to experiments in man;
- the *Zeitgeist* – the spirit of the times in which they worked, i.e. the cultural and, in the present case, in particular the scientific views, prevailing in a specific time and in a specific society;
- the availability of basic knowledge from several related disciplines.

At first sight we are quite willing to accept the importance of all four factors stated by Jeste *et al.*, but closer consideration raises several questions. There is no doubt that the discoverers of lithium, chlorpromazine, imipramine etc.

(Cade, Delay and Deniker, Kuhn) were highly motivated investigators and doctors, but there were also many highly motivated investigators at other times in psychiatry who were ready and able to check laboratory observations in clinical trials. The first two points put forward by Jeste *et al.* (1979) are thus quite non-specific. What characterized the scientific *Zeitgeist* of the late 1940s, and how did this differ from that of the 1920s and 1930s? The question cannot be answered in this general form, but in the case of psychiatry it should be remembered that physical and pharmacological methods of therapy had already been introduced in earlier times without leading to the discovery of chlorpromazine, and that the idea that mental illnesses could be caused or promoted by physical factors is a very old concept. What was decisive here was rather the circumstance that several pharmaceutical companies had started research and development programmes after the Second World War which, although aimed in different directions, resulted in pharmacologically active and relatively well-tolerated compounds that could be clinically tested in various, sometimes even speculative indications.

The fourth point in the analysis by Jeste *et al.* (basic knowledge from allied disciplines) is also unconvincing: Has the improvement in basic knowledge really made a decisive contribution? Lithium was already known and in medical use in the nineteenth century, without its antimanic properties and prophylactic effect in depression being discovered. The synthesis of the chemical structures of phenothiazine and iminodibenzyl, from which chlorpromazine and imipramine respectively were developed, had also been known since the nineteenth century (Caldwell, 1978) and, whilst the benzodiazepine structure was new, it was by no means so complicated that it could not have been synthesized far earlier. Finally, the pharmacological methods used to characterize the compounds in the laboratory were also not based on newly acquired basic knowledge, despite the fact that the scientists at Rhône–Poulenc had to develop several new tests.

It follows that newly acquired basic knowledge in psychiatry, e.g. about the biochemistry of psychoses (which was essentially unknown), cannot be shown to have had a direct impact on the discovery of modern psychopharmaceuticals. The neurophysiological, neurosurgical and neurochemical methods developed in the twentieth century played no part, either in the pharmacological or in the clinical characterization of lithium, chlorpromazine, imipramine, etc., and the minds of the then leading psychiatrists were directed to psychoanalysis and not to the biological basis of psychiatry. On the contrary, major fresh impetus was given to neurophysiology, neuropharmacology, neurochemistry, and to clinical research methodology *in the wake* of the discovery of these psychopharmaceuticals in the 1950s and 1960s.

2.5.3   Quantitative aspects

Possibly too little attention is paid in the historical accounts of psychopharmacology to one quantitative factor: the number of research workers in the field of natural science who have at various times grappled with problems in psychiatry, and the numbers of substances which have been used on the mentally ill at various periods in time. Both these figures have grown very appreciably over the last 100 years, especially after the First and Second World Wars. It is probably no coincidence that the major discoveries – the shock therapies on the one hand and the psychopharmaceuticals on the other – fall within these periods. It is evident that the prospects of finding a suitable medication for an illness of unknown pathogenic mechanism increase with the number of novel substances tested – always assuming that the pharmacological and clinical pharmacological work is properly conducted.

On the other hand, quantitative viewpoints alone are not sufficient to explain the sudden advance in the 1950s and the subsequent striking stagnation of psychopharmacology, with few new principles of action discovered since that time. In the 1960s and 1970s the number of researchers involved with psychopharmacology in hospitals, universities and industry increased considerably and an enormous number of substances were tested during that period without awakening decisive advances in the pharmacotherapy of schizophrenia, depression and other mental disorders. Therefore, this historically orientated chapter can suitably end with the affirmation that past results provide no recipe for future success except in one respect: it clearly requires a high 'suffering pressure' ('Leidensdruck'), the pressure of a major unresolved therapeutic problem, to release the required material resources and to motivate preclinical and clinical researchers to the tireless and at the same time original activity that then gives the lucky chance its opportunity. The partial therapeutic solutions available today in the form of neuroleptics, antidepressants and tranquillizers reduce this suffering pressure and in the final analysis may stand in the way of further pharmacological research in this area. Material incentives alone, the prospects of economic gain, are apparently insufficient to initiate research leading to novel principles of activity.

CHAPTER 3

Effects of psychopharmaceuticals on healthy subjects: perception and behaviour

3.1 THE SUBJECT OF PHARMACOPSYCHOLOGY

The topic of this chapter, namely the study of the effects of psychopharmaceuticals on healthy subjects, is termed *pharmacopsychology*. A typical pharmacopsychological experiment involves the administration of one or more doses of a psychotropic drug under 'controlled conditions', i.e., in a double-blind, balanced trial versus placebo, with determination of the pharmacological actions by empirical psychology methods (questioning, observation, counting, measurement). How is it then that psychopharmaceuticals are administered to healthy subjects, and what conclusions do we hope to draw from experiments such as these? In outline, the following objectives can be differentiated:

(1) Substance-orientated: The interest lies primarily in the drugs being studied, the common features and especially the differences between their actions, and the similarities and differences between their spectra of action in healthy subjects and the mentally ill. This field of investigation is also termed *human pharmacology*.

(2) Method-orientated: Interest is directed primarily to the test methods and their sensitivity and specificity with regard to drug effects. The actions of the drugs used are presumed to be known and they serve as readily usable tools for modifying the mental state of the subjects.

(3) Theory-orientated: Questions of theoretical interest form the centrepoint, e.g. the relationship between dopaminergic activity in the brain and a mental 'function' such as attention. Here also, drugs whose action on the brain is known from other studies, e.g. neuroleptics, can be used as instruments to induce the desired modifications in healthy subjects. It is also assumed that sensitive and specific psychological test methods are available to assess a function such as 'attention' (refer to Janke and Erdmann, 1992, on this topic).

(4) Testing of new drugs: Trials of this type are again substance orientated but involve new compounds that are in the development stage and not yet extensively tested in humans. They are generally performed in Phase I of the clinical development of new medicines (see Chapter 6).

(5) Practice-orientated: Pharmacopsychology also includes experiments to assess the action of psychopharmaceuticals on vehicle driving behaviour (see review by Hobi, 1992) or, for example, the ability to operate complicated apparatus. These studies are based on the assumption that results from experiments in healthy test subjects can be extrapolated to the conditions prevailing in patients.

Who are 'healthy test subjects'? In almost all publications on pharmacopsychology this means subjects who are medically and psychiatrically healthy at the time of the experiment and who are not taking any medicines; health therefore means 'the absence of a detectable illness' and generally implies that the subjects have also not previously suffered from severe mental disturbances. Since pharmacopsychological experiments are often conducted in university laboratories, the healthy subjects in many cases are students, i.e., a group that is not representative of the general population in various respects. Drug experiments are increasingly also being performed by commercially directed private institutes, especially in the testing of new substances. The healthy subjects in these cases are often unemployed, sometimes destitute tourists passing through the country, or pensioners, all of whom wish to improve their financial situation by participating in drug trials.

The term 'healthy subjects' can thus mean a number of different things, and the necessary attention has to be paid to the normally precisely stated selection criteria when interpreting experimental results.

3.2   STUDIES CONDUCTED BY KRAEPELIN

Pharmacopsychology in the present-day sense of the word has been referred to since the time of Kraepelin (1892) and yet this field of research only really began to acquire importance in the years following the discovery of chlorpromazine (see Uhr and Miller, 1964). Kraepelin's studies 'Ueber die Beeinflussung einfacher psychischer Vorgänge durch einige Arzneimittel' (The influence of some drugs on simple mental processes) related in particular to the psychotropic effects of alcohol. In addition, Kraepelin studied the hypnotics paraldehyde and chloral hydrate as well as the 'inhalation poisons' ether and chloroform. The stimulants he used were caffeine and tea and some of his experiments related to morphine. Kraepelin's hopes in connection with his studies were twofold. On the one hand he regarded it as a forward step 'to be able to set out, in numerical terms, those changes in our spiritual life which we could otherwise only describe in quite general terms using the deceptive method of self-observation and to attribute these to certain very simple, elementary disturbances through the use of experimental methods' (1892, p. 227). On the other hand, he hoped to gain knowledge for psychology, since drugs can be used to act repeatedly on normal mental processes and thus enable one to better study their 'true nature'.

Kraepelin performed his studies in W. Wundt's laboratory in Leipzig, using the objective methods newly developed there. He measured reaction times to serve as indicators of 'mental performance in general', reading speed with the aid of standardized texts and calculation performance by means of the addition of single-figure numbers over 5-minute periods. Sequences of 12-digit numbers had to be learnt off by heart, whereby the number of repetitions before a sequence could be recited without error served as a criterion of memory performance. Time-estimation trials were intended to indicate inner mental speed and association experiments were used to record the speed and wealth of word associations.

Apart from minor technical modifications, almost all the methods described by Kraepelin are still used today in pharmacopsychological and other psychological experiments. What has been very considerably improved in the intervening period is the experimental design of such studies. Kraepelin's trials were mostly conducted in the evenings since he himself and some of his colleagues served as test persons at the end of the normal working day. Kraepelin was often his own experimenter and in all cases the subjects knew what dosage of which substance they were taking. Quite a number of blank trials (without medication) were run in order to obtain reference values and yet no-substance and active-ingredient days were not balanced, and the use of a placebo for experimental purposes was unknown. Kraepelin ensured that no subject consumed tea, coffee or alcohol for 5–6 hours preceding the trial and saw that the last meal was taken 2–3 hours before the trial commenced. What he could not prevent, however, was that many of the experiments took place under unfavourable circumstances. His subjects and he himself were occasionally overtired or indisposed for other reasons, which may explain why one in a number of instances reads references to the difficulty of establishing the drug effects over and above spontaneous fluctuations. A further obvious difference in comparison to present-day experiments is the absence of formal statistical comparisons: Kraepelin confined himself to the elucidation of mean or median values and to descriptive comparisons. Tests of significance and statistical test procedures in the present-day sense were unknown at the end of the 19th century.

Whereas in Kraepelin's work the care devoted to the individual measurement methods was in contrast to the somewhat freely handled experimental design, great importance is nowadays laid on the planning and evaluation of pharmacological studies on subjects. The most important elements in the organization of pharmacopsychological studies are: selection of persons commensurate with the purpose of the study; standardization of experimental conditions (time of day, personnel, room used); balanced administration of test substances and placebo without knowledge on the part of the subjects and experimenter of the nature of the treatment given (double-blind technique); consideration of the constitution and disposition of the subjects (age, sex, body weight; sleep during the preceding night; health condition during preceding days; meals on the day of the study; etc.) as well as use of statistical methods appropriate to the data level. These are the same criteria as those applied in psychological experiments in general and are thoroughly discussed in textbooks on experimental psychology.

Despite many shortcomings in the design, the results of Kraepelin's trials remain interesting: after 30–50 g *alcohol*, corresponding to 70–110 ml of cognac or whisky or 250–400 ml of wine, a biphasic action was observed. Some 30–45 minutes after the alcohol had been consumed simpler activities such as reading and speed of reaction were often improved, whilst there was no change in the more difficult tasks. Later on, i.e., more than 45 minutes after intake, performance was in general reduced, particularly in the case of higher doses of alcohol and of the more complex activities (choice reaction times, wealth of word associations). After 3–5 g of the hypnotic *paraldehyde* a qualitatively similar pattern of action was observed as after alcohol, whereby the stimulation phase was briefer and less pronounced whilst the 'paralysing' action of the preparation was more pronounced. Following the intake of *chloral hydrate* and with the inhalation poisons the paralysing effect was still more pronounced. Only very few experiments were conducted using morphine (10 mg subcutaneously) owing to poor tolerability and no conclusions could be drawn. Following 500 mg *caffeine* and after tea (10 g yellow China and black East Indian tea, allowed to infuse for 5 minutes) improved performance was observed in a number of areas: there was an increase in the number of additions in the arithmetic test and in the number of word associations, but not in the latter's inventiveness.

Kraepelin made the following comments in his 'Summary of the results', which is formulated with great caution:

(1) He was 'very gratified' to note that 'the results of our studies show that each of the substances discussed herein exert an entirely characteristic effect on our spiritual life' (p. 228).
(2) His 'aim was exclusively to develop methods for a precise determination of the actions of drugs on the mind, and to demonstrate the possibility of their practical application and the utility of their results in selected examples' (pp. 229–230). This aim could be achieved, even though some questions could not be definitively answered, such as that concerning 'individual differences' (in response to drugs).
(3) In addition, it was possible to link the results achieved experimentally with everyday experience in the use of alcohol, and to gain a better understanding of the mode of action of these substances.

An appreciation of Kraepelin's pharmacopsychological work is given in a volume edited by Oldigs-Kerber and Leonard (1992) on the 100th anniversary of the Kraepelin monograph. The impact of these studies is particularly discussed in the chapter by Debus (pp. 44–68), where the discipline of pharmacopsychology is defined in terms of organization and methods.

- Interest centres on the effect exerted by psychopharmaceuticals in healthy subjects in an experimental situation not influenced by factors which are typical for the therapeutic use of psychopharmaceuticals in patients: a specific illness, the relationship to the doctor, and the therapeutic environment.
- In order to record such effects, use is made of sensitive, objective, reliable and valid methods. These methods today include procedures which reliably demonstrate subjective aspects of the effects of pharmaceuticals.

The following paragraphs begin with a survey of methods of assessment used in pharmacopsychology today. A review is then given of the most important experimental results, and the end of the chapter deals with a few theoretical and practical consequences of pharmacopsychological investigations.

3.3   METHODS USED IN PHARMACOPSYCHOLOGY

Psychotropic drugs exert effects which the subject or patient feels after their administration and which he can describe in words – for simplicity's sake we speak in terms of subjective effects. In addition, effects are triggered which are apparent to an observer – the subject appears to slow down, his speech sounds slurred, and his thoughts seem to wander; such changes can be objectively defined and quantified using appropriate methods. They are termed objective effects.

3.3.1   Methods for recording subjective drug effects

The method which, at first sight, appears to be the simplest one for recording subjective drug effects is to ask the subject how he feels before a substance is given and then to repeat the question after its administration. In the course of those *freely formulated questions*, the subject describes his current condition in his own words. The experimenter can then ask questions designed to help the subject to compare his current state after ingestion of the medicament with his state before its ingestion, provided he is still able to recall this. By means of *freely formulated descriptions of actions*, one can record individually felt, and qualitatively possibly very differentiated, subjective drug effects. The problems posed by this approach lie in the semantic and measurement areas: what is the meaning of such remarks as 'I feel all closed up' or 'it is like being behind a smoke-screen' to the individual subject? What do they mean to the investigator and how can one collate and quantify such individual declarations into standardized dimensions?

A more standardized method for determining subjective effects is that of *structured questioning*: here the subject is asked specific questions as to his mood, wakefulness and physical freshness (or other aspects of his condition of interest in the context of the study) and should then quantify his answers wherever possible into 'somewhat', 'slight', 'of medium intensity', etc. An advantage of this procedure is that unclear answers can be clarified by further questioning – a disadvantage is that the experimenter loses much time and may get bored in trials with larger groups of subjects and several repetitions per test day after taking the medicine. Moreover, it cannot be avoided that the experimenter's questions and assessment may be biased, as may his personal impressions of the real or presumed state of the subject. From the point of view of data analysis, fewer difficulties arise than with freely formulated questions since the dimensions governing the questions are laid down in advance so that intra- and inter-individual comparisons become possible.

For reasons of expediency and objectivity, and particularly in the case of more extensive studies, questions are preferably submitted in writing, i.e., in some form of *self-rating scale*. Here one distinguishes between symptom checklists, adjective checklists and semantic differentials.

Symptom checklists can be formulated as alternatives, i.e., the subject is asked whether or not he is experiencing a symptom, e.g. headache, at a given point in time. The list of predetermined symptoms can either be compiled on the basis of previous knowledge of the substances being tested, or a published symptom list can be used, such as the B–L and B–L′ symptom lists in German-speaking areas, each with 24 items (Zerssen, 1986a). Symptom checklists may also be formulated in grades; i.e., the subject is asked if a stated symptom is absent, mild, moderate, severe or intolerable. An example for this format is the SCL-90 (see *ECDEU Assessment Manual*, 1976). There is no general agreement as to which procedure is preferable, but short lists are best in principle if several determinations are to be made per test day. It is also considered that methods not requiring a yes–no decision but offering graded answers are advantageous.

Adjective checklists can be formulated as alternatives or grades. In both cases the subjects seek to describe their current mental state by means of predetermined adjectives. The EWL (Eigenschaftswörterliste = adjective checklist) of Janke and Debus (1981) is known in German-speaking areas, containing 123 adjectives that each have to be answered as 'applies' or 'does not apply'. The Bf–S and Bf–S′ scales of subjective feeling (Befindlichkeits-skalen; Zerssen, 1986b) are also known, each containing 28 contrasting pairs of terms. Similar instruments for use in English-speaking countries are the Clyde Mood Scale (Clyde, 1963) and the POMS (Profile of Mood States) by McNair *et al.* (see *ECDEU Assessment Manual*, 1976).

A *semantic differential* (polarities profile) compiled some 20 years ago on the basis of the EWL available at that time and similar methods of Heimann (1967, 1969) has proved very sensitive for drug effect in our own studies (Fig. 3.1). This semantic differential covers four dimensions with each of four pairs of contrasting terms:

(1) Concentration (pairs 1, 5, 12, 15).
(2) Fatigue (pairs 2, 8, 11, 14).
(3) Extroversion (pairs 3, 7, 10, 13).
(4) Negative mood (pairs 4, 6, 9, 16).

The words below can be used to describe an individual's mood. Please rate yourself according to what you are feeling *at this moment*, using the extreme terms given and placing a cross in the appropriate box: ☒

At this moment I feel . . .

	very					very	
concentrated	☐	☐	☐	☐	☐	☐	absent-minded
sleepy	☐	☐	☐	☐	☐	☐	wide-awake
talkative	☐	☐	☐	☐	☐	☐	silent
sad	☐	☐	☐	☐	☐	☐	cheerful
attentive	☐	☐	☐	☐	☐	☐	inattentive
anxious	☐	☐	☐	☐	☐	☐	confident
interested	☐	☐	☐	☐	☐	☐	uninterested
confused	☐	☐	☐	☐	☐	☐	lucid
irritable	☐	☐	☐	☐	☐	☐	well-balanced
sociable	☐	☐	☐	☐	☐	☐	withdrawn
over-worked	☐	☐	☐	☐	☐	☐	refreshed
serious	☐	☐	☐	☐	☐	☐	frivolous
active	☐	☐	☐	☐	☐	☐	passive
tired	☐	☐	☐	☐	☐	☐	fresh
self-controlled	☐	☐	☐	☐	☐	☐	boisterous
bad-tempered	☐	☐	☐	☐	☐	☐	good-tempered

Should you wish to provide additional information on your condition, please do so here:

Figure 3.1. Example of a semantic differential

For evaluation, the scores (left-hand column = 1 point, to right-hand column = 6 points) for the four pairs of a dimension are summed so that scores from 4 to 24 are obtained per dimension and are then processed statistically.

Together with U. Ferner we have sought to clarify the factorial structure of this semantic differential but the results of these efforts were unsatisfactory, since different factorial solutions are obtained depending on the data set used (only initial values of drug trials, initial values plus values after medication, daytime experiments, studies after sleep recordings). As a pragmatic way out in this case we evaluate the semantic differential according to the four originally defined dimensions and have thus obtained readily interpretable results in most experiments.

In this context mention should be made of the so-called *visual analogue scales* (Aitken, 1969) which have become popular and which can be individually adapted to suit specific experimental questions. These enable the subject to pinpoint his current condition somewhere along a 10 cm line, the ends of which denote extreme states (see Maxwell, 1978). The method is an extension of the principle of semantic differentials, which should permit a more finely graded self-assessment (some critical aspects are set out in Nicholson, 1978).

In general, greater standardization of questionnaire items simplifies quantitative comparisons between individuals and conditions, but simultaneously curtails each individual statement and forces it into what may be inappropriate categories. Moreover, giving the same degree of importance to all the items in a questionnaire, such as all 16 pairs of concepts in a semantic differential, may iron out the effects of substances and obscure interesting individual effects. A freely formulated description of drug action, be it in oral or written form, will therefore continue to be indispensable for the majority of drug studies.

3.3.2   Methods for recording objective drug effects

In principle any form of human activity capable of being observed and recorded can serve as a parameter indicating the effect of a psychopharmaceutical, provided that the situation within which the behaviour manifests itself can be sufficiently standardized. Behaviour in social situations, for example in groups, behaviour in situations where a certain level of performance is required, as well as times of relaxation or pleasure – all these activities can vary according to the degree of wakefulness and motivation of the individual and thus provide an opportunity for observations to be made. A review of the pharmacopsychological literature shows, however, that considerable overemphasis has been placed on studies of performance-orientated behaviour in the last 15 years, whereas there have been very few studies of drug effects on social behaviour and virtually none on the way in which they influence behaviour during relaxation and pleasure. There are various reasons for this one-sidedness (see Kohnen, 1992), and it is also a result of the difficulty in creating standardized, relevant and at the same ethically acceptable situations in which specific forms of social behaviour can be studied. Several older studies, which are summarized by McGuire *et al.* (1982), provide only minimal yield with regard to definable pharmacological effects.

In the following description the emphasis has consequently been laid on studies using *performance tests*, adhering to a classification of methods according to Janke (1977). He distinguishes between procedures which record:

- general performance;
- characteristics of perception;
- aspects of thought and intelligence;
- characteristics of memory;
- characteristics of motor function.

Table 3.1.   General performance tests (a selection)

Name	Nature of test	Task set	Duration	Remarks
Pauli test	Arithmetical	Adding long columns of single-digit numbers	60 min	Very simple task
K-L-T after Düker	Arithmetical	Calculation of two partial results and, depending on partial results, subtraction or addition of these	20 min	Difficult and tiring test
d2 after Brickenkamp	Cancellation	Picking out and marking of symbols according to a given criterion	4 min 40 s	Measures short-term concentration
Cancellation after Meili	Cancellation	ditto	2–4 min	ditto
Digit symbol substitution test (DSST) taken from WAIS	Coding	Allocation of given symbols to numbers	90 s	Complex performance test
Continuous performance test	Continuous performance	Calculation or discrimination task	20–60 min	Determines consistency of performance
Mackworth Clock	Vigilance	A second-hand travels round a dial, sometimes jumping over 2 s; these jumps have to be reported	15–60 min	Very boring, especially when of long duration
Acoustic vigilance test after Wilkinson	Vigilance	Single, slightly longer tones are interspersed in a sequence of tones of identical length; these have to be reported	60 min	ditto

It should be mentioned in this context that the borderline between the individual areas of performance are not sharply drawn (components of motor function and perception are involved in all forms of performance) and that allocation to a specific area is a matter for discussion in several of the tests. When studies are planned in practice this overlap will be considered by compiling a battery of tests containing some duplication whilst still retaining parameters from various areas of performance (in this context, see Debus and Janke, 1978, p. 2194 ff.).

Tests of general performance

This term designates procedures calling for neither special abilities such as verbal intelligence, nor motor dexterity, but simply recording the degree of alertness, concentration or exertion. General performance tests include simple arithmetical tasks, and cancellation and coding tests, as well as tasks designed to test vigilance (Table 3.1). A more detailed description of performance and vigilance tests may be found in Buros (1978) and Koelega (1989).

As Table 3.1 shows, general performance tests not only differ as regards the nature and difficulty of the tasks to be performed, they differ also in respect of their duration. Thus, cancellation tasks, such as the d2 test, last only a few minutes, whereas the Pauli test and the majority of vigilance tests normally last 1 hour or longer. By carefully selecting appropriate tests it is consequently also possible to measure characteristics of performance consistency. It should, however, be said that long and tedious tests such as the Mackworth Clock or the Pauli test cannot be repeated more than two or three times on the same experimental day.

Assessing processes of perception

The term 'perception' is used to designate those processes which serve to absorb and classify information from our surroundings. Speed, extent and quality of perception not only depend on the condition of the sensory organs, but are also a function of such factors as wakefulness, attentiveness or concentration, and emotional and motivational state as well as of cognitive processes, particularly of memory and thinking. In general, a distinction may be made between procedures for the determination of:

– thresholds of perception;
– speed of perception and of extent of perception;
– qualitative characteristics of perception.

Only a small proportion of the methods available (e.g. Lezak, 1983) are regularly used in pharmacopsychological experiments. Special mention should be made of the determination of critical flicker fusion frequency and of tachistoscopic trials, i.e. of methods which are directed at characteristics of visual perception. In contrast, drug effects on hearing have rarely, and those influencing senses of touch, smell and taste have hardly ever, been investigated (see Turner, 1971).

In studies of *critical flicker fusion frequency* (CFF) the frequency of a discontinuous light source is increased until the subject has the impression of seeing a continuous light. The corresponding frequency is termed the critical flicker fusion frequency. Another procedure, which may be combined with the first, consists in gradually reducing the frequency of a light source until that threshold is attained at which the continuous light begins to flicker. CFF serves as an indicator of wakefulness or tiredness, even though the underlying neuronal mechanisms are poorly understood (reviews by Smith and Misiak, 1976; *Pharmacopsychiatry*, 1982).

Tachistoscopic trials serve to record speed and extent of perception. In the course of such experiments, pictures, letters, numbers, etc. are shown for a very short time and the subject has to name the items presented as far as he has recognized them. Tests with simple configurations of stimuli (colours, single letters or objects) primarily record speed of perception, whilst experiments with more varied content investigate the extent of perception and hence also components of short-term memory. In contrast to the 1960s, when tachistoscopic experiments were undertaken frequently, they are nowadays hardly used at all in pharmacopsychology, presumably because of their low sensitivity to the effects of substances. The same applies in the case of methods used to record qualitative characteristics of perception (Gestalt tendencies).

Assessing aspects of thought and intelligence

Psychologists have at their disposal many intelligence and aptitude tests which have been developed for applications in the school and training sector, in personnel selection and for diagnostic purposes. Some of these tests, such as the well-known Wechsler Adult Intelligence Scale (WAIS) and its revisions, consist of subtests some of which are also used in pharmacopsychology. The Digit Symbol Substitution Test (DSST) from the WAIS in particular has been used in many studies, as have also the Block Design and Figure Completion Tests. Their frequent use may be attributed to the brevity of these tests and to the fact that it is easy to devise parallel forms. These WAIS subtests, which are all taken from the so-called performance part, are generally used in pharmacopsychological studies in the sense of general performance tests rather than as indicators of intelligence (Table 3.1).

Methods which tend to relate to verbal aspects of intelligence are also used in pharmacopsychological experiments. In vocabulary and word fluency tests the subject is, for example, given an initial letter for which he should name as many nouns as possible, or he is asked to name as many four-legged animals as possible within a specific time limit. Other tasks tend rather to call for powers of logic, such as the solution of syllogisms and finding communalities, similarities and contradictions. Tasks of this nature are above all suitable for trials in which the same subject is tested once or only a few times. When trials involve the repeated testing of the same subject on the same day or over several days, the problem arises of devising equivalent parallel forms of the same type of task – a problem which cannot always be satisfactorily solved.

Assessing memory performance

The processes of learning and remembering can be broken down into the following stages, which follow each other in time: information intake (registration), processing (encoding), storage and retention, and retrieval (reproduction). In addition, a division into memory files or 'stores' has been proposed, involving, depending on the author, two or more components: ultrashort-term, short-term and long-term stores are constructs which can be operationalized and quantified in suitable experimental designs. For pharmacopsychological experiments the time at which a product is administered and develops its action is decisive (Fig. 3.2):

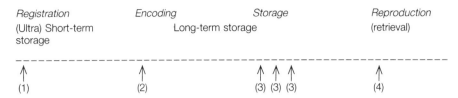

(1) Administration of a drug before the registration phase.
(2) Administration after the registration phase, at the time of encoding.
(3) Chronic administration during long-term storage.
(4) Administration before the retrieval phase.
(1) and (4): Experiments on state-dependent learning and remembering.

Figure 3.2. Possible timing of drug administration during the learning and memory process

(1) If a drug is administered *before the registration phase*, its general effects on wakefulness, alertness and motivation are confounded with its possible specific effects on memory processes, e.g. on the encoding that is closely linked with registration. It is therefore to be expected that stimulant substances administered before the registration phase will have a 'memory-promoting' effect as a result of their action on attentiveness, whereas sedative compounds will have the opposite effect.

(2) A drug can be administered *after the registration phase* with the purpose of studying its actions on encoding processes. Trials of this type in humans supply ambiguous results (see Section 7.1 in Chapter 7) since encoding processes of various types and various hierarchical grades last for seconds, minutes and hours, whereas the time at which a drug reaches and affects the relevant brain structures cannot be controlled precisely. In addition, positive and negative interferences are possible in this experimental design: as in case (1), in parallel with its possible action on encoding the initially registered material, a drug can affect the registration and encoding of subsequent information and thus increase or reduce the tendency of the later information to interfere with the earlier information.

(3) A drug may be administered *after the likely conclusion of the encoding processes*, i.e., at a time when the acquired information is stored in the long-term store, and may therefore counteract or promote the spontaneous decay of previously learned information. This is a particularly interesting question in long-term drug administration. Restrictions similar to those in case (2) exist with regard to the specificity of pharmacological action, and restrictions similar to those in case (4) exist if retrieval is tested under the influence of the drug.

(4) A drug may be administered *before the reproduction phase* in order to study its action on the retrieval of stored information. As in case (1), the general effects of the substance on wakefulness, motivation, etc. are confounded with its possible specific effects on retrieval.

Table 3.2.   Methods for testing learning and memory performances

Method	Type of task	Duration	Comments
Digit span (Lezak, 1983)	Repetition forwards or backwards of a series of single-digit numbers of increasing length: short-term memory	About 5 min	Sub-test of WAIS and of the Wechsler Memory Scale
Rey's 15-word test (Lezak, 1983)	Repetition of a series of 15 words, 5 repetitions: short-term memory	About 5 min	Parallel forms are available
Selective reminding task (Buschke and Fuld, 1974)	Repetition of a series of 10–12 words; only omitted words are repeated by the tester	About 10 min	Complex test for the tester and test subject
Benton visual retention test (Lezak, 1983)	Geometric shapes are shown for 10 s each and then have to be drawn from memory (drawing version) or picked out from several similar shapes (multiple-choice version)	5 min	Motor handicaps interfere with the drawing version but not with the multiple-choice version
Paired associate learning	Words, numbers, etc., each belonging to a stimulus word or number, shape, etc., have to be learned	5–10 min	Recall of the associated words, etc. may be tested after minutes, hours or days
Logical memory	Recall of a story with a specific number of elements	5 min	E.g. as part of the Wechsler Memory Scale

Also of interest are studies on *state-dependent learning and memory*, which may be considered as a combination of cases (1) and (4): registration and retrieval occur after administrations of one and the same substance. This is a special case of context-dependent learning and memory, i.e. concerning the question of whether information acquired under the influence of a drug (case (1)) can be retrieved better or worse when this same substance or placebo are administered before the retrieval phase (case (4)).

Studies of the actions of drugs on memory performance are attractive in several respects, yet they make particularly great demands on the planning and interpretation of a trial. Some well-known test methods for learning and memory are summarized in Table 3.2, only a few of which are regularly used in pharmacopsychology, (e.g. digit span, word list learning and paired associate learning tests).

Assessing motor performance

According to Janke (1977, p. 31 ff.), 'contrary to the generally accepted view, characteristics of motor activity constitute an extremely differentiated system', an opinion that is illustrated by the fact that various motor tests show

Table 3.3.   Methods for testing motor performance (selection)

Name of test	Nature of test	Type of task	Duration
Tapping	Straightforward speed test	Subject taps on a pad as quickly as possible	≤30 s
Aiming	Tests speed and accuracy	Subject inserts a dot into circles or squares arranged in various patterns	≤2 min
Visual tracking	Tracking movements with the eyes	A regularly or irregularly oscillating light spot is tracked with the eyes	≤5 min
Purdue Peg Board	Motor dexterity	Pegs have to be inserted into rows of holes in a board	≤3 min
Pursuit rotor	Visuo-motor coordination (now mostly VDUs)	Subject follows a point affixed to a rotating disc	≤5 min
Measurements of reaction times	Alertness; psychomotor coordination	Reactions to simple or more complex acoustic and optical stimuli	2–10 min
Dynamometer	Strength and fatigability	A handle has to be pressed repeatedly against resistance provided by a spring	15–60 s

only low correlations with one another. There is a large number of methods for recording motor performance (Table 3.3), drawn mainly from occupational and traffic psychology. More comprehensive accounts are given in Fleishman (1964, 1972) and Kunsman *et al.* (1992). Some of these methods are subject to a pronounced practice effect when the tests are repeated and thus increasingly acquire the character of general performance tests.

The test times quoted in Table 3.3 can be varied according to the questions covered and it is consequently possible to investigate fluctuations in motor speed and quality of performance as a function of time.

3.4   RESULTS OF PHARMACOPSYCHOLOGICAL TRIALS

The following paragraphs summarize old and new results obtained from drug experiments in healthy subjects, with the emphasis initially on the question of *specificity of action*. As drug types with different clinical indications, do neuroleptics, antidepressants, tranquillizers and psychostimulants also have different actions in healthy subjects? Complying with this line of enquiry, Sections 3.4.1–3.4.4 are arranged per drug type. Even in this single sector of pharmacopsychology the number of individual studies is so great that only a selection of references can be given, where possible with a reference to review articles.

3.4.1   Effects of neuroleptics (see Table 3.4)

There are several older publications which cover the *subjective effect* of neuroleptics in higher doses. It is known from the trials conducted by Delay *et al.*

Table 3.4. Effects of neuroleptics in healthy subjects (selection)

Dimension	Product	Dose (mg) p.o.	Parameters investigated: type of effect
Subjective effects	Chlorpromazine	25–200	Dose-dependent unpleasant sedation, need to sleep, mood deterioration
	Clozapine	5–10	Tiredness, need to sleep
	Flupenthixol	1.0–2.0	No significant effects
	Fluphenazine	1	Mild increase in drive in emotionally labile subjects
	Haloperidol	1–4	Inner unrest from 2 mg, combined with external inhibition
	Perphenazine	2–16	No marked effects up to 8 mg; mood deterioration with 16 mg
	Pimozide	1–2	No clear action in emotionally labile subjects
	Remoxipride	30–60	No significant effects
	Sulpiride	400	No significant effects
General performance	Chlorpromazine	50–200	Cancellation, calculation, digit-symbol tests: reduced performance
	Flupenthixol	1–2	DST, cancellation test: not significant
	Haloperidol	3	Continuous attention test: deterioration
	Perphenazine	2–16	No significant effects
	Remoxipride	30–60	Continuous attention, vigilance: deterioration
	Sulpiride	400	Continuous attention: deterioration (late effect)
	Trifluoperazine	2–16	No significant effects
Perception	Chlorpromazine	25–100	CFF: reduced (also after 20–40 mg dipiperon and other neuroleptics)
	Chlorpromazine	200	Tachistoscope: slight slowing (with other neuroleptics also)
	Flupenthixol	1–2	CFF: not significant
	Haloperidol	3	CFF: decrease
	Remoxipride	30–60	CFF: decrease
	Sulpiride	400	CFF: not significant

Table 3.4. *Continued*

Dimension	Product	Dose (mg) p.o.	Parameters investigated: type of effect
Thought, intelligence	Chlorpromazine	12.5–25	Hanoi tower puzzle: worse (Danion *et al.*, 1992)
		100	Analytical thought: no significant effect
	Haloperidol	1–2	Word fluency: no significant effect
Learning, memory	Chlorpromazine	100–200	Verbal learning: worse
			Digit span: no significant effect up to 50 mg
	Flupenthixol	1–2	Digit span: no significant effect
	Haloperidol	3	Digit span: no significant effect
	Sulpiride	400	Digit span: no significant effect
	Trifluoperazine	8–15	Verbal learning: worse
Motor function	Chlorpromazine	50–200	Tapping, reaction time, pursuit rotor: performance impaired
	Flupenthixol	1–2	Tapping, tracking: performance impaired
	Fluphenazine	1	Reaction time, pursuit rotor, etc.: no significant effect
	Haloperidol	3	Tapping, choice reaction time: no significant effect
	Perphenazine	2–16	Tapping, pursuit rotor, precision movements: no significant effect
	Remoxipride	30–60	Choice reaction time, decision test: no significant effect
	Sulpiride	400	Motor manipulation test: performance impaired
	Thioridazine	100	Reaction time, pursuit rotor: performance impaired

See DiMascio *et al.* (1965), Wittenborn (1978), Janke (1980) and Spiegel (1980) for references to older studies and information on other products. See text for references to recent works.

(1959) and Di Mascio *et al.* (1963) that chlorpromazine has a pronounced sedative effect in healthy subjects. Single doses of 100–200 mg gave rise to the following effects:

- pronounced tiredness, need to sleep, but no agreeable relaxed feeling;
- slower and confused thinking, difficulties in concentrating, feelings of clumsiness;
- dejection, anxiety, irritability.

Lower doses of chlorpromazine (12.5 and 25 mg) lead to milder sedation (Danion *et al.*, 1992). The vegetative effects (dryness of the mouth, visual disturbances, sweating) seen when chlorpromazine is used therapeutically were also experienced by the subjects with single doses of 50 mg or more and contributed to the subjectively quite disagreeable state.

Neuroleptics which have no initial sleep-inducing effect when used therapeutically have a different pattern of action in healthy subjects from that of chlorpromazine. Perphenazine and trifluoperazine, which were administered in rather high doses in the early study conducted by Di Mascio *et al.*, and haloperidol which has been tested in up to 4 mg single doses, are neither sleep-inducing nor clearly sedating. After each of the three preparations, some of the subjects felt dysphoric; after doses of more than 2 mg haloperidol or after 30 or 60 mg of remoxipride a state arose which was simultaneously characterized by inner restlessness and external sedation (Eiff and Jesdinsky, 1960; McClelland *et al.*, 1990; Fagan *et al.*, 1991). The subjects felt the urge to do something, to move around, but were at the same time inhibited and felt restrained. When given to healthy subjects, clozapine, a clinically highly sedating medicament, produces tiredness and a desire to sleep, even in low doses. No significant subjective effects were reported after 1.0 or 2.0 mg of flupenthixol or after 400 mg of sulpiride (Mattila *et al.*, 1988; McClelland *et al.*, 1990).

Whilst the effects of chlorpromazine on *functions of performance* have been studied very thoroughly and over a wide dosage range, only fragmentary results are available for other neuroleptics. When given in doses of 50 mg or more, chlorpromazine may cause a drop in performance in several test parameters (general performance tests, perception, motor functions), whereas learning and memory functions are not significantly affected up to 50 mg (McClelland *et al.*, 1990). Neuroleptics with marked antipsychotic activity but little sleep-inducing properties (flupenthixol, haloperidol, perphenazine, trifluoperazine) reduce performance in individual tests but do not display a uniform pattern of activity, which may be partly due to the low doses investigated compared to the doses commonly used in clinical practice. Remoxipride, an experimental neuroleptic, also has only slight effects on performance parameters.

There is generally very good agreement between subjective perceptions and objective effects of neuroleptics since preparations or doses which test subjects which are perceived to be highly sedating also lead to significant declines in performance tests. Improvements in performance after neuroleptics were found in only one study (improved reaction time after 1 mg of haloperidol; King and Henry, 1992).

3.4.2 Effects of antidepressants (Table 3.5)

Subjective effects: Whereas Bye *et al.* (1978) describe a calming action of amitriptyline in small doses, and various authors have described a sleep-inducing effect with doses over 25 mg, imipramine, although in much larger doses, leads to a subjectively unpleasant state of sedation associated with pronounced vegetative symptoms (Pöldinger, 1963; DiMascio *et al.*, 1964; Heimann, 1969). Desipramine, which was also investigated by Pöldinger (1963) and DiMascio *et al.* (1964), showed qualitatively similar, albeit less pronounced, subjective effects. A few reports are on hand relating to the administration in subject trials of newer antidepressants which have a less pronounced sedative action when used therapeutically (binedaline: Jones *et al.*, 1986; bupropion: Hamilton *et al.*, 1983, paroxetine: Hindmarch, 1988); there seems to be good agreement between healthy subjects and patients with regard to the acute sedating and sleep-inducing effects. Antidepressants which are more markedly sedating in clinical use (maprotiline, mianserin, trimipramine) also induce tiredness or drowsiness in healthy subjects (Warot *et al.*, 1989a, 1989b).

Most antidepressants have been tested in healthy subjects with regard to their actions on various areas of *performance*; Table 3.5 presents only a selection of results. It is clear from this summary that, as representatives of the more sedating antidepressants, amitriptyline, mianserin and trimipramine inhibit almost all areas of performance in healthy subjects even in low doses, whereas the mainly newer and less sedating antidepressants binedaline (Jones *et al.*, 1986), bupropion (Hamilton *et al.*, 1983), fluoxetine (Moskowitz and Burns, 1988), moclobemide (Tiller, 1990) and paroxetine (Hindmarch, 1988; Deijen *et al.*, 1989) do not impair performance after the administration of single doses to healthy subjects. Here again the good agreement between subjective perceptions and the changes detected by objective methods is striking. Only in one study with sertraline (Hindmarch and Bhatti, 1988) is there a discrepancy between subjectively perceived drowsiness and signs of stimulation in some test areas (CFF, choice reaction time).

The effect of *lithium* in healthy subjects has been studied on a number of occasions. According to results collected to date, the effects of a single dose of lithium are small and closely related to personality and motivation of the subject, and this also holds true when the substance is given over a period of several weeks: Pflug *et al.* (1980) found no noticeable effects either on subjective or on several objective parameters after daily doses of 30 mEq, whereas Kropf and Müller-Oerlinghausen (1979) as well as Herrmann *et al.* (1980) recorded slightly disturbed well-being and vigilance after somewhat higher doses. Ulrich and Kriebitzsch (1987) also reported significant effects on performance in a visual-motor tracking task.

Table 3.5. Effects of antidepressants on healthy subjects

Dimension	Product	Dose (mg) p.o.	Parameters investigated: type of effect
Subjective effects	Amitriptyline	6.25–25	Feeling of calmness, relaxation; drowsiness with larger doses
	Binedaline	50–100	No significant effect
	Desipramine	50–200	Similar to imipramine, but less pronounced
	Imipramine	50–200	Unpleasant sedation, feeling of passivity, dullness, lethargy, confused thought
	Maprotiline	25–75	Tiredness, lack of energy
	Nortriptyline	12.5–25	Relaxation
	Paroxetine	30	No significant effects
	Sertraline	25–100	Dose-dependent drowsiness
	Trimipramine	25–100	Dose-dependent drowsiness
General performance	Amitriptyline	6.75–75	Vigilance test, arithmetical test and DSST: impaired performance
	Binedaline	100	Cancellation test: no significant effect
	Fluoxetine	60	Attentiveness, vigilance: no significant effect
	Imipramine	200	Arithmetical test and DSST: impaired performance
	Mianserin	10–15	Continuous attention test, vigilance test: impaired performance
	Moclobemide	100–300	DSST: no significant effect
	Nortriptyline	12.5–25	Vigilance test: impaired performance
	Trimipramine	25–100	DSST: no significant effect
Perception	Amitriptyline	50–75	Critical flicker fusion frequency (CFF): reduced
	Binedaline	50–100	Stroop interference test: no significant effect
	Imipramine	75	Stroop interference test: no significant effect
	Maprotiline	25–75	CFF: reduced after 50 or 75 mg
	Mianserin	15	CFF reduced
	Moclobemide	100–300	CFF: no significant effect

Table 3.5. *Continued*

Dimension	Product	Dose (mg) p.o.	Parameters investigated: type of effect
	Paroxetine	30	Eye movements: no significant effect
	Sertraline	25–100	CFF: dose-dependent increase
	Trimipramine	25–100	CFF: dose-dependent increase
Thought, intelligence	Binedaline	50–100	Relational thought ('logical reasoning'): no significant effect
	Imipramine	75	Relational thought ('logical reasoning'): slowed
Learning, memory	Amitriptyline	25	Digit span: performance impaired
	Fluoxetine	60	Word list learning: no significant effect
	Maprotiline	25–75	Various tests: all with no significant effect
	Trimipramine	25–100	Various tests: all with no significant effect
Motor function	Amitriptyline	12.5–25	Tapping, reaction time: performance impaired
	Fluoxetine	60	Tracking: no significant effect
	Imipramine	200	Pursuit rotor: performance impaired
	Maprotiline	25–75	Choice reaction time: no significant effect
	Moclobemide	300–600	Choice reaction time: no significant effect
	Nortriptyline	12.5–25	Tapping, reaction time: performance impaired
	Paroxetine	30	Various tests: no significant effect
	Sertraline	25–100	Choice reaction time: improved
	Trimipramine	25–100	Reaction time: performance impaired

For references to the cited older studies and information on other products, see Spiegel (1980), Smiley (1987) and Curran *et al.* (1988). See text for references to more recent works.

Table 3.6. Effects of tranquillizers on healthy subjects (selection)

Dimension	Product	Dose (mg) p.o.	Parameters investigated: type of effect
Subjective effects	Chlordiazepoxide	10–60	Relaxation up to 30 mg, tiredness with higher doses
	Diazepam	5–20	Pattern of action qualitatively similar to that of chlordiazepoxide;
	Lorazepam,	2–10	differences with regard to strength, onset and duration of effect
	Oxazepam, etc.		
	Buspirone	5–20	Doses over 10 mg: sedation
	Suriclone	0.2–0.4	Few subjective effects
	Zopiclone	7.5	Sedation
General performance	Chlordiazepoxide	40–60	Arithmetical tests: no significant effect
	Oxazepam	7–20	Arithmetical and cancellation tests: performance impaired; contradictory results in DSST
	Lorazepam	5–10	Cancellation tests: performance impaired
	Buspirone	5–20	Variable results, mostly no effect
	Suriclone	0.2–0.4	DSST, copying test: performance impaired
	Zopiclone	7.5	DSST: performance impaired
Perception	Chlordiazepoxide	20–60	CFF: reduced
	Diazepam	5–10	CFF: reduced
	Lorazepam	2	CFF: reduced (Subhan et al., 1986)
	Buspirone	5–20	CFF, eye tracking movements: no effects
	Suriclone	0.2–0.4	CFF: slight reduction after 0.4 mg
	Zopiclone	7.5	CFF: reduced

Table 3.6. *Continued*

Dimension	Product	Dose (mg) p.o.	Parameters investigated: type of effect
Thought, intelligence	Chlordiazepoxide	20–60	See McNair (1973): variable results with different tests
	Diazepam	7–20	Sequence completion: no significant effect; spatial thinking: impaired
Learning, memory (see Chapter 7)	Diazepam	7–20	Digit span, word list learning: performance impaired
	Lorazepam	4 (i.v.)	Picture recollection: performance impaired
	Buspirone	5–10	No amnestic effect; attentiveness: no effect
Motor function	Chlordiazepoxide	40–60	Tapping, reaction times: performance impaired
	Diazepam	5–20	Numerous motor and reaction tasks: performance impaired from 10 mg
	Lorazepam	2	Motor and reaction tasks: performance impaired (Subhan *et al.*, 1986)
	Buspirone	5–20	Reaction time, tracking, divided attention: no effect
	Suriclone	0.2–0.4	Tapping: slower
	Zopiclone	7.5	Tracking: more errors; reaction time: slower

See Wittenborn (1979), Hindmarch (1980), Johnson and Chernik (1982) and Taylor and Tinklenberg (1987) for references to the cited studies and information on other products (including hypnotics). See text for references to more recent works.

3.4.3 Effects of tranquillizers (Table 3.6)

Subjective effects: Depending on the experimental situation and other factors, benzodiazepines can have a relaxing effect even in healthy subjects (review by Debus and Janke, 1986). However, this effect has not been confirmed in all studies (e.g. Ghoneim *et al.*, 1984b) and seems to be restricted to a narrow dose range: just a slight increase in dose leads to feelings of tiredness, drowsiness and languor. Similar effects are felt after taking sleep-inducing agents of the benzodiazepine group. Meprobamate, a tranquillizer hardly used any more today (and not shown in the table), produces relaxation in healthy subjects without inducing a feeling of diminished activity or reduced performance with increasing dose. Healthy subjects may feel bored or indifferent after doses over 800 mg, but not tired or sleepy (Janke and Debus, 1968).

Instead of relaxation, either no effect (suriclone) or general sedation is obtained after some newer non-benzodiazepine preparations (buspirone: various authors; suriclone: Allen and Lader, 1992; zopiclone: Kuitunen *et al.*, 1990).

Hundreds of studies have been published on the effects of tranquillizers and hypnotics on *performance parameters* in healthy subjects; the older works are summarized in the reviews mentioned in the last two lines of Table 3.6. Whereas meprobamate has no effects on performance parameters even in large single doses (Berger and Potterfield, 1969) and although not confirmed in each and every individual study, all benzodiazepines cause a dose-related reduction in practically all examined areas of performance.

Tests which appear to be particularly sensitive to the effects of tranquillizers and hypnotics – apart from the critical flicker fusion frequency – are those calling for complex motor or psychomotor coordination, such as simulated traffic situations (O'Hanlon *et al.*, 1982; Smiley, 1987). Vigilance tests of longer duration are also considered to be very sensitive (Koelega, 1989). In contrast, reaction times to different configurations of stimuli were only slowed in a few individual studies. Even in large doses, benzodiazepines have not been shown to have any distinctly negative influence on tasks calling for a certain intellectual effort. In the case of buspirone, no adverse effects on performance were detected after single doses corresponding to therapeutically used doses (review by O'Hanlon, 1991), whereas the sedating action of the non-benzodiazepines suriclone (Allen and Lader, 1992) and zopiclone (Kuitunnen *et al.*, 1990) was expressed in various areas of performance. In general there is very good agreement between the subjectively perceived effects of the tranquillizers and their action on performance parameters with respect both to the nature of the effect and the effective dose.

Great interest has been shown in the amnestic effects of the benzodiazepines which are utilized in anaesthesiology. When given prior to surgery, higher doses of diazepam and other preparations lead to amnesia covering the period immediately preceding, during, and – depending on the dose and the duration of action of the preparation – after operation (anterograde amnesia, see Chapter 7). Since diazepam and other benzodiazepines are mainly used as tranquillizers and hypnotics, the question arises as to whether amnestic effects occur in their everyday use and at non-anaesthetic doses. A number of trials on healthy subjects involving dosages typical for use as tranquillizers yielded no clear indications as to impairment of memory, although the amnestic effect of these preparations can be demonstrated easily in higher doses.

The question of whether the amnestic action of benzodiazepines is specific or is part of a general 'sedation syndrome' will be taken up again in Chapter 7.

3.4.4   Effects of psychostimulants (Table 3.7) **and other medicaments enhancing cerebral performance (nootropics)**

Subjective effects: In healthy subjects, amphetamines and related psycho-stimulants as well as caffeine produce a feeling of energy and activity (Weiss and Laties, 1962; Spiegel, 1979). Such effects can generally also be demonstrated in subjects not suffering from overtiredness and they are particularly pronounced in the case of strenuous or monotonous activities of longer duration. Which method of assessment is employed appears to be of no great importance since, after reviewing about 200 controlled studies using stimulants in healthy subjects, it is apparent that quite widely differing subjective evaluation scales have been applied. There is, however, a minority of subjects who show a negative response to stimulants and feel tired, listless and occasionally also depressed.

Few results are available of experiments in healthy volunteers involving the use of medicaments, such as co-dergocrine mesylate, piracetam or vincamine, which are used in mentally deteriorating geriatric patients; experience collected to date suggests that a single dose of these preparations corresponding to therapeutic levels has no subjective stimulant or other effect in young test subjects (see Spiegel, 1992).

The effects of stimulants on *performance criteria* have been studied extensively (reviews of older works by Weiss and Laties, 1962; Spiegel, 1979) and may be summarized as follows:

(1) Improvements in performance after amphetamine in dosages of 2.5–20 mg are particularly marked in tasks where prolonged attentiveness and concentration are called for. With increasing test duration the effect of amphetamine on cancellation, arithmetical and vigilance tasks becomes more pronounced.

(2) Performance involving a motor component is also improved. Motor performance is stepped up only slightly in rested subjects, but improvements are more pronounced when the test persons are overtired.

(3) A few studies involving amphetamine revealed improved learning and memory performance. These effects may presumably be attributed to improved alertness during the acquisition phase (Chapter 7), and the

Table 3.7. Effects of psychostimulants on healthy subjects (selection)

Dimension	Product	Dose (mg) p.o.	Parameters investigated: type of effect
Subjective effects	d-Amphetamine	5–20	Feelings of energy, activity, interest, well-being
	Caffeine	56–600	Activity and energy increased. 'Nervousness' with larger doses
	Pyritinol	600, 1200	No significant effects
General performance	d-Amphetamine	2.5–15	Prolonged arithmetical, cancellation and vigilance tests: performance improved
	Captagon	50	Concentration-performance tests (CPT): performance improved
	Caffeine	32–750	Cancellation tests: performance improved after 750 mg
			Vigilance test: performance improved after 32–300 mg
			Complex reaction times: performance improved after 32–250 mg (Lieberman et al., 1987)
		125, 250	Stroop test: slowed (Foreman et al., 1989)
Perception	d-Amphetamine	5–15	CFF: occasionally increased, generally no significant effect
	Captagon	50	CFF: no significant effect
	Methylphenidate	10–20	Tachistoscope: performance improved
	Modafinil	200	CFF: increased (after sleep deprivation)
	Pyritinol	600, 1200	CFF: slightly increased
Thought, intelligence	d-Amphetamine	5–10	Simple tasks: performance improved. Intelligence tests: performance improved
	Caffeine	300	Free word association: improved (Pons et al., 1988)

Table 3.7. *Continued*

Dimension	Product	Dose (mg) p.o.	Parameters investigated: type of effect
Learning, memory	*d*-Amphetamine	10–15	Acquisition of motor skills, paired associate learning, long-term retention: performance improved
	Caffeine	70–300	Free memory: improved, depending on test conditions (Gupta, 1991)
		125, 250	Word lists: no significant effects
	Modafinil	200	Paired associates learning: improved (after sleep deprivation)
	Pyritinol	600, 1200	Short-term memory: no significant effect
Motor function	Amphetamine	10–20	Physical strength and endurance improved; Tapping, aiming: variable results
	d-Amphetamine	10–20	Reaction times: reduced in tests of longer duration
	Caffeine	75–300	Tapping: performance improved after 150, 300 mg; Reaction time reduced after 75, 150 mg
		125, 250	Reaction times: no significant effect
	Methylphenidate	20–40	Reaction times: reduced
	Modafinil	200	Reaction times: reduced (after sleep deprivation)
	Pyritinol	600, 1200	Reaction times: no significant effect

See Weiss and Laties (1962), Spiegel (1979, 1980) and Murray (1988) for references and further information on the cited studies.

improved performance in intelligence tests found in various trials is very likely due to a similar mechanism.

After caffeine which, in contrast to amphetamines, has been studied repeatedly in the last 10 years, improved performance has been observed in various domains, although the stimulating effect of this preparation is of shorter duration than that of amphetamine. Doses tested and found to be effective lay between 75 mg (corresponding to two cups of coffee) and 750 mg. The higher doses can, however, lead to quite unpleasant vegetative side effects (for review see Murray, 1988).

In a study by H.R. Lieberman *et al.* (1987) in 20 healthy subjects, significant improvements in performance were obtained in the Wilkinson vigilance test and in a complex reaction test after just 32 mg caffeine, i.e., after an amount corresponding to a cola drink or a cup of coffee. No additional improvements beyond the effect of 32 mg were observed after larger doses (64, 128, 256 mg).

Bensimon *et al.* (1991) observed an improvement in performance after modafinil, a new catecholaminergic stimulant not available in all countries, in subjects who had previously been fatigued by sleep deprivation.

Results of pharmacopsychological experiments with *nootropics* have only rarely been published. However, on the basis of a study by Hindmarch *et al.* (1990) with pyritinol and our own results with co-dergocrine mesylate, piracetam and vincamine (Spiegel, 1992) it is safe to assume that a single administration of these products in normal therapeutic doses has no effect on the performance of healthy subjects.

3.5 DISCUSSION: THE SIGNIFICANCE OF PHARMACOPSYCHOLOGICAL EXPERIMENTS

3.5.1 Specificity of action of the various classes of substances

From the results mentioned in the preceding paragraphs it emerges that most psychopharmaceuticals induce subjective and objective effects in healthy subjects that can be detected and quantified by psychometric methods. Within the context of substance-orientated objectives (p. 50) it now remains to be discussed whether and to what extent the various clinically used drugs (neuroleptics, antidepressants, etc.) differ in experiments in healthy subjects. For this purpose, the most important substance effects shown in the preceding tables are summarized and compared across drug classes, in Table 3.8. The following points emerge clearly:

(1) In doses far below their therapeutically used daily doses, the initially sleep-inducing neuroleptics of the chlorpromazine type induce subjective and objective sedation and a reduction in performance, which is a state not perceived to be pleasant by the test subjects.

Table 3.8. Summary of the effects of psychopharmaceuticals in healthy subjects

Dimension	Neuroleptics[a]	Antidepressants[b]	Tranquillizers[c], hypnotics	Stimulants[a] and similar
Subjective effects	Unpleasant sedation, mood deteriorated, indifference	Relaxation, sedation tiredness, drowsiness	Relaxation; in higher doses tiredness, need for sleep	Alertness, activity, interest, mood, sociability improved
General performance tests	Cancellation ↓ Arithmetics ↓ DSST (↓)	Arithmetics ↓ DSST ↓ Vigilance ↓	Cancellation ↓ Arithmetics ↓ DSST (↓) Vigilance ↓	Cancellation ↑ Arithmetics ↑ Stroop ↓ Vigilance ↑
Perception	CFF ↓ Tachistoscope ∅	CFF ↓	CFF ↓	CFF ∅ Tachistoscope ∅
Thought, intelligence	Analytical thought ∅ Intelligence tests ∅	Relational thought ↓ (Imipramine)	Analytical thought ∅ Verbal fluency ∅	Word association ↑ Intelligence tests ↑
Memory	Acquisition phase ↓ Digit recall ∅	Digit recall ∅ Various tests ∅	Digit recall, picture recognition, list learning ↓	Various learning and memory tasks ↑
Motor function	Tapping ↓ Tracking ↓ Reaction time ↓	Tapping ↓ Tracking ↓ Reaction time ↓	Tapping ↓ Reaction time ↓	Tapping (↑) Reaction time (↑) Tasks requiring physical strength ↑

[a] Applies in particular to sedating neuroleptics such as chlorpromazine.
[b] Applies to sedative preparations such as amitriptyline, trimipramine and mianserin. Binedaline, bupropion, fluoxetine, moclobemide, etc. have hardly any effects.
[c] Applies to benzodiazepines; a rather different pattern after buspirone.
[a] Improvements in particular in lengthier tasks.
↓ = performance deteriorated; ↑ = improved performance; ∅ = no significant effects; ( ) = only a few studies show significant changes.

(2) The spectrum of action of the sedating antidepressants (amitriptyline type) in healthy subjects is similar to that of the initially sleep-inducing neuroleptics. Although there have been no recent comparative trials, there is no evidence that these two classes of preparations can be reliably differentiated by studies in healthy subjects.

(3) Neuroleptics of the haloperidol type (initially not sleep-inducing) and non-sedating antidepressants (such as binedaline and several SSRIs (selective serotonin reuptake inhibitor)) do not induce notable or specific actions in experiments on healthy subjects that would clearly indicate the specific therapeutic class to which they belong.

(4) With regard to performance parameters, tranquillizers of the benzodiazepine class exhibit more similarities than differences from initially sleep-inducing neuroleptics and sedating antidepressants, so that here again a reliable classification is not possible. There is some difference in subjective effects in that, unlike neuroleptics, benzodiazepines are perceived by many subjects as being pleasantly relaxing, although nuances of this type have not yet been studied in direct comparative trials. In its actions in healthy subjects, buspirone resembles neuroleptics of the haloperidol type rather than benzodiazepines, but here again there have been no detailed comparative trials.

(5) Stimulants of the amphetamine type (which have been little studied in the last 10 years) as well as caffeine can be delimited from the other substance classes on the basis of their subjective and objective effects: in no other group is there the pervasive pattern of subjective and objective improvements in drive, mood and performance as in the case of stimulants. On the other hand, so-called nootropics have no actions that characterize them as clearly active on the central nervous system or even as an independent class of substances.

On the basis of this knowledge, the following conclusions may be drawn:

(1) Stimulant and sedative drugs can be reliably described and differentiated in experiments with healthy subjects.

(2) Many psychopharmaceuticals are 'drive neutral' in experiments with healthy subjects; i.e., they fall neither in the stimulant group nor in the sedating group of substances, and do not differ clearly from placebo. This group includes some neuroleptics, antidepressants and the nootropics.

(3) Since neither neuroleptics in general nor antidepressants (both at low doses) and nootropics are distinguished by specific patterns of activity in experiments on healthy subjects, their therapeutic actions must either be disease-specific or be expressed only after prolonged use. It is also possible that their specific effects are revealed only after prolonged use in appropriate patients.

(4) In any event, unlike Kraepelin (1892), we could not claim that each of the substance classes discussed here has 'a clear and specific action on mental life' (see p. 53).

3.5.2   Sensitivity and specificity of the test methods

The sensitivity and specificity of the instruments used in pharmacopsychological experiments may now be discussed in the sense of the method-orientated objectives mentioned on p. 53. Since neuroleptics, antidepressants and other psychopharmaceuticals do not exhibit specific patterns of action encompassing their entire classes, the following discussion of the objective measurement instruments concentrates on the dimension of stimulation–sedation and then deals with a comparison between subjective and objective methods of determination.

Kraepelin (1892, p. 88) assumed 'that the course of very simple mental processes which have furthermore become almost automatic through long practice is less changed by the influence of medicaments than are those more complex processes which always represent a special mental performance'. A complex task such as driving a car in a driving simulator should accordingly be a more sensitive indicator of drug effects than the simple tapping task. However, a study of Tables 3.4–3.7 shows that Kraepelin's assumption is not so generally applicable: for example, in experiments with neuroleptics, doses that induced clear effects on several other parameters of performance had no effect on complex intelligence tasks, and the relative insensitivity of intelligence tests to sedative drug effects has also been found in studies with tranquillizers. On the basis of a detailed analysis of all experiments with amphetamines and caffeine known at the time, Weiss and Laties (1962) stressed that the performance-improving effect of stimulants is clearer in simple and repetitive than in more intellectually demanding tasks, and Latz (1968, p. 87) reached the following conclusion in his review – a conclusion also differing considerably from that of Kraepelin: 'There is an inverse relationship between test difficulty and performance change after drugs, especially impairment of performance . . . performance on cognitively simple tests is changed (usually impaired) by drugs which affect the central nervous system, but the same drugs do not affect performance in cognitively more complex tests'.

The question of the sensitivity of various objective assessment methods has been discussed extensively in earlier editions of this volume (Spiegel and Aebi, 1983, p. 75 ff; Spiegel, 1989, p. 72 ff.) so that only a few conclusions will be considered here. These are:

(1) Methods of the general performance test type are particularly sensitive to the actions of drugs even though impairments caused by sedating substances are not always detected in tests of short duration. Vigilance tests and continuous performance tests (Table 3.1), which usually last for more than 15 minutes, take first place with regard to sensitivity (Koelega, 1989; 1993).

(2) Except for the CFF test, perception tests have found little use in recent studies. The CFF seems to respond highly sensitively to sedating substances, especially benzodiazepines.

(3) Procedures that assess thought processes or aspects of intelligence are also being used less; as Latz (1968) has remarked, their sensitivity to the effects of psychopharmaceuticals seems to be low.

(4) Learning and memory processes are impaired by sedating substances, especially benzodiazepine tranquillizers, and are promoted by psychostimulants; this topic will be further discussed in Chapter 7.

(5) Motor and so-called psychomotor tasks, e.g. reaction tests of varying complexity, also respond to sedative and stimulant drug effects (Kunsman *et al.*, 1992), but no specific procedure shows particularly great sensitivity.

The relative sensitivity of subjective and objective test methods to stimulant and sedative actions of psychopharmaceuticals was studied systematically in the 1970s by an English group (Bye *et al.*, 1973, 1978; Clubley *et al.*, 1979; Peck *et al.*, 1979). Among subjective methods, visual analogue scales (VAS) stood out as particularly sensitive; among the objective procedures the Wilkinson vigilance test was the most sensitive one. At very low doses of sedating or stimulating substances, both these methods were equal in terms of sensitivity (Spiegel, 1989, p. 75), but it must be said that the completion of a VAS takes about 30 seconds whereas it takes up to 1 hour to perform the Wilkinson vigilance test. In terms of economy of time, therefore, subjective methods offer clear advantages and, in addition, they make it possible to determine substance effects outside the stimulation–sedation continuum.

3.5.3   Theory-orientated objectives

Various authors, but particularly Wilhelm Janke, have referred to the possibility of using drugs experimentally for theory-orientated objectives: 'The administration of drugs represents a central research strategy for physiological psychology. It is distinguished from other classical methods, such as lesions, by the reversibility and quantifiability (by using different doses) of the effects achieved. In humans, the administration of drugs is often the only feasible method for modifying somatic processes directly and thus to study them as independent variables' (Janke and Erdmann, 1992, p. 121). An example of the use of psychopharmaceuticals in physiological psychology would be the administration of a neuroleptic of the haloperidol type (as a dopamine antagonist) and of *d*-amphetamine (as an indirect dopamine agonist) to study relationships between the dopaminergic activity of the brain and psychological constructs such as attentiveness, mood, etc. Prerequisites for projects of this type are (a) access to pharmacologically well-characterized and well-tolerated drugs with the most specific actions possible, and (b) confidence that suitable instruments are available to determine complex mental functions such as attentiveness or mood (see King, 1990).

Theory-orientated objectives in the context of differential psychology concern the relationships between so-called personality features (e.g. neuroticism or extraversion according to Eysenck, 1962) and drug actions, a topic of great interest in the 1960s (reviewed by Janke, 1964). It was repeatedly shown that subjects with higher levels of 'anxiety' could respond to sedating substances such as tranquillizers in a different way from less anxious test subjects. This was explained on the basis of an activation theory proposed by Claridge (1967), i.e., as the consequence of different 'levels of arousal' of anxious and less anxious subjects (Heimann, 1974). Janke, Debus, Kohnen and other authors have also examined the question of how far the test situation in pharmacopsychological experiments can be modified in the directions of 'stress accentuation' or 'relaxation', and how manipulations of this type may influence the responses of healthy subjects to drugs. Studies of this kind are discussed extensively and with the appropriate literature references by Debus and Janke (1986), Janke and Erdmann (1992) and Kohnen (1992).

This concludes Chapter 3. Other topics of a theory-orientated type (relationships between specific drug actions, such as actions on the cholinergic system, and learning and memory performances) will be discussed in Chapter 7. Pharmacopsychological studies as part of the testing of new medicines will be discussed in Chapter 6, and we shall return to some practice-orientated topics of pharmacopsychology in Chapter 9.

CHAPTER 4

Effects of psychopharmaceuticals on healthy subjects: electrical correlates of brain activity

4.1 INTRODUCTION

Psychopharmaceuticals exert their desired actions on subjective experience and behaviour in the brain. It therefore seems logical to study the brain and its functions as directly as possible with a view to understanding the actions of psychopharmaceuticals. However, the possibilities for studying cerebral functions *in situ* in the human brain are very limited. The so-called invasive techniques which are common in physiological psychology (removal of tissues, insertion of electrodes or cannulas) cannot be considered for purely research purposes in humans, and newer non-invasive procedures such as positron emission tomography (PET) and nuclear magnetic resonance imaging or spectroscopy techniques (NMR, MRS) do not provide time-related information over hours and days. This chapter will therefore concentrate on some neurophysiological techniques which have been available for some decades now.

The discovery of the human electroencephalogram (EEG) by H. Berger almost 70 years ago (see Gloor, 1969) made it possible for the first time to record electrical correlates of brain activity in human subjects objectively and non-invasively. Berger himself established that the pattern of the EEG curves alters in relation to the degree of wakefulness and alertness of the test subject, and in his earliest studies he used drugs such as cocaine, scopolamine and chloroform in order to manipulate the degree of wakefulness and consciousness of his subjects and to investigate the EEG correlates of the conditions brought about in this manner (Berger, 1931). Nowadays electroencephalography is still an important diagnostic method in neurology and related fields and also plays a role as a research tool in vigilance and sleep research. Since most psychopharmaceuticals act on vigilance, i.e., on the degree of wakefulness and reactivity, the technique can also be usefully applied to psychopharmacological studies.

Berger and almost all authors before 1960 conducted their EEG studies 'by eye and hand'; i.e., they evaluated the recordings, which were written out on paper strips by hand. Automatic evaluation procedures arose later, allowing longer EEG traces to be analysed objectively and with good reproducibility, thus also permitting the execution of more extensive pharmacological experiments. Since experiments of this type are performed on waking subjects and include the administration of drugs, we speak of *pharmaco-EEG*. Section 4.2 gives a description of the methods and results of pharmaco-EEG studies.

Running parallel to, but initially independent of, psychopharmacological developments, the 1950s and 1960s saw the growth of psychophysiological sleep research – a field of study also making use of neurophysiological methods. It was discovered early on in studies of patients and healthy subjects that psychotropic drugs not only change the wake EEG but also alter the electrophysiological correlates of the sleep state, the so-called sleep polygram. As a result, it became possible to study the actions of pharmaceuticals on the brain over a broad range of vigilance states from deep sleep to active waking states. The results of polygraphic sleep studies with psychopharmaceuticals are summarized in Section 4.3.

Another part of this chapter (Section 4.4) is devoted to the effects of drugs on *evoked potentials* (EPs). EPs are electrical correlates of brain responses to stimuli. As in the case of the EEG in wake and sleep, these can be recorded from the surface of the skull and provide information on reactions of the brain to standardized sensory stimuli (tactile, visual, auditory).

Recordings of wake EEG, sleep polygrams and EPs are all based on the possibility of suitably sampling and amplifying the tiny changes in electrical tension arising on the cranial surface as a result of brain activity. Apart from some common technical features, however, the three methods differ in essential characteristics, especially with regard to the time dimension:

– As a basis for pharmaco-EEGs, wake EEGs usually are recorded for just a few minutes. The automatic evaluation techniques commonly used today are based on the averaging (determination of the mean) of several artefact-free EEG segments, each lasting several seconds. They therefore do not take into account the brief single features (so-called grapho-elements) of interest in clinical electroencephalography. They also assume that the subject's state of vigilance does not change significantly during the studied interval of time.

– Sleep polygrams usually last for several hours, generally the whole night. The visual evaluation processes still used in almost all sleep laboratories divide the hour-long traces into discrete segments of 20 or 30 seconds and take account of the EEG features only insofar as they are necessary for determining the sleep stages (see Section 4.3.1).

– In the case of EPs, the time interval of interest lasts for less than 1 second, often only a few tenths of a second. As in the case of the wake EEG, evaluation is based on the averaging of several segments of a recording, involving some tens or hundreds (depending on the type of EPs) of single potentials over a period of some minutes.

On the other hand, these three neurophysiological procedures exhibit several advantages in common which recommend their use in human psychopharmacology.

(1) They are non-invasive and inconvenience the subject only slightly or not at all.
(2) Once the subjects have become adapted, the methods show virtually no purely time-related fluctuations.
(3) They require no effort or attention on the part of the subject and consequently do not alter the processes which they are designed to study (event related potentials are an exception in this respect; see Section 4.4.2).
(4) Since they require neither effort nor attention, their application is largely independent of motivational factors on the part of the test subject.
(5) Recordings can be made whilst the subject is engaged in other activities and it is thus also possible to relate aspects of ongoing performance and well-being to neurophysiological parameters (Rösler, 1992).
(6) EEG studies can in principle be conducted over hours, days and even weeks, particularly when telemetric instrumentation is available.

4.2 PSYCHOPHARMACEUTICALS AND THE WAKE EEG

4.2.1 General information on the EEG

The function of nerve cells in animals and man is accompanied by electrical activity which can be recorded, using the appropriate methods, from individual cells, cell clusters and brain regions, as well as from the surface of the entire brain. The variations in electrical potential which constitute the EEG are produced by the simultaneous activity of thousands of neurons within the range of the recording electrodes. The generators of this activity are, however, probably not located in the cortex, but presumably in the thalamus – an important sensorimotor relay station situated deeper in the brain (Creutzfeldt, 1983, p. 145 ff.). EEG recordings on the surface of the skull, which are the rule in man, depend on massive amplification and filtering of the original activity since, in their unprocessed state, the signals sought correspond to electrical potentials in the microvolt range and are mixed with other potentials stemming from muscle activity, eye movements and other interfering factors. EEG signals are characterized by frequency (cycles per second = cps (Hz)) and electrical potential or amplitude (in microvolts (μV)). In man, the EEG spectrum covers a range between 0.5 and about 40 Hz (Table 4.1). EEG recordings from the surface of the skull do not permit precise localization of the processes taking place deep within the brain and for this reason so-called depth electrodes have to be used for certain clinical purposes (further details in Kooi, 1971; Birbaumer and Schmidt, 1991, Chapter 24).

Table 4.1.   EEG rhythms in man (see Shagass, 1972)

Name, frequency amplitude	Localization	Appear under the following conditions
Alpha activity 8–13 Hz 20–60 μV	Occipital, Parietal (posterior area of the skull)	Eyes closed, relaxed wake state Disappears when eyes are opened and when subject concentrates on a task. Often in the form of spindles of 1–2 s duration
Beta activity 14–30 Hz >20 μV	Central, Frontal (upper, anterior area of the skull)	Eyes open, alertness, concentration on a task. Often in combination with low-amplitude theta waves
Delta activity 0.5–3.5 Hz up to 300 μV	All regions	During wake only isolated and of low amplitude. During sleep with higher amplitude and pronounced synchronization. Delta waves are an expression of an extremely low level of activation
Theta activity 4–7.5 Hz up to 150 μV	Central, Temporal (upper and temporal regions)	Sleepiness, light sleep; also during wakefulness in children. Generally in combination with (superimposed by) beta waves

4.2.2   The EEG as a psychophysiological indicator

With eyes closed and in a state of relaxation, a so-called alpha rhythm is encountered in the majority of people. This has a frequency of 8–13 Hz and is particularly pronounced in recordings from regions at the back of the head (parietal, occipital). About 10–15% of all people fail to show alpha activity, even in a relaxed state and with eyes closed; this is not considered as a pathological characteristic. The frequency of the alpha rhythm in young adults generally lies between 9 and 11 Hz; in older subjects it normally drops by an average of 1–2 Hz. It has, however, been known for some old people to display alpha activity in the region of 10 Hz.

There are vast inter-individual differences in respect of the amplitude of the alpha rhythm and of its share of total EEG activity. The question consequently arises as to whether there are any relationships between EEG characteristics, particularly the alpha rhythm, and other characteristics of an individual. Many older and methodologically imperfect studies have been devoted to the relationships between EEG variables (usually calculated from one or a few derivations), mental disorders and personality characteristics, the majority of which concluded with negative findings: neither patients with functional psychoses (depression, schizophrenia), nor those with neuroses were distinguished by specific EEG characteristics (Itil, 1981, did not share this opinion). Moreover, no reliable correlations were found in early studies between those personality characteristics which can be measured using psychodiagnostic tests (neuroticism, extraversion, variables of the Rorschach

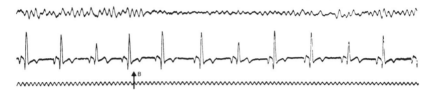

Figure 4.1. Desynchronization of the EEG on sensory stimulation. An extract from a historical experiment by Berger (1930, p. 167 ff.). At point B the volunteer, who had been lying with closed eyes on a deckchair, had the back of his right hand touched with a glass rod; 0.27 s later the EEG (upper tracing) flattened out and the alpha rhythm was replaced by more rapid activity of lower amplitude which lasted for several seconds. Middle tracing: ECG recording; lower tracing: time scale in 1/10 s

test) and EEG criteria (review in Robinson, 1974). Likewise, conventional parameters of intelligence showed no reproducible correlations with EEG characteristics (Oswald and Roth, 1974).

The alpha rhythm is interrupted when the eyes are opened (alpha blocking) and also disappears when a subject with eyes closed is confronted with an unexpected stimulus or when his thoughts are concentrated on accomplishing a task. In such circumstances, alpha activity is then replaced by an EEG pattern in which lower-amplitude beta and theta waves predominate. This is termed a desynchronized or activated EEG (Fig. 4.1). A desynchronized EEG pattern also appears when a subject is very sleepy and drops off to sleep. It is consequently not always easy to distinguish between an alert EEG and a sleepy EEG without drawing on other characteristics. In general, however, the incidence and amplitude of the theta waves increase steadily when a subject is sleepy or drowsy and the wake EEG gives way to a sleep EEG.

Whereas the EEG very reliably reflects changes in alertness and variations in vigilance, it has not been possible to correlate affect states with EEG patterns (Berkhout *et al.*, 1969; Schacter, 1977). The conventionally quantified EEG is also unsuitable as a research instrument for other psychophysiological questions: 'the mean power spectrum of the spontaneous EEG . . . always reflects activity over a long time, i.e. the state of the system over one or several minutes. This sets the limits to the specificity of the relationships between EEG variables and psychological constructs or variables of subjective experience and behaviour. A measure which reflects mean activity over several minutes cannot be coupled with very specific psychological constructs, e.g. individual steps of information processing or subjectively distinguishable epochs in the evaluation of an event' (Rösler, 1992, p. 250). Event-related potentials are better for questions of this type (Section 4.4).

The 'topographic EEG' represents a more recent development of quantitative EEG methods. It has been called 'neurometry' by John *et al.* (1988) and is termed EEG mapping or brain mapping by other authors. This imaging procedure is concerned with the distribution of EEG frequency components over the entire cranial surface and not just at individual lead points. After extensive processing of signals from usually 16 conventional leads, 'maps' in black and white or in colour are created to show the distribution of frequency fractions over various brain regions. EEG mapping can be used for diagnostic purposes, e.g. in neurology and psychiatry (Szelies, 1992), but a definitive judgement cannot yet be made on its advantages over other procedures or its uses apart from diagnostics (John *et al.*, 1994).

4.2.3 Actions of drugs on the EEG (pharmaco-EEG)

Early studies by Bente (1961) led to the assumption that there are 'regular correlations' between the changes occurring in the EEG of healthy subjects after a single dose of psychopharmaceuticals and those occurring in patients under therapeutic conditions. This aspect was studied more systematically by Fink (1968) and led to the division of psychopharmaceuticals into four classes and nine subclasses on the basis of EEG characteristics; however, this scheme has not become widely accepted (Spiegel and Aebi, 1983, p. 108 ff.). Fink, Itil (both 1981) and other authors subsequently published a number of studies concerning the reliable classification of psychopharmaceuticals on the basis of EEG criteria, derived from two hypotheses:

(1) that the different therapeutic effects of neuroleptics, antidepressants, tranquillizers, etc. are expressed in the form of different EEG effects in patients as well as in healthy persons;
(2) that it must therefore be possible to allocate new and clinically as yet unknown substances hypothetically to a therapeutic class on the basis of their EEG effect in healthy subjects, and then to confirm this classification in clinical trials.

Table 4.2 summarizes some of the findings published in the last 20 years on the topic of pharmaco-EEG. These are exclusively the results of placebo-controlled experiments in healthy subjects given a single dose of a substance. However, as can be seen from columns 4 and 5 in Table 4.2, these studies also show important differences with regard to the circumstances of EEG recording and evaluation:

– In the case of EEG recording with *vigilance control* (VC), it is ensured that the subject does not fall asleep during the recording even when feeling sleepy as a result of taking the test product. VC can be accomplished by entrusting the subject with a (generally simple) task during recording (Leonard *et al.*, 1992) or by calling him out loud at the first signs of sleepiness. In the case of the spontaneous resting EEG (spon), events are allowed to take their own course.
– With regard to EEG analysis, differentiation is made between the now dated procedures such as amplitude integration and interval analysis and newer, computer-assisted methods (spectral analysis or power spectrum

analysis) that allow a more thorough and finer utilization of the information contained in the EEG.

Some systematic relationships between the administered substances and the EEG effect can be seen in Table 4.2:

(1) *Neuroleptics* such as chlorpromazine and clozapine lead to an increase in slow waves (delta, theta) in healthy subjects even in small doses, with a decrease in alpha activity: these changes can be interpreted as an expression of the initial sleep-inducing action of the compounds. After haloperidol, a potent antipsychotic neuroleptic without initial sleep-inducing action, Matejcek (personal communication) found an increase in delta plus theta as well as a decrease in the alpha and beta component, i.e., a pattern of action similar to that of chlorpromazine and clozapine. Rohloff *et al.* (1992) also observed an increase in slow frequency components after 4.0 mg of haloperidol, whereas Matejcek found not a decrease but an increase in the beta region. An EEG profile similar to that induced by clozapine was observed after fluperlapine, an experimental (and later abandoned) clozapine-like neuroleptic, whereas savoxepine (also abandoned) produced an EEG pattern comparable to that of conventional neuroleptics such as chlorpromazine and haloperidol. Although all the neuroleptics listed in Table 4.2 increase the slow EEG components, and cannot speak of a uniform EEG pattern.

(2) After the administration of *antidepressants* such as amitriptyline, imipramine and mianserin, an increase in the slow wave fraction and a decrease in the alpha fraction are observed. Variable results have been reported for the fast frequency fraction, probably due to the different methods used in the individual studies. However, an increase in the median beta region (20 Hz) seems to be typical for the conventional antidepressants. The experimental product levoprotiline has a pharmaco-EEG effect similar to but weaker than that of imipramine (Herrmann *et al.*, 1991b) whereas little or no effect is seen after some modern antidepressants such as bupropion, fluvoxamine or viloxazine. Overall, a common pharmaco-EEG pattern cannot be detected for antidepressants known to be clinically active. After a single administration within the therapeutic dose range, lithium has no significant effects on the wake EEG of healthy subjects; after repeated administration for two weeks, an increase in slow waves at the expense of alpha waves has been detected (Herrmann *et al.*, 1980). In another study, there was an increase in anterior alpha activity combined with slowing of alpha activity recorded from posterior skull localizations (Ulrich *et al.*, 1987).

(3) *Tranquillizers* and hypnotics of the benzodiazepine group led to a decrease in alpha waves and an increase in beta activity in practically all studies. With regard to the theta and delta waves, the results of different studies vary. Meprobamate, a tranquillizer with only a slight sedative

Table 4.2. Effects of psychopharmaceuticals on quantitative EEG parameters

Substances class	Compound	Dose (mg, p.o.)	Methods Analysis[1]	Controls[2]	Effects on frequency bands				Authors
					Delta[3]	Theta[3]	Alpha[3]	Beta[3,4]	
Neuroleptics	Chlorpromazine	50	IA	spon	↑	↑	↓	→	Saletu (1976)
	Clozapine	5, 10	SA	spon	↑	↑	↓	B1 ø, B2 ↑	Matejcek et al. (1984)
	Fluperlapine	5, 10	SA	spon	↑	↑	↓	B1 ↓, B2 ↑	Matejcek et al. (1984)
	Haloperidol	2.5, 5	SA	spon	↑	↑	↓	→	Matejcek et al. (unpublished)
	Haloperidol	4	SA	VC, spon	↑	↑	↓	B, ↑	Rohloff et al. (1992)
	Savoxepine	0.5	SA	VC	↑	↑	ø	B, ↑	Herrmann et al. (1991a)
Antidepressants	Amitriptyline	25	FI	spon	↑	ø	↓	ø	Peck et al. (1979)
	Buspirone	50, 100	FI	spon	ø	ø	↓	ø	Peck et al. (1979)
	Fluvoxamine	50	FI	n.d.	ø	ø	↓	ø	Curran and Lader (1986)
	Imipramine	35	IA	spon	↑	ø	→	↑	Saletu (1976)
	Imipramine	0.5/kg	FI	VC	n.d.	ø	↑	↑	Karniol et al. (1976)
	Mianserin	15	IA	spon	↑	ø	↓	B1 ↓, B2 ↑	Itil et al. (1974)
	Viloxazine	100	SA	spon, VC	ø	ø	ø	↑	Bente (1979)
	Lithium	40 mEq	IA	VC	ø	ø	ø	ø	Herrmann et al. (1980)
Tranquillizers, hypnotics	Buspirone	10, 20	FI, SA	spon	ø	ø	ø	(↑)	Bond and Lader (1981)
	Cloxazolam	1, 3, 6	SA	spon	↑	↑	→	↑	Matejcek (1979)
	Diazepam	0.067/kg	FI	VC	n.d.	↑	↓	↑	Karniol et al. (1976)
	Diverse BZD	diverse	IA	VC	↓	ø	→	↑	Saletu (1976)
	Meprobamate	600	IA	VC	↓	ø	ø	↑	Saletu (1976)
	Chloral hydrate	500	IA	spon	ø	ø	ø	→	Saletu (1976)
Psycho-stimulants	d-Amphetamine	5, 10	FI	spon	ø	ø	ø	ø	Peck et al. (1979)
	d-Amphetamine	10	FI	spon	↑	↑	(↑)	(↑)	Montagu (1968)
	Caffeine	100	FI	spon	↑	ø	ø	ø	Clubley et al. (1979)
	Caffeine	250, 500	SA	VC	n.d.	↓	↓	↓	Bruce et al. (1986)
	Methylphenidate	30	IA	n.d.	↓	↓	↓	↑	Saletu (1976)

[1] n.d. = not stated; FI = filter integration; IA = interval analysis; SA = power spectrum analysis.
[2] spon = spontaneous EEG; VC = EEG with vigilance control.
[3] ↑ = significant increase; ↓ = significant decrease; ø = no significant effect; ( ) = trend.
[4] B1 = beta frequencies 12–20 Hz; B2 = beta frequencies >20 Hz.

effect, showed the same pattern of EEG activity as benzodiazepines in an early study by Saletu. In contrast, Bond and Lader (1981) established that the tranquillizer buspirone induces only a very weak EEG effect and is thus differentiated from the benzodiazepines.

(4) *Psychostimulants* present a non-uniform picture: whereas two studies with *d*-amphetamine and one study with methylphenidate reported a reduction in delta and theta waves, other authors report either an increase in slow activity or no effect at all. There is also no agreement in the case of changes in the alpha band and in beta frequencies. *Nootropics* induce very weak or no EEG effects at all in acute experiments in healthy subjects (Spiegel, 1992).

What can be concluded from these findings? First, it can be recognized that sedative products, irrespective of their therapeutic use, exhibit common aspects of EEG action: after almost all neuroleptics, after sedative antidepressants such as amitriptyline, imipramine and mianserin, and after all tranquillizers there is a decrease in the proportion of alpha frequencies and generally an increase in the proportion of slower frequencies (delta, theta). This is not a surprising finding since an increase in slow waves in the EEG at the expense of the alpha component is typical for a decrease in alertness or an increase in drowsiness (Table 4.1). It is, however, difficult to understand the decrease in slow frequencies that has been described after several of the benzodiazepine tranquillizers; since these observations all derive from studies performed under vigilance control (Saletu, 1976), they probably represent exceptions due to the methods used. An increase in (slow) beta activity is characteristic for tranquillizers, whereas the beta increases after some neuroleptics and antidepressants concern faster beta frequencies.

Antidepressants are not characterized by a common pattern of EEG effects (Saletu, 1982): products such as bupropion, fluvoxamine and viloxazine, which are not sedative and have no anticholinergic effects, show very weak or no effects in the wake EEG of healthy subjects. The claim of earlier authors such as Fink (1978) and Itil (1981) of being able to predict the antidepressant effects of new, unknown compounds on the basis of EEG studies has thus not been substantiated.

Of interest in this connection are the results reported by Herrmann *et al.* (1991c) concerning a study with the experimental product maroxepine, which showed evidence of possible antipsychotic and antidepressant action in pre-clinical trials. The vigilance-controlled pharmaco-EEG showed an increase in delta, theta and frontal beta frequency fractions with a concomitant fall in the alpha fraction, a pattern which, in the authors' opinion, suggests more of a sedating and antipsychotic action than an antidepressant effect. However, initial clinical trials in acute schizophrenia patients have refuted the hypothesis of a chlorpromazine-like profile of action, whereas pilot studies in chronic schizophrenics with so-called negative symptoms have shown some drive-enhancing action of the product. The authors admit that in this case the

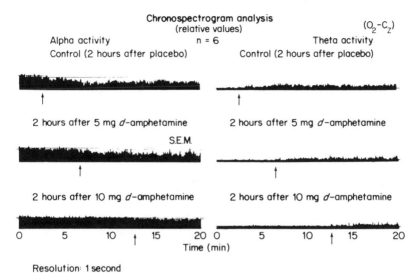

Figure 4.2. Effects of d-amphetamine on the wake EEG. Mean EEG spectral values for six healthy male subjects who took placebo, 5 mg and 10 mg d-amphetamine, each on one occasion, in a balanced cross-over trial are shown. Whereas the EEG trace 2 hours after placebo shows a rapid decline in alpha waves and an increase in theta waves (upper third, the arrows show the alpha decrease and the theta increase), the corresponding changes occurred later after 5 mg (middle third) and 10 mg (lower third) d-amphetamine. A decrease in vigilance occurred after 2 minutes (placebo), but only after 7 (on 5 mg d-amphetamine) or 12 minutes (on 10 mg d-amphetamine) (Matejcek, 1979, with permission)

pharmaco-EEG study had led them along a false path, and they subsequently discussed the predictive validity of the pharmaco-EEG model (Section 4.5.2).

The absence of a uniform EEG pattern after psychostimulants in various studies is surprising in view of the unequivocal subjective and objective actions of these substances, and must be due to the methods used: in short-lasting experiments, small amphetamine doses lead only to modest subjective and behavioural effects (Chapter 3), so that no massive effects can be expected in EEG recordings covering a period of a few minutes. In contrast, EEG trials lasting 15 minutes or more very clearly show the effects even of small amphetamine doses (Matejcek, 1979): alertness, expressed by the ratio of alpha and theta waves, falls rapidly with placebo once the subjects are accustomed to the experimental conditions, but vigilance is retained longer with amphetamine. This difference can be represented in so-called chronospectrograms (Fig. 4.2).

Thus, experience from these mostly older pharmaco-EEG studies lead to the following conclusions:

(1) Stimulant and sedative drug effects can be identified in studies with healthy subjects; small groups of subjects are adequate under properly standardized experimental conditions.

(2) Some groups of substances may be characterized by specific EEG features but these features cannot be clearly correlated with any specific therapeutic use. Examples are the increase in slow frequencies after sedating substances, the increase in slower frequencies of the beta range after benzodiazepines and the increase in faster beta waves after substances such as clozapine and some antidepressants.

(3) The prediction of possible therapeutic applications of new and clinically still unknown compounds from their EEG effects is a very uncertain process. Nevertheless, pharmaco-EEG studies can be of practical use in human psychopharmacology: studies of the correlation between blood levels of a substance and its action on the brain, delineation of the time of onset of action, peak action and duration of action of single doses (Fink, 1981) are of interest within the context of clinical testing of new compounds (see Chapter 6).

4.3 PSYCHOPHARMACEUTICALS AND THE SLEEP POLYGRAM

4.3.1 General information on sleep polygrams

The EEG wave pattern changes in a characteristic way on transition from waking to sleeping: generally speaking, the average frequency of the waves decreases with the onset of sleep and the EEG amplitude then increases with increasing depth of sleep. On the basis of the EEG pattern and other physiological indicators, several *sleep stages* can be differentiated. These differ with respect to the strength of stimulus required to wake a sleeping person and with regard to other physiological and psychological features. The classification of sleep into stages is done on the basis of polygrams, i.e., simultaneous recordings of the EEG, eye movements (electro-oculogram, EOG) and the activity of representative muscles (electromyogram, EMG). The electrophysiological features of the sleep stages are shown in Table 4.3; instead of 'by eye and hand', the analysis of sleep polygrams can also be made computer-assisted. The currently accepted sleep stage classification (Rechtschaffen and Kales, 1968) is a convention that primarily serves practical purposes; other and finer subdivisions are also possible with computer-assisted procedures.

The sleep of man and of many species of animal is a cyclical process, the individual segments of which – the sleep stages – follow a regular sequence in time: sleep onset is characterized in the ideal situation by gradual transition from the wake state into stage 1, which is followed by stage 2, deep sleep stages 3 and 4 and, finally, by REM sleep. The term REM (rapid eye movement) sleep denotes those segments of sleep characterized by rapid horizontal

Table 4.3. Classification of sleep stages on the basis of sleep polygrams

State	Electroencephalogram (EEG)	Electro-oculogram (EOG)	Electromyogram (EMG)
Awake: eyes closed, relaxed	Alpha activity; in non-alpha-dominant individuals there is beta-theta activity of low amplitude	Fast and/or slow eye movement	High amplitude, movement artefacts
Stage 1: drowsiness, transition to sleep	Less than 50% alpha activity, predominantly theta waves of low amplitude, mixed with beta waves; sharp vertex waves	Slow 'rolling' eye movements	Relatively high amplitude which decrease with the onset of sleep
Stage 2: sleep	Background rhythm theta waves, appearance of spindles (groups of 14 Hz waves of about 1 s duration) and K-complexes (slow, large amplitude potentials with positive and negative components)	No eye movements; K-complexes also visible in the EOG	Low amplitude
Stage 3, 4: deep sleep, slow wave sleep	Delta waves (0.5–3 Hz, amplitude >75 µV) predominate; 20–50% delta waves in stage 3, >50% delta waves in stage 4	No eye movements; delta waves are visible in the EOG also	Low amplitude
REM sleep: rapid eye movement sleep, paradoxical sleep	Similar to stage 1: in many individuals distinct alpha activity occipitally, occasional 'saw-tooth waves'	Single or groups of rapid eye movements	Very low amplitude, occasional brief increases in amplitude ('twitches')

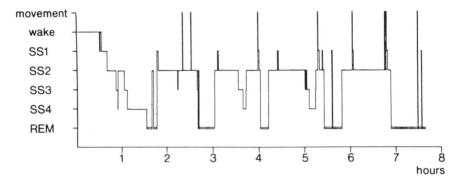

Figure 4.3. Schematic representation (hypnogram) of the course of sleep. The hypnogram of a 25-year-old healthy subject illustrates the chronological sequence of polygraphic sleep stages in a single night (SS = sleep stage). Each NREM–REM cycle begins with NREM sleep (stages 2, 3 and 4) and ends with an REM period that lasts from a few up to 40 or more minutes. Deep sleep stages 3 and 4 mainly occur during the first two to three NREM–REM cycles; as the night wears on, sleep becomes more superficial. In contradistinction to this schematic representation, the transition from lighter to deeper sleep stages, e.g., from SS 1 to SS 2, does not occur in the form of steps, but smoothly. Upward 'shifts', however, are predominantly abrupt as a result of body movements or brief awakenings (from Spiegel, 1981b, p. 41)

and vertical eye movements, accompanied by the features of stage 1 in the EEG, while the EMG shows an almost total relaxation of the musculature. When subjects are woken out of REM sleep and asked appropriate questions, they will give a detailed report of a dream in 80% of all cases, whilst reports of dreams are rarer and less detailed when subjects are woken from other stages of sleep.

Sleep stages 1, 2, 3 and 4 are collectively referred to as NREM (non-rapid eye-movement) sleep; taken together with the REM phase which follows each NREM sleep segment they constitute NREM–REM cycles which are of from 80 to 120 minutes in duration. The majority of people pass through between three and five NREM–REM cycles each night, whereby the proportion of deep sleep stages 3 and 4 in the individual cycles decreases in the course of the night with a corresponding lengthening of the proportion taken up by stage 2 (Fig. 4.3).

4.3.2 The sleep polygram as a psychophysiological indicator

The relationships between polygraphic characteristics of sleep and subjective criteria such as the feeling of depth of sleep, recovery and mood in the following morning have been investigated in many studies without fully clarifying the biological and psychological relevance of sleep and the sleep stages (review by Borbély, 1991; Koella, 1988). In the case of REM sleep it is known that it designates periodically appearing phases of 10–40 minutes duration that are generally accompanied by dreams, although dreams also occur in other sleep segments, primarily in stages 1 and 2. Deep sleep (or slow wave sleep) depends mainly on the prior time spent awake: the longer a subject has been kept awake, the greater is the deep sleep fraction of total sleep when the subject is again allowed to sleep undisturbed. Sleep that is considered deep on the basis of EEG amplitudes and frequencies is generally also perceived subjectively as particularly deep sleep.

Clear correlations between personality variables and polygraphic features of sleep do not seem to exist in healthy subjects; in the mentally ill and especially in depressive patients, however, severe disorders of the sleep process are the rule and can also be represented polygraphically (review by Reynolds and Kupfer, 1987). Patients with chronic insomnia usually do not display a lack of one or more specific sleep stages in the sleep polygram; their sleep is, however, generally interrupted more frequently than that of good sleepers. Similarly, nights with subjectively disturbed sleep experienced by otherwise normal sleepers are characterized by more polygraphically demonstrable sleep interruptions than are nights with deep and refreshing sleep. With advancing age the proportion of sleep taken up by deep sleep stages 3 and 4 drops, particularly in men, whereas frequency and duration of sleep interruptions increase. This development is accompanied in many elderly people by a subjective impression of shallower sleep, and, in the older age groups, more people complain of sleep disorders than do the young (Spiegel *et al.*, 1991).

4.3.3 Pharmacological studies in man

I. Oswald is to be considered the pioneer in this field of research, having taken up the sleep-polygraphic study of the actions of barbiturates, amphetamines, antidepressants, benzodiazepines and other substances in the early 1960s, originally having been interested in questions of barbiturate and stimulant dependency (Oswald, 1968). He established that almost all psychotropic substances have objective effects on the sleep of healthy subjects and mentally ill patients after single and repeated administrations, and that there are systematic correlations between the assumed mechanism of action of a substance and its effects on the sleep polygram.

Table 4.4 gives a summary of the results of sleep-polygraphic drug studies in healthy subjects: in all cases the drugs were administered shortly before the start of recording, i.e., in the evening hours before retiring to bed. The experimental designs were not uniform but the studies were generally double-blind and placebo-controlled. With regard to the classes of substances studied, the following statements can be made.

(1) *Neuroleptics* have no striking effects on sleep when given in small doses: sleep-inducing drugs such as chlorpromazine and clozapine stabilize sleep (decrease in 'unrest', i.e., fewer interruptions of the course of sleep) and, in larger doses, prolong the duration of sleep; products with potent

Table 4.4. Effects of drugs on polygraphic sleep parameters

Substance class	Compound (mg, p.o.)	Dose	Effects on sleep parameters						Authors
			Duration of sleep	Stage 1	Stage 2	Slow wave sleep	REM sleep	Sleep unrest	
Neuroleptics	Chlorpromazine	12.5–150	↑	→↓	←	(↑)	↑, →	→↓	Hartmann (1978)
	Clozapine	5, 10	(↑)	→↓	(↑)	0	0	→↓	Spiegel (unpublished)
	Haloperidol	1.0	0	0	0	0	0	0	Spiegel (unpublished)
	Mesoridazine	10, 20	0	0	0	0	(↑)	→	Adam et al. (1976)
	Pimozide	1, 4	0	0	0	0	0	→	Sagales and Erril (1975)
Antidepressants	Amitriptyline	12.5–100	0, ↓	0, ↓	n.d.	0, ↓	→↓	→↓	Chen (1979); Kay et al. (1976)
	Chlorimipramine	75	0	←	n.d.	0, ↓	→	←	Dunleavy et al. (1972)
	Clovoxamine	50, 150	0, (↓)	0, ←	0, →	0, →	→	←	Wilson et al. (1986)
	Dibenzepine	40–160	0	(↑)	↑←	n.d.	→↓	↑	Spiegel and Dixon (1982)
	Doxepin	75	0	n.d.	n.d.	n.d.	→↓	(↓)	Dunleavy et al. (1972)
	Fluoxetine	20–60	0, ↓	0, ↑	n.d.	n.d.	0, →↓	0, ←	Nicholson and Pascoe (1986)
	Imipramine	25–100	0	↑←	0	0, (↑)	→↓	↑←	Chen (1979); Kay et al. (1976)
	Mianserin	5, 10	0	(↑)	↑←	0	(↓) →	(↑), 0	Spiegel and Dixon (1982)
	Moclobemide	4, 6.5 mg/kg	0, ↓	↑↑	↑←	0	←↑	↑↑	Blois and Gaillard (1990)
	Nefazodone	100 + 100	(↑)	0	0	0	→	n.d.	Sharpley et al. (1992)
	Paroxetine	15, 30	0, ↓	↑←	0	0, ←	0	0, ↑	Oswald and Adam (1986)
	Trazodone	50–200	0	0	0	←	0	(↓)	Ware and Pittard (1990)
	Trimipramine	25–75	↑↑	→	←	n.d.	→	→	Nicholson and Pascoe (1988)

Table 4.4. *Continued*

Substance class	Compound (mg, p.o.)	Dose	Duration of sleep	Stage 1	Stage 2	Slow wave sleep	REM sleep	Sleep unrest	Authors
Tranquillizers, hypnotics	Alprazolam	0.25–1.0	(↑)	↓→	↑↑	→	↓→	→→	Bonnet *et al.* (1981)
	Chlordiazepoxide	20–100	0	→→	↑←	0	0	→→	cf. Kay *et al.* (1976)
	Diazepam	5–15	↑←	→→	↑←	0	0,→	→→	cf. Kay *et al.* (1976)
	Flurazepam	7.5–60	↑←	→→	↑←	0,→	0,→	↓→	cf. Kay *et al.* (1976)
	Barbiturates	div.	↑←	↓→	↑←	0	↓→	→→	cf. Kay *et al.* (1976)
	Meprobamate	400–1200	n.d.	→	←	n.d.	0,→	→→	cf. Kay *et al.* (1976)
Psycho-stimulants	*d*-Amphetamine	2.5–15	↓↓	↑,0	0,→	0,→	↓→	↑,0	cf. Spiegel (1979)
	l-Amphetamine	2.5–10	0,(↓)	0,(↑)	0	0	↓→	0,↑	cf. Spiegel (1979)
	Caffeine	200–450	0,→	↑←	0,→	0	0→	n.d.	cf. Kay *et al.* (1976)
	Methylphenidate	5–20	0,→	n.d.	0	n.d.	→→	n.d.	cf. Kay *et al.* (1976)
	Modafinil	100, 200	→	(↑)	0	0	→→	0	Saletu *et al.* (1989)

n.d. = no published data; 0 = no significant effect; ↑ = increase; ↑↑ = dose-dependent increase; ↓ = decrease; ↓↓ = dose-dependent decrease; ( ) = trend.

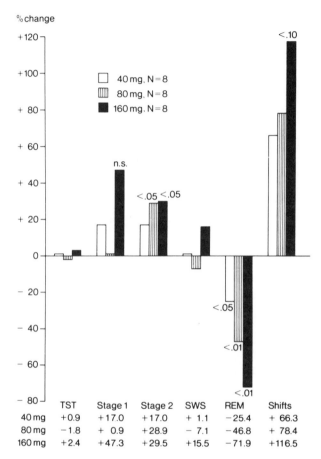

	TST	Stage 1	Stage 2	SWS	REM	Shifts
40 mg	+0.9	+17.0	+17.0	+ 1.1	−25.4	+ 66.3
80 mg	−1.8	+ 0.9	+28.9	− 7.1	−46.8	+ 78.4
160 mg	+2.4	+47.3	+29.5	+15.5	−71.9	+116.5

Figure 4.4.   Effect of a tricyclic antidepressant on polygraphic sleep stages. A characteristic effect of many antidepressants is the dosage-dependent reduction in REM sleep without simultaneous change in total sleep time (TST). The present trial covered eight healthy male volunteers who slept in the laboratory for five successive nights. After allowing one night for adaptation, they received placebo, 40, 80 and 160 mg of the antidepressant dibenzepine (Noveril®) according to a balanced Latin square experimental plan. They subsequently went to bed and their sleep was recorded polygraphically for 7½ hours. The figure shows the mean percentage deviations from the individual placebo values after three doses of the drug; statistical comparisons were performed by means of three-way analyses of variance and subsequent pair comparisons (from Spiegel, 1981b, p. 50)

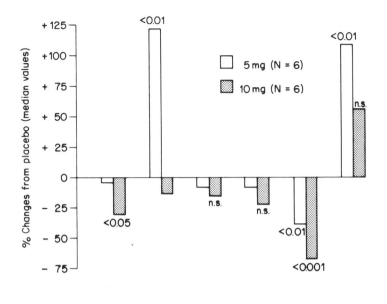

Change in % (median)	TST	Stage 1	Stage 2	SWS	REM	Shifts
5 mg	− 3.5	+122.5	− 7.5	− 7.5	−38.0	+109.0
10 mg	−30.5	− 13.0	−14.5	−22.0	−67.0	+ 55.5

Figure 4.5. Effects of the psychostimulant *d*-amphetamine on poly-graphic sleep stages. A decrease in REM sleep, an increase in sleep unrest ('shifts': changes from sleep stages 2, 3 and 4 into the waking state and into stage 1) and an increase in stage 1 are typical for amphetamine-like stimulants given in small doses. With larger doses, amphetamine reduces REM sleep even more markedly and also reduces the duration of sleep (TST, total sleep time) (reproduced from Spiegel, 1982 with permission from S. Karger AG, Basel)

'antipsychotic' action such as haloperidol and pimozide are unremarkable with regard to their subjective and objective effects on sleep. The effects of neuroleptics on REM sleep are not uniform, and the effects on other sleep stages are slight.

(2) Polygraphic sleep studies with *antidepressants* have proved to be of great interest since certain forms of depression are characterized by specific features in the sleep polygram (Reynolds and Kupfer, 1987) and since it was found early on that the actions of some antidepressants precisely counteract the sleep pattern observed in depression (Vogel *et al.*, 1990). Almost all known antidepressants lead to a dose-dependent prolongation of REM latency (time until appearance of first REM phase), a reduction in REM sleep and, depending on the clinical pattern of action, to other changes also. Sedative products such as amitriptyline, doxepine and trimipramine stabilize sleep (decrease in 'unrest') and, in larger doses,

prolong its duration; antidepressants which tend to increase drive, such as dibenzepine, moclobemide and paroxetine, intensify sleep unrest in normal subjects and can lead to a decrease in the duration of sleep when given in larger doses (Fig. 4.4).

(3) Like barbiturates, tranquillizers and hypnotics of the benzodiazepine group also increase the duration of sleep when given in larger doses, whereas meprobamate, in accordance with its only weak sedative action in the waking state, also has little effect on sleep. In larger doses, benzodiazepines reduce the proportion of REM sleep, but the interval between sleep-inducing doses and those suppressing REM sleep is greater than in the case of barbiturates. An increase in spindle activity, i.e., groups of waves arising phasically in the 12–14 Hz region, is observed both after benzodiazepines and after certain barbiturates.

(4) Stimulants impair sleep; i.e., they delay sleep onset, reduce sleep continuity in low doses, and curtail sleep duration in higher doses (Fig. 4.5). Amphetamine-like stimulants and caffeine have different effects on REM sleep, which is unchanged after caffeine, whilst amphetamine produces a dose-dependent reduction. Modafinil, a new stimulant, has only weak effects on the sleep polygram in the tested doses, but its pattern of effects is more like that of amphetamine than caffeine. Nootropics have shown no marked effects in sleep polygraphic studies in healthy subjects (Maggini *et al.*, 1988; Spiegel, 1992).

4.3.4   Comment

Inspection of the results in Table 4.4 shows that the majority of modern psychopharmaceuticals modify the sleep of healthy subjects even in small doses: irrespective of their clinical indications, sedative products reduce sleep unrest and, in larger doses, lead to a prolongation of sleep, whereas stimulant substances have the opposite effect. As in pharmaco-EEG studies in awake subjects, sedative and stimulant drug effects can be characterized in the sleep polygram. The observation that the results of polygraphic sleep studies are highly reproducible is important, being attributable to the uniform methods used in these studies (Rechtschaffen and Kales, 1968) and to the fact that, after suitable acclimatization in the sleep laboratory, the subjects are hardly exposed to external disturbing factors.

Many drugs modify not only sleep continuity and the duration of sleep but also have an effect on other polygraphic parameters, particularly REM sleep: the majority of antidepressants and some psychostimulants reduce the proportion of this stage in a dose-dependent manner; small doses of barbiturates and large doses of benzodiazepines also lead to a decrease in REM sleep, giving the impression that REM sleep shortening is a highly non-specific action of many centrally acting drugs. This impression is supported by the knowledge that clonidine, a centrally effective hypotensive medicine, as well as opiates and anticholinergics, greatly reduce REM sleep. On the other hand, not all psychopharmaceuticals affect REM sleep, and even the phenomenon of REM sleep suppression is not uniform in itself: some compounds act primarily on the eye movements, and others on the muscle tone as partial aspects of polygraphically defined REM sleep (Passouant *et al.*, 1972). In the present context it can be stated that there is no firm correlation between the therapeutic use of a drug and its action on REM sleep. There is also no clear relationship between the action of a substance on REM sleep and its effects in waking subjects, since both stimulants such as amphetamine and sedative drugs (barbiturates, some antidepressants, clonidine) reduce REM sleep.

Drug effects on *deep sleep* (slow wave sleep, stages 3 and 4) are also of interest: as can be seen from Table 4.4, a decrease of these sleep stages occurs with some substances, primarily after repeated administration of benzodiazepine derivatives and after the use of certain antidepressants. The physiological significance of this change is unknown and, in the case of benzodiazepines, could be a purely EEG amplitude phenomenon (Feinberg *et al.*, 1979). On the other hand, some years ago we observed a prolongation of slow wave sleep after some serotonin receptor antagonists and a shortening of slow wave sleep after mixed serotonin receptor agonist/antagonist products (Spiegel, 1981a; Oswald *et al.*, 1982); the relevance of this finding remained an open question at that time. It has been established since then that an increase in deep sleep occurs only after certain serotonin antagonists, the so-called 5-HT_2 antagonists (Adam and Oswald, 1989; Sharpley *et al.*, 1990) whereas the so-called 5-HT_3 antagonists have no effect on the sleep EEG of healthy subjects (Guldner *et al.*, 1991). These relationships will no doubt become clearer as advances are being made in serotonin receptor pharmacology, and new insights can also be expected in relation to the 'sleep pharmacology' of benzodiazepine receptors. Irrespective of that, however, it must be stated that, as in the case of REM sleep, there is no detectable correlation between the therapeutic uses of a substance and its effects on slow wave sleep.

4.4 PSYCHOPHARMACEUTICALS AND EVOKED POTENTIALS

4.4.1 General information on evoked potentials

When a subject is exposed to sensory stimuli it is possible to use electroencephalographic leads in order to record evoked potentials, i.e., changes in electric tension which arise as a function of the nature and intensity of the stimulation and some other conditions of the experiment. In the wake EEG, the naked eye is hardly able to detect sensory evoked potentials (EPs) individually since they are concealed by spontaneous EEG rhythms which have a higher amplitude. However, EPs can be made visible by consecutively presenting several identical stimuli and then graphically or mathematically averaging the respective EEG segments. In this manner it is possible to 'average out' spontaneous EEG activity, and the EP, the amplitude of which lies

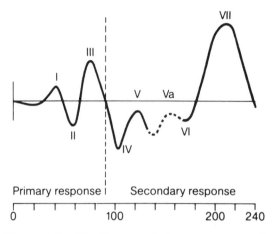

Figure 4.6. Classification of the components of visually evoked potentials (VEPs). The two negative peaks I and III and the positive peak II are termed the primary response by Cigánek (1961), peaks IV–VII (negative peaks = 'upwards' pointing peaks) being termed the secondary response. The amplitude of these peaks lies in the region of 10–30 μV and is normally obscured by the underlying EEG activity. In addition to amplitudes (e.g. between peaks I and II) calculations are carried out to determine latencies, i.e., the time in milliseconds between the stimulus and the appearance of a peak, e.g. peak IV

between 5 and 30 μV, emerges. EPs consist of several components: in respect of visual EPs (Fig. 4.6) and, similarly, in respect of EPs of other sensory modalities, a distinction is made between a primary response, i.e., changes in potential which appear with particular clarity above those parts of the cortex onto which the stimulus in question is projected, and secondary responses which may be observed somewhat later and which are presumably phenomena linked to the cognitive processing of the stimulus in the brain (Hillyard and Kutas, 1983).

Unfortunately, the EP nomenclature used by different authors is not quite uniform, which hampers an understanding of the relevant literature: instead of primary responses, some authors speak of exogenous components or of stimulus-correlated potentials, thus emphasizing that the latency and amplitude of early EPs with a latency of up to about 100 ms depend largely on the objective features of the stimulus. Secondary responses are also called endogenous components or, more frequently, event-related potentials (ERPs): their properties depend primarily on the mental disposition of the subjects, i.e., their expectations, state of consciousness and alertness at the time of the experiment.

4.4.2   Evoked potentials as psychophysiological indicators

According to an early statement by Guttmann (1972, p. 135) it is possible to 'regard the sensory evoked potential as the last direct consequence of a stimulus in the central nervous system . . ., which is a modality-, quality-, and intensity-specific correlate of the objective reality. The applications illustrate the consequences of such direct access to the effects of central nervous system stimulation: by means of bypassing self-observation and verbal communication it is possible to conduct objective tests of sensory ability and thus, to study subjective reality on the basis of the physiological correlates.'

EPs with latencies below 100 ms are actually used for functional testing of the optic, auditory and various somatosensory nerve pathways (see Chiappa, 1983). This procedure has the advantage of providing information on the function of sensory afferents independently of factors such as motivation and tiredness (including drug-induced tiredness). On the other hand, EPs are most certainly not 'physiological correlates of subjective reality' (Guttmann) since the early potentials (short-latency potentials) used for neurological function testing also arise in altered states of consciousness, e.g. during sleep, and therefore provide no conclusions regarding subjective reality. Accordingly, EPs with latencies below 100 ms are considered uninteresting for psychological questions.

The situation is different with EPs or ERPs having longer latencies, especially waves N200 and P300. The N200 wave (now also called N2) appears about 200 ms after a suitable stimulus (hence its original name), and the P300 wave (now P3) after about 300 ms on average. Consequently, both potentials lie in a time region familiar to experimental psychologists from experiments with simple and complex reaction tests. N2 and P3 can be observed in so-called odd ball (two-stimuli differentiation) paradigms: the subject is presented with a sequence of frequent and rare stimuli, e.g. frequent high tones and rare low tones, and is given the task of noting and counting only the low tones (= rare stimuli). In these experiments, N2 and P3 arise only after the noted rare stimuli; their amplitude depends on the stimulus probability (the lower the probability, the greater the amplitude) and the relevance of the stimulus in the experiment. P3 can also be induced by creating an expectancy in the subjects that is then not fulfilled, e.g. by omitting a stimulus in an otherwise unchanged repetition of a stimulus sequence (see Hillyard and Kutes, 1983, for further information).

P3 latency is age-dependent: older subjects have a longer mean latency than young subjects, and abnormally prolonged P3 latencies are observed in patients with mild to moderate dementia. A decrease in P3 amplitude has been found in schizophrenic patients, a finding that has been hypothetically related to a (qualitatively undefined) disturbance of information processing (Barrett et al., 1986). According to some authors (see review by Nuechterlein and Dawson, 1995), non-psychotic twins and children of schizophrenics also show similar differences compared with normal subjects. Olbrich (1987) has, however, indicated that the P3 decrease in schizophrenics is not great enough to be useful as a diagnostic tool in the evaluation of individual cases (Friedman and Squires-Wheeler, 1994). Finally, systematic correlations between personality features and EP parameters have so far not been found in experiments with healthy subjects.

4.4.3 Pharmacological studies in man

Saletu (1976) performed a series of EP experiments in healthy subjects to study the action of what were standard psychopharmaceuticals at that time (three neuroleptics, three antidepressants, four tranquillizers, two psychostimulants). Systematic changes in EP latency were observed after somatosensory stimulation and can be summarized schematically as follows:

Single doses of	Latency of primary response	Latency of secondary response
Neuroleptics	prolonged	prolonged
Antidepressants	shortened	prolonged
Tranquillizers	prolonged	shortened
Stimulants	shortened	shortened

According to these results, class-specific short-latency evoked potential profiles would arise after all psychopharmaceuticals, which would be an astonishing statement if, as mentioned above, the primary EP responses are independent of intrinsic factors such as tiredness and motivation. Herrmann *et al.* (1981) and other groups subsequently were unable to reproduce most of the results published by Saletu so that it must now be concluded that there are no 'pharmaco-EP profiles' of neuroleptics, antidepressants etc. which are generally valid and independent of specific sensory modalities.

Since the studies by Saletu and by Herrmann *et al.* there have been no further publications of systematic studies of the actions of psychopharmaceuticals on EPs. Bartel *et al.* (1990) reported results for chlorpromazine which demonstrate part of the complexity of EP studies with psychopharmaceuticals. After 100 mg of this neuroleptic they observed a significant increase in latency of early VEP components (50–100 ms), but attributed this not to any action of the substance in the brain but to a 'peripheral' effect (inhibition of dopaminergic synapses in the retina). If this concept is taken further, EP studies, although not useful for the classification of psychopharmaceuticals according to therapeutic classes, could well contribute to the micro-analysis of the course of drug actions within the context of stimulus-response studies.

4.4.4 Actions of psychopharmaceuticals on late potentials

In a review article published in 1986, Münte *et al.* expressed their surprise at the fact that the effects of psychopharmaceuticals on ERPs had still not been greatly studied at that time. The few studies of P300 cited by Münte *et al.* did, however, show that compounds such as methylphenidate and scopolamine could influence certain components of the P300 complex. However, since the corresponding experiments were mostly performed with specific experimental–psychological rather than pharmacological orientation, it is not possible to assess the sensitivities and specificities of the various P300 paradigms for pharmacological questions. Newer studies with the sedating antihypertensive substance clonidine (Joseph and Sitaram, 1989) and with various antihistamines (Swire *et al.*, 1989) do not allow definitive statements to be made concerning the possible contribution of P300 studies to the characterization of CNS-active substances in healthy persons.

Another electric signal recorded from the surface of the skull is termed *contingent negative variation (CNV)*. This is a very late negative potential fluctuation in the parietal region which arises when a subject participating in a reaction experiment is advised, through a warning stimulus, of the imminence of another stimulus to which he or she has to react (Haider *et al.*, 1981). In psychological terminology the CNV is also called the expectancy wave. It is terminated as soon as the subject reacts to the second stimulus and the anticipatory phase is concluded. There exist only a few isolated studies of drug effects in normal subjects on the CNV; according to an early review by Tecce *et al.* (1978) the following results have been recorded during controlled trials on volunteers:

– Sedatives such as alcohol, tranquillizers, and hypnotics led to a reduction in CNV amplitude. The same result was found in a study involving 50 mg chlorpromazine.
– CNV amplitude was generally increased after stimulants, although the opposite effect has occasionally also been observed. Moreover, interindividual differences were surprisingly large. No reports have been published to our knowledge in respect of the effect of antidepressants on CNV.

It would be premature to say, on the basis of these findings, whether and to what extent CNV recordings may be of use as an assessment parameter in psychopharmacological experiments. However, the compounds and doses which Tecce *et al.* (1978) cited as showing an effect do suggest that CNV is neither particularly sensitive nor very specific as a measure of the effects of drugs. This assumption is supported by the results of a study by Heinze *et al.* (1985), which revealed a statistically significant decrease in CNV amplitude after 8 mg of diazepam in healthy subjects, but also a similar if weaker effect after 200 mg of caffeine, i.e. after a stimulant compound. Since a decrease in CNV amplitude was also reported in a study by Matejcek *et al.* as a response to the neuroleptic haloperidol (Fig. 4.7), this parameter does not appear to be a specific indicator of psychopharmaceutical actions.

106

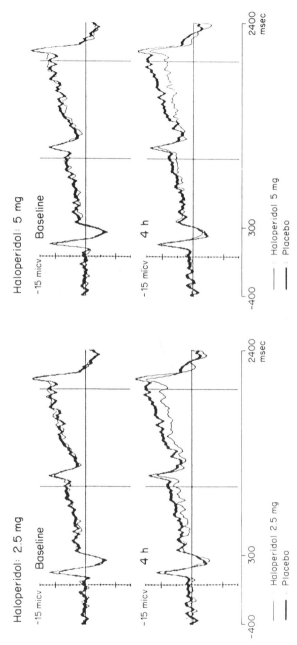

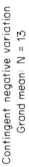

Figure 4.7. Changes in contingent negative variation (CNV) after haloperidol. The CNV paradigm used here involves three stimuli (a warning stimulus, a decision stimulus and an imperative stimulus) presented at 1000 ms intervals and which are indicated by vertical lines in the figure. As a result of the warning stimulus (far left) there is a response composed of negative and positive components with a latency of 150–250 ms. In expectation of the decision stimulus, this overlaps with a slowly rising negative potential, the first CNV. The first CNV ends with a further negative shift as a result of the decision stimulus, arising in expectation of the imperative stimulus (loud noise which the subject has to switch off by pressing a button) and declining rapidly after the imperative stimulus. In this experiment haloperidol leads to a slightly dose-dependent decrease in CNV amplitude 4 hours after medication, detectable by comparing the thick (placebo) and thin (haloperidol) lines (figure kindly made available by M. Matejcek and H. Klee)

4.5   DISCUSSION: THE SIGNIFICANCE OF NEUROPHYSIOLOGICAL INVESTIGATIONS IN HUMAN PSYCHOPHARMACOLOGY

The foregoing sections show that single doses of most psychopharmaceuticals have significant effects on neurophysiological parameters in healthy subjects. Nootropics and some neuroleptics represent exceptions since they produce detectable modifications neither in waking nor in sleeping subjects; interestingly, the same compounds are also found to be inactive in experiments with psychological methods (Chapter 3). In the same way as at the end of Chapter 3, questions concerning the sensitivity, specificity and, finally, the relevance of neurophysiological studies in human psychopharmacology are posed in the following pages.

4.5.1   Sensitivity

The sensitivity of a method to determine drug effects can be assessed in *dose–effect studies*: The lowest dose of a product leading to significant changes in the studied parameters serves as a measure of sensitivity of the method. A method is particularly sensitive when the substance effect is detected at doses which do not yet induce effects on other parameters. In the case of electrophysiological methods it is difficult to reach a definitive evaluation of sensitivity since several parallel assessment techniques, including neurophysiological methods, where various doses of one or more products have only been used in a few studies in healthy subjects.

Nevertheless, in order to provide an overview, we have set out in Table 4.5 those doses of psychopharmaceuticals showing statistically significant effects in controlled studies with psychological (Chapter 3) and electrophysiological (Chapter 4) measurement methods. The picture that arises in this way is certainly incomplete (particularly in the absence of usable information concerning EPs and ERPs) but does reveal that electrophysiological and psychological parameters generally respond to drug doses of the same order of magnitude. In the case of sedative substances, i.e., some neuroleptics, antidepressants and tranquillizers, the minimum effective doses with the various levels of measurement are very similar, and the same applies to psychostimulants. Sleep polygraphic studies are relatively sensitive to the actions of many antidepressants. In some wake EEG studies the authors concentrated primarily on qualitative profiles of activity and less on the sensitivity of the methods. Despite this fact, diazepam and amphetamine had distinct effects on quantitative parameters of wake EEG, even after relatively low doses. Viewed as a whole, electrophysiological methods respond as sensitively to the acute effects of psychotropic drugs as do traditional experimental–psychological procedures; decisive differences in this respect cannot be discerned. An advantage worthy of mention is that electrophysiological trials, in particular sleep studies, can generally be

Table 4.5. Sensitivity of psychological and electrophysiological parameters to the effects of psychopharmaceuticals

Substance class	Compound	Subjective criteria	Psychological performance parameters		Wake EEG	Sleep polygram
Neuroleptics	Chlorpromazine	25–50 mg	25–50 mg	→	50 mg	12.5 mg
	Clozapine	5 mg	n.d.		5, 10 mg	5, 10 mg
	Haloperidol	2 mg	up to 4 mg	0	up to 4 mg	1 mg
Antidepressants	Amitriptyline	6.25–12.5 mg	6.25–12.5 mg	→	25 mg	12.5 mg
	Imipramine	50 mg	75 mg	→	35 mg	25 mg
	Mianserin	n.d.	15 mg	→	15 mg	5, 10 mg
Tranquillizers, hypnotics	Chlordiazepoxide	10–30 mg	20 mg	→	n.d.	35 mg
	Diazepam	5–10 mg	5 mg	→	5 mg	5 mg
	Meprobamate	up to 800 mg	up to 800 mg	0	600 mg	400 mg
Psychostimulants	d-Amphetamine	5 mg	2.5 mg	←	5 mg	2.5–5 mg
	Caffeine	75 mg	75 mg	←	100 mg (?)	200 mg
	Methylphenidate	n.d.	10–20 mg	←	30 mg	5 mg

The smallest single doses of the respective drug leading to significant changes are shown in the table; references to the respective studies are given in Tables 3.4–3.8 and 4.2–4.4. n.d. = no data; 0 = no significant effects; ↑ and ↓ = improvement or deterioration (only for performance parameters).

conducted using small subject samples, thanks to the high standardization of the experimental procedures.

4.5.2   Specificity

In the present context, a test method is considered specific if it characterizes psychopharmaceuticals of different therapeutic groups by means of typical and unmistakable profiles of action.

The presentation of results of wake EEG studies (Table 4.2) leads to the conclusion that we cannot speak of specific profiles of action of neuroleptics, antidepressants, etc. On the other hand, stimulant and sedative substances can be reliably differentiated, especially when the EEG recordings last longer than the usual 5–10 minutes. In addition, benzodiazepines and, as older studies show, barbiturates are characterized in the wake EEG by an increase in beta activity around 14–20 Hz, i.e. by an effect not described for other compounds and which is possibly specific. From all this it emerges that EEG studies in awake subjects do not reveal specific profiles of action of currently known psychopharmaceuticals but can provide information on other features of a substance.

In an extensive study, Herrmann (1982) concentrated on the problem of specific profiles of action of neuroleptics, antidepressants, etc. in the wake EEG. Twenty substances were each tested against placebo in five separate but methodologically comparable experimental series with a total of 75 subjects. The central question was how reliably the individual substances could be detected as a neuroleptic, etc. on the basis of quantitative EEG parameters. According to the information given by the author, the hit rate for correct identification was 3/5 for neuroleptics, antidepressants and tranquillizers and 2/5 for psychostimulants and placebo, i.e., about 50% overall. If the results of psychological performance measurements were also taken into account, the hit rate improved to over 90%. Unfortunately, the results of this important study are published in such a way that the effects of individual substances and classes are unrecognizable and comparisons with other investigations are not possible (see also Herrmann and Schärer, 1987).

Sedative and stimulant substances can also be reliably characterized and differentiated from each other in polygraphic sleep recordings, but again one cannot speak of specific profiles of actions of different drug classes (Table 4.4). The curtailment of REM sleep seen after numerous antidepressants is not a specific feature of this class of substances (Section 4.3.4) and a striking effect of benzodiazepines in the sleep polygram, namely the increase in spindle activity around 14 Hz, is also found with other sedative substances, e.g. with some barbiturates (Kay *et al.*, 1976). In all, sleep polygraphic studies with psychopharmaceuticals can therefore claim no specificity in the sense that is of interest here.

Owing to a lack of reliable published findings, no conclusions can be drawn regarding the specificity of drug effects in various EP paradigms.

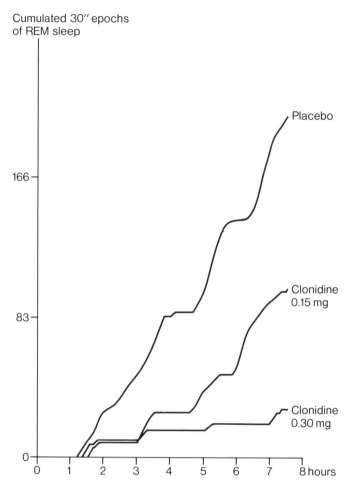

Figure 4.8. Effect of clonidine on REM sleep. Clonidine, an anti-hypertensive drug acting on alpha-2-adrenergic receptors, curtails REM sleep in a dose-dependent manner. The three curves show the mean duration of REM sleep in six subjects in relation to recording time. With 0.15 mg clonidine, REM sleep is greatly curtailed for about 5 hours; after 0.30 mg clonidine REM sleep is almost completely suppressed throughout the recording period. The curves allow a very precise estimation of the duration of action of clonidine on the brain (reproduced by permission of Blackwell Science Ltd from Spiegel and Devos, 1980)

4.5.3   Relevance

According to the foregoing, the relevance of drug studies with recording and analysis of wake EEGs of healthy subjects is primarily of a practical nature: stimulant and sedative substance effects can be detected even after small doses; the timing of the onset, peak and duration of an action on the brain can be determined with precision; in addition, correlations between blood levels of a substance and its effects, as well as pharmacodynamic interactions between several concomitantly or successively administered compounds, can be studied (Matejcek et al., 1984, 1985). Thus, drug–EEG studies in healthy subjects are potentially useful in both the early and later stages of drug development (see Chapter 6): in early stages as so-called screening methods, i.e., to roughly characterize clinically still unknown substances in healthy subjects; and in later stages as procedures for studying aspects of drug safety and for the investigation of other major practical questions.

The relevance of polygraphic sleep studies may be considered from both the practical and the theoretical aspects. Of practical value is the finding that most psychopharmaceuticals affect the polygraphically recorded course of sleep: thus, many centrally acting substances can be, as in the wake EEG, characterized by their type, intensity and duration of action (see Fig. 4.8). Apart from their effects on vigilance, many substances also affect so-called sleep architecture, i.e. the time sequence and proportions of the various sleep stages, especially the NREM–REM cycle and the proportions of REM sleep and slow wave sleep. These effects initially allow the formulation of hypotheses, often still very non-specific, concerning the effects of the tested compounds on neurotransmission in the brain (Chapter 5). In some cases, as demonstrated by the following example, they can also give rise to novel questions and studies:

It has long been known that substances with anticholinergic action, such as scopolamine and some antidepressants, adversely affect REM sleep, whereas compounds which promote cholinergic neurotransmission, such as physostigmine, favour the appearance of REM sleep (Gillin and Sitaram, 1984). Use can be made of this knowledge when studying new substances, especially potential cholinergics. Sleep-polygraphic study of two cholinergic drugs demonstrated that a direct cholinergic agonist, the experimental compound RS 86, promoted the onset of REM sleep, i.e. shortened REM latency (Spiegel, 1984a) but had no effect on REM density; in contrast, the brain-selective acetylcholinesterase inhibitor ENA 713 increased REM density but did not shorten REM latency (Holsboer-Trachsler et al., 1993). At present, the significance of this differential effect of two cholinergic compounds with different mechanisms of action can only be guessed at (Holsboer-Trachsler et al., 1993); however, due to the great interest currently being shown in cholinergic compounds (Chapter 7), at least the clinical correlates of these observations should be known soon.

Many of the hypotheses and theories based on polygraphic sleep studies, and especially those concerning the physiological and psychological relevance of REM sleep and the consequences of its suppression or reduction, have proved to be premature generalizations and have not withstood careful appraisal (Borbély, 1991, p. 211 ff.). Nevertheless, the linking of pharmacological, sleep-physiological and psychopathological objectives has proved very fruitful, both theoretically, especially with regard to our current models for understanding the regulation of sleep and wakefulness (Borbély, 1991), and practically in the form of contributions to the development of drugs with more specific action and of a better founded therapeutic approach to sleep disorders of varied genesis (Berger, 1992).

With the presentation of the actions of psychopharmaceuticals on electrophysiological parameters we have come closer to the biological substrate on which the clinically observable actions of these drugs are based. These biological aspects and the assumed mechanisms of actions of psychopharmaceuticals are dealt with in Chapter 5.

CHAPTER 5

Mechanisms of action of psychopharmaceuticals*

5.1 WHERE AND HOW DO PSYCHOPHARMACEUTICALS WORK?

This chapter deals with a fact that is hard to understand at first sight, namely that psychopharmaceuticals i.e., chemical compounds administered in the form of tablets, capsules or injections can act on mental phenomena such as feelings, mood, behaviour, symptoms. The term *mechanism of action* expresses the fact that the action of psychopharmaceuticals on mental processes occurs not *directly* but via a chain of intermediate links. Some of these links, i.e., biochemical, neurobiological and electrophysiological processes, are discussed in the following text.

Psychopharmaceuticals are mostly taken in the form of tablets, capsules or dragees: in these cases we speak of oral forms of administration or oral presentations. Parenteral presentations are also available for some psychopharmaceuticals, i.e., injection or infusion solutions which can be administered directly into the bloodstream and thus circumvent the gastrointestinal tract. Psychopharmaceuticals exert their intended effects in the central nervous system (CNS), where they primarily affect those processes which are involved in the transmission of information between nerve cells (neurons).

In a schematic and highly simplified manner, Fig. 5.1 illustrates the passage through and effects of a psychopharmaceutical ('active substance') in the body. After oral or parenteral administration, the active substance reaches the bloodstream and is transported to the target organ. In many cases the orally administered substances are modified to such an extent during their absorption from the gastrointestinal tract and during their first passage through the liver that only small amounts of the original substance circulate in the body. It can also happen that an absorbed compound is first converted into the actual active substance by enzymes in the body; the initial compound is then called a prodrug. In the majority of cases, what is excreted is not the original active substance but one or more breakdown products (= metabolites) which generally have attenuated biological activity.

There is a constant exchange of gases, nutrients, building materials and metabolic products between the blood circulating in the body and the CNS.

---

* Sections 5.1–5.3 in collaboration with R. Markstein.

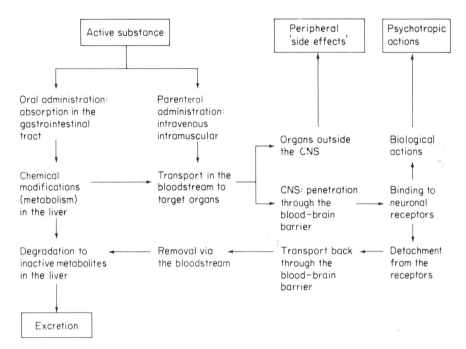

Figure 5.1.   Passage through and effects of a psychopharmaceutical in the body

As a consequence of this exchange, some of the administered active substance molecules cross over into the brain, provided that they can penetrate the *blood–brain barrier* (BBB). The BBB screens the nerve cells of the brain from disturbing chemical factors of all types; the term 'barrier' witnesses the fact that the fine blood vessels in the brain (= brain capillaries) have a structure different from that of capillaries in other organs and that only a fraction of the substances transported in the blood can pass through the capillary walls into the surrounding brain tissues. Brain capillaries are hardly permeable at all to fat-insoluble and very large molecules, a circumstance which has to be taken into account in the synthesis and development of new psychopharmaceuticals.

At no time during their passage through the body do psychopharmaceuticals come into direct contact with mental processes but their actions are mediated via numerous biochemical and biological steps. In common with all drugs, psychopharmaceuticals are chemical compounds which trigger or modify physicochemical processes in the body, and these effects can lead to biological and, finally, mental changes. Psychopharmaceuticals can influence nerve cell functions and the exchange of information between neurons at several levels: by acting on the cell wall (= cell membrane) or by penetrating into the cell and altering the biochemical processes taking place there.

The actions of most psychopharmaceuticals are exerted on the neuron membrane, where large molecules (macromolecules) are embedded and either provide for the transport of nutrients and ions into and out of the cell or serve as information receivers and converters. The macromolecules specializing in the recognition of information are called *receptors*. Receptors have two important functional features:

- Firstly they recognize and bind only very specific structures from among the many molecules present in the intercellular compartment; they thus have a structure-selective action.
- Secondly, when activated by a suitable molecule, they trigger a specific biological reaction in the cells; they thus exhibit selectivity of action.

The modern view is that receptors are the primary site of action of psychopharmaceuticals. Receptors can be isolated and studied in large amounts by means of molecular biological methods, mainly physicochemical techniques. This makes it possible to synthesize and test drugs with improved, more specific actions, and also creates an approach to the mechanistic understanding of mental illnesses.

The emphasis on the molecular level of action and on the significance of physicochemical processes introduces an essential assumption underlying the concept of mechanisms of action, which can be set out as follows: *if chemical compounds have a symptomatic or curative action on psychoses and other mental disorders, then these disorders must emanate from chemical deviations from the norm or, alternatively, chemical processes must play a decisive role in the mechanism which gives rise to, and/or maintains, the mental disturbance.*

In order to avoid any misunderstanding, it should be added here that the emphasis placed on chemical processes as the foundation or causal elements of mental disorders does not imply a disregard for other aetiological or intervening factors: genetic, sociopsychological, psychodynamic and other explanatory viewpoints are not negated by a biochemical approach to psychopathology, any more than these viewpoints cancel each other out.

In the early 1950s, when the modern psychopharmaceuticals were discovered, pathophysiological knowledge and hypotheses that could have been used for goal-directed development of antipsychotic or antidepressant drugs were lacking. 'Mechanistic concepts', i.e., in this context the synthesis of compounds based on a model of chemical mechanisms of the disease being treated, played no role in these early developments (Chapter 2). Instead of this, hypotheses concerning the disturbances of brain function underlying schizophrenia, depression, anxiety states, etc. were largely based on the effects of neuroleptics, antidepressants and other drugs that were detectable in suitable pharmacological models.

Neuroleptics, antidepressants, tranquillizers and the mechanisms of action attributed to them will be discussed separately in this chapter also, preceded by a brief introduction to the main basic neurobiological terms; these are discussed in more detail in Chapter 1 in Leonard (1992) and in textbooks of biological psychology (e.g. for German readers: Birbaumer and Schmidt, 1991).

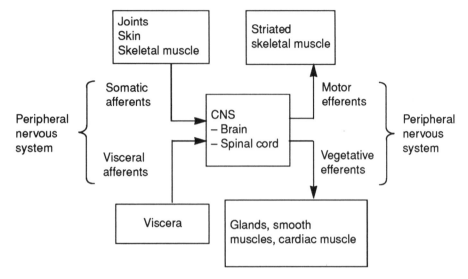

Figure 5.2. Schematic division of the peripheral and
central nervous system

5.2 BASIC NEUROBIOLOGICAL TERMS

5.2.1 The nervous system

Anatomically, distinction is made between a central and a peripheral nervous system: the central nervous system (CNS) consists of brain and spinal cord, the peripheral nervous system comprising all the nerves lying outside these two structures. In the peripheral nervous system (Fig. 5.2) a distinction is made between an afferent and an efferent portion. The afferent portion brings in information (nerve impulses) from the body periphery and from the viscera to the CNS. The efferent portion is that which carries information from the CNS to the periphery. In the afferent portion one distinguishes between the *somatic afferents*, i.e., those nerves which bring to the CNS information from the joints, from the skin and from the skeletal muscles, and *visceral afferents*, i.e., nerve fibres which carry the flow of information from the viscera to the CNS. Similarly one distinguishes on the efferent side between a motor and a vegetative component: *motor efferents* link the CNS to the skeletal musculature; *vegetative efferents* form the link between CNS and glands, smooth muscle and cardiac muscle.

5.2.2 Neurons, resting potentials and action potentials

In common with all organs, the nervous system is built up of cells, the most important of which are the nerve cells or *neurons*. These are capable of taking

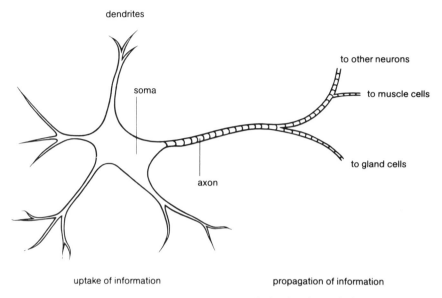

Figure 5.3. Schematic diagram of a neuron. A distinction is made between an entry side (dendrites, soma) and an exit side (axon). The axon is surrounded by an insulating sheath which is interrupted by gaps ('nodes of Ranvier') at regular intervals

up chemical and electrical signals, of processing, storing and transmitting them. In the case of neurons it is impressive to note the variety of forms which may be observed in the individual regions of the nervous system. Despite this variety, most neurons have the same basic structure (Fig. 5.3). Two kinds of processes emerge from a cell body (soma): there are generally several shorter processes, which in the majority of cases are highly branched and known as *dendrites*, and one longer process, *the axon*, the end of which is generally branched.

The uptake of signals occurs mainly on the side of the dendrites and soma, whereas the further transmission of a signal generally occurs through the axon. This is a connecting cable which links the neuron to other cells, e.g. to other neurons, muscle or glandular cells. In addition to neurons, the nervous system also comprises another type of cell, so-called glia cells. Although not specialized in passing on signals, they play an important role by assuming supportive and nutritional functions for the neurons and also by forming insulating sheaths (myelin sheaths) around the axons and so prevent cross-talk between nerve cells.

Electric processes are involved in the transmission of information within the nervous system. Every nerve cell is able to produce electrical impulses itself, or to convert and retransmit signals received into electric impulses. In the resting state, a negative electrical potential exists between the inside of the nerve cell and the extracellular space. This *resting potential* arises in the following manner: within the cell there is a lower concentration of positively charged sodium (Na+) and negatively charged chloride (Cl-) ions and a greater concentration of positively charged potassium (K+) ions and of large organic anions than in the extracellular space. The K+ ions pass to the outside by means of passive diffusion. Since the larger, negatively charged anions are unable to follow (they do not pass through the cell membrane), there arises a separation of charge along the cell membrane, which is the basis for the so-called resting potential. Na+ ions entering the cell passively from the outside are, with the consumption of energy, pumped out again in exchange for K+ ions, so that the concentration gradient and therefore the resting potential are maintained. The electric resting potential is the prerequisite for the formation of action potentials, i.e., short-term depolarizations and repolarizations, which affect the entire neuron. Action potentials which may be looked upon as units of information operate on the basis of the all-or-nothing principle; i.e., they either occur or fail to occur and move at high speed on the surface of the neuron. The transmission of action potentials from one neuron to the next, or from a nerve cell to a muscle cell, occurs at what are known as synapses.

5.2.3   Synapses

Synapses are points of contact between nerve cells or between nerve cells and the effector cells which they control, e.g. glandular cells, sensory cells or muscle cells. Synapses serve to transfer information and, depending on the nature of the information carrier, differentiation is made between electrical and chemical synapses. In the case of electrical synapses, the membranes of two cells touch each other directly and thus make it possible for an electrical current to be transferred, which leads to a rapid signal transfer in both directions. Electrical synapses have previously been studied mainly in lower animals but also occur in humans. It is uncertain whether they have relevance to psychopharmacology and we shall not discuss them further here.

In chemical synapses, electrical signals are converted into chemical signals and these are in turn converted into electrical impulses. Together with receptors, they are considered to be the most important sites of action of psychopharmaceuticals.

In a chemical synapse, the membrane of the nerve ending is separated from the subsynaptic membrane by a cleft of about 100–300 Å (mm^{-6}) (Fig. 5.4). An electrical impulse arriving at the nerve ending, known as the action potential, is unable simply to jump across this cleft; instead there occurs a chemical process which leads to the secretion of chemical compounds known as *neurotransmitters*. Neurotransmitters are messenger substances which, after being liberated by an electrical impulse, travel to the postsynaptic membrane where they trigger several effects.

– Firstly, there is interaction with chemical receptors, i.e., macromolecules that specifically bind the transmitter in question.

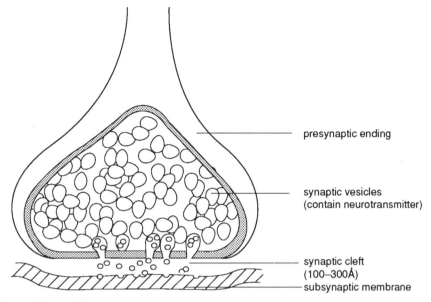

presynaptic ending

synaptic vesicles
(contain neurotransmitter)

synaptic cleft
(100–300Å)
subsynaptic membrane

Figure 5.4. Diagram of a chemical synapse. The electrical potential arriving at the presynaptic nerve ending is not passed on directly. The transmission of information occurs chemically with the aid of a neurotransmitter stored in vesicles located in the presynaptic nerve ending

– When the transmitter binds with its receptor it triggers subsequent reactions on the surface of the postsynaptic cell and, for example, may cause a local change in the electrical potential of the postsynaptic membrane. Depending on the type of transmitter and on the properties of the postsynaptic receptors, the membrane potential of the affected cell is shifted in either a negative (hyperpolarization) or positive (depolarization) direction. When the postsynaptic membrane potential is depolarized down to a specific critical value, termed the threshold, an action potential arises in the second neuron and is transmitted by the axon. With this, the membrane potential spontaneously depolarizes to positive values, but returns to its initial value after a very short time.

The activities of enzymes inside the cells that are important in the production of energy and in maintaining cell structures can also be modified via postsynaptic receptors. Intracellular messenger substances, the so-called 'second messengers' such as cyclic AMP, cyclic GMP and cleavage products of phosphatidylinositol, play an important role in this respect. These molecules are formed at the cell membrane and migrate into the cell, where they affect the activities of other enzymes.

As a rule, receptors specific for the secreted transmitter are present in the presynaptic membrane. These *autoreceptors* on the presynaptic side regulate the further release and synthesis of the neurotransmitter and therefore are

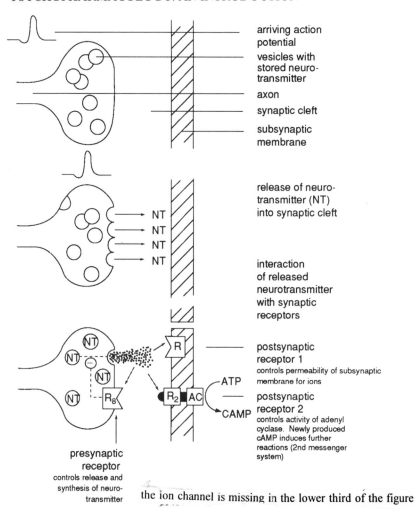

arriving action potential

vesicles with stored neuro-transmitter

axon

synaptic cleft

subsynaptic membrane

release of neuro-transmitter (NT) into synaptic cleft

interaction of released neurotransmitter with synaptic receptors

postsynaptic receptor 1
controls permeability of subsynaptic membrane for ions

postsynaptic receptor 2
controls activity of adenyl cyclase. Newly produced cAMP induces further reactions (2nd messenger system)

presynaptic receptor
controls release and synthesis of neuro-transmitter

the ion channel is missing in the lower third of the figure

Figure 5.5. Processes occurring at the chemical synapse. The action potential (upper third of the figure) arriving at the presynaptic nerve ending releases the neurotransmitter (NT) stored within the vesicles, which then travels to the synaptic cleft (middle third). Here it produces a number of effects:

- On the postsynaptic receptor 1 which regulates the ion permeability of the subsynaptic membrane. This part of the activity is important for the further transmission of the electric signal in the downstream neuron.
- On postsynaptic receptor 2 which is linked to an enzyme system of the subsequent nerve cell. This may trigger a number of different intracellular enzymatic processes, such as an increase of glucose metabolism and of protein synthesis as well as phosphorylation reactions.
- On the presynaptic receptors which regulate the further synthesis and release of the neurotransmitter. Stimulation of the presynaptic receptor by the released transmitter generally leads to a reduction in the further release of transmitter: the system consequently operates on the principle of negative feedback.

part of a biological feedback system (Fig. 5.5, lower third). Neurons in the CNS have between a few dozen to a few thousand synaptic connections with other neurons. Each individual neuron in the CNS thus simultaneously receives dozens to thousands of stimulating and inhibiting influences from other cells. What it transmits is a function of the sum of the impulses received and also depends on the functional state of the neuron at a particular time. Viewed in this context, the nerve cell has an integrating function. When we consider the number of neurons in the human brain ($50-100 \cdot 10^9$ in the cerebral cortex alone), at least some idea can be obtained of the complexity of neuronal circuitry.

5.2.4   Neurotransmitters

The neurotransmitters acting at the chemical synapses are chemical compounds which are formed in the organism in a number of sites, including the nervous system. The best-known neurotransmitters are noradrenaline, dopamine, serotonin, acetylcholine and GABA (gamma-aminobutyric acid) (see Table 5.1). It was assumed for decades that each neuron could synthesize, store and release only one type of neurotransmitter, e.g. noradrenaline (see Bloom, 1980, p. 246). This concept, named Dale's principle after its author, no longer applies unrestrictedly; some nerve cells can be affected by more than one neurotransmitter, and various types of molecules with transmitter functions can also occur within the same neuron.

It has long been known which neurotransmitters act on which synapses of the peripheral nervous system. Synapses between motor nerve cells and

Table 5.1.   Known and putative neurotransmitters

Name	Class		Localization in the CNS
Adrenaline	⎫	⎫	Subcortical
Noradrenaline	⎬ Catecholamines	⎬	Practically everywhere
Dopamine	⎭		Several systems,
		⎬ Monoamines	especially mesolimbic and nigrostriatal
Serotonin			Everywhere
Acetylcholine		⎭	Everywhere
GABA	⎫		Supraspinal
Glycine	⎬ Amino acids		interneurons
Glutamic acid	⎭		Spinal interneurons
			Interneurons generally
Enkephalins	⎫		
Substance P			
Vasopressin			In numerous CNS
	⎬ Neuropeptides		regions, sometimes together with other
Angiotensin			neurotransmitters
Somatostatin	⎭		

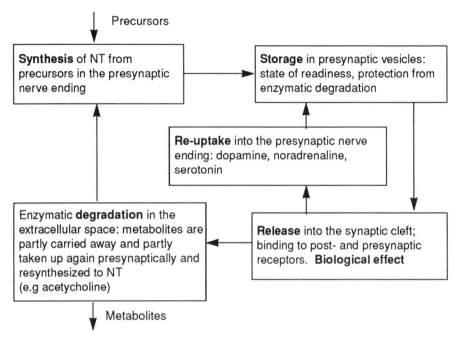

Figure 5.6. Life cycle of neurotransmitters (NT)

muscle cells of striated musculature – the neuromuscular junctions – are cholinergic; i.e., it is at this site that the stimulation is transmitted with the aid of acetylcholine. Acetylcholine is also a neurotransmitter in certain parts of the vegetative nervous system as well as playing an important role as a transmitter substance in the brain. About 10% of the synapses in the CNS are cholinergic. Significant parts of the vegetative nervous system are noradrenergically innervated and noradrenaline (NA; also known as norepinephrine, NE) is also present as a neurotransmitter in the CNS but amounts to less than 1% of the total amount of neurotransmitters there. Serotonin is also a neurotransmitter in the CNS, but only in small amounts, and is also present in the vascular system, in connective tissue and in the platelets. The presence and functions of these neurotransmitters are thus by no means restricted to the CNS.

It follows that many drugs which influence noradrenergic, serotoninergic and cholinergic neurotransmission develop effects not only – as intended – in the CNS, but also in the peripheral nervous system and, in addition, in many other systems of the organism. Such effects often become apparent clinically in the form of side effects or 'adverse events'.

GABA is the major inhibitory neurotransmitter in the CNS, and is mainly found in small interneurons, i.e., nerve cells which are located between dopaminergic, serotoninergic or other neurons and connect with them so that any overactivity on their part can be prevented. GABAergic neurons are found at all levels in the CNS, from the spinal cord to the cortex, but not in structures outside the CNS, so that drugs which affect GABAergic neurotransmission selectively cannot be expected to have direct vegetative side effects.

Apart from their information-transmitting functions, nerve cells have the ability to synthesize, store and metabolize neurotransmitters from their biological precursors as well as to reuse them following their reuptake from the synaptic cleft (Fig. 5.6). These processes are regulated by the functional demands existing at a specific point in time of neurotransmission and by factors which determine the functional level of an organism in the broader sense: circadian (about one day long) and other biological rhythms, the degree of fatigue and the state of health.

All the processes mentioned above, i.e., synthesis, storage, release, reuptake, degradation and postsynaptic effects of neurotransmitters, can be influenced by drugs. As Table 5.2 shows, of all the numerous conceivable possibilities for influencing neurotransmission, the following are used in practice today:

– postsynaptic blockade in the case of neuroleptics (Section 5.3.3);
– inhibition of reuptake in the case of antidepressants (Section 5.4);
– inhibition of enzymatic breakdown in the synaptic cleft (some antidepressants, Section 5.4.1);
– enhancement of the neurotransmitter action on postsynaptic receptors in the case of benzodiazepine anxiolytics (Section 5.5).

5.2.5   Receptors, agonists and antagonists

The name *receptors* is given to macromolecules which possess regions to which certain chemical molecules can bind in specific ways, thereby triggering a characteristic secondary reaction in a cell (p. 115). In principle, two types of compounds which bind to receptors can be differentiated:

– If the bound molecule triggers an action specific for the receptor, we speak of an *agonist*;
– If, on the other hand, a molecule binds to the receptor without triggering an action, but thereby preventing the binding of an agonist, we speak of an *antagonist*.

The strength with which both agonists and antagonists are bound can vary greatly; the binding ability is called *affinity* and is described quantitatively by the dissociation constant for the specific binding site. Agonists can be characterized by two constants, their affinity and their potency of action, often called efficacy or intrinsic activity. The potency of action is mostly stated as a value relative to that of the natural agonist, i.e., the corresponding transmitter.

Thanks to the use of modern molecular biology methods, our knowledge of the structures and molecular processes involved in signal transmission via

Table 5.2. Possible points of attack on neurotransmission

Site of action	Type of action	Effect on neurotransmission	Examples	Therapeutic uses
NT synthesis	Supply of NT precursors	Promotion: more NT available	L-Dopa → dopamine	Treatment of Parkinson's disease
	Interference with NT synthesis	Inhibition: less NT available	AMPT	None known
NT storage	Disturbance of storage	Inhibition: less NT available	**Reserpine**	Treatment of schizophrenia (outdated)
NT release	Increased release	Promotion: more NT available	**Amphetamine**	Hyperkinetic syndrome narcolepsy
NT degradation	Inhibition of degradation	Promotion: more NT available	**Monoamine oxidase inhibitors**	Treatment of depressions
NT reuptake	Inhibition of re-uptake	Promotion: more NT available	**Antidepressants**	Treatment of depressions
Postsynaptic receptors	Stimulation	Promotion	Bromocriptine	Treatment of Parkinson's disease
	Blockade	Inhibition	**Neuroleptics**	Treatment of schizophrenias
Presynaptic receptors	Stimulation	Inhibition	Clonidine	Reduction of blood pressure
	Blockade	Promotion	?	Antidepressive principle?

NT = neurotransmitter; AMPT = alpha-methyl-paratyrosine. **Bold face**: possibilities used today (psychopharmaceuticals).

receptors is much greater now than it was just a few years ago. Thus, receptors can now be classified according to structure instead of the previously used differentiation according to pharmacological and functional properties only. Dopamine receptors were originally divided into two types, D-1 and D-2, but three more types have now been discovered. On the basis of functional, structural and pharmacological similarities, the dopamine receptors known today are divided into D-1 and D-2 'families'. The D-1 family includes the D-1 and D-5 receptors, and the D-2 family includes the D-2, D-3 and D-4 receptors. The D-1 and D-5 receptors of the D-1 family activate the enzymes adenylate cyclase or phospholipase C. The D-2 receptor of the D-2 family either inhibits adenylate cyclase or opens the calcium channel, whereas the functional activities of the D-3 and D-4 receptors are not known at present (Sibley and Monsma, 1992).

The situation is similarly complex in the field of serotonin receptors. New types and particularly new species variants have been discovered in recent years. The serotonin receptors known today are divided into seven families, a detailed description of which is given by Hoyer *et al.* (1994). In the case of noradrenaline, alpha and beta receptors were originally distinguished, but here also there have been several subtypes discovered. The same applies to acetylcholine, with not only nicotinic receptors but also at least five subtypes of muscarinic receptors present in man, some of them with unknown functional significance.

5.3   HYPOTHESES REGARDING THE MODE OF ACTION OF NEUROLEPTICS

The 'antipsychotic' action of chlorpromazine discovered in the years 1952/53 could not be explained in terms of the pathophysiological concepts of schizophrenia prevailing at that time. The foremost authors assumed that genetic, social and individual psychodynamic factors and life experience factors contributed to various degrees to the development of schizophrenic psychoses. Speculation certainly concerned possible biological or biochemical disturbance in the brain, but analytical methods necessary to check these assumptions were not available. Two of the pathophysiological hypotheses of the time that proved quite fruitful in stimulating research but which have no direct connection with the action of neuroleptics will be mentioned here briefly.

5.3.1   The serotonin hypothesis of schizophrenia

In 1954, i.e., about two years after the discovery of chlorpromazine in Europe, two American biochemists (Woolley and Shaw) published the hypothesis that schizophrenia and similar psychoses could be based on a disturbance of serotoninergic neurotransmission in the brain. This hypothesis was supported by some facts that had become known shortly beforehand:

(1) The spectacular psychotropic actions of LSD (lysergic acid diethylamide), which causes disturbances in perception, thought and feelings as well as hallucinations in healthy subjects (Stoll, 1947).

(2) The serotonin-antagonistic effects of LSD, i.e., the ability of this psychotomimetic drug to block the actions of serotonin in various pharmacological tests.

Although it was still unknown that serotonin occurs in the brain and acts as a neurotransmitter, Woolley and Shaw speculated that the psychotropic effects of LSD were the result of its ability to block serotonin in the brain; they then suggested that a disturbance in serotoninergic transmission in the brain underlies schizophrenic psychoses which, among other things, are characterized by disorders in perception and thought processes. This hypothesis could be tested by giving schizophrenic patients serotonin or a longer-acting serotonin analogue: an improvement in the state of the patient would support the correctness of the serotonin hypothesis.

It became known in the same year (1954) that a substance derived from the Indian plant *Rauwolfia serpentina*, reserpine, had antipsychotic effects. This finding was of interest for the serotonin hypothesis of schizophrenia for two reasons: firstly, the molecular structure of reserpine has a partial similarity to that of serotonin and LSD; secondly, it was found that reserpine liberates serotonin in the CNS from presynaptic stores and thus produces a short-lived excess supply of functionally available serotonin at the synapse. In the context of a serotonin hypothesis it could therefore be postulated that the antipsychotic effect of reserpine was due to its ability to liberate serotonin presynaptically and make it functionally available.

The serotonin hypothesis of schizophrenia could not last long since it was in conflict both with psychopathological and with pharmacological findings:

(1) The 'psychotic' symptoms produced by LSD in healthy persons differ qualitatively and quantitatively from the symptoms typical of schizophrenia (Bleuler, 1956). Thus, for example, the hallucinations experienced by schizophrenic patients are predominantly acoustic in nature, whereas LSD mainly gives rise to visual phenomena.

(2) LSD is not a specific serotonin antagonist, but also exerts agonistic effects on serotonin receptors. On the other hand, many serotonin antagonists, which are more effective than LSD, are not hallucinogenic.

(3) In addition to serotonin, reserpine releases other neurotransmitters, especially dopamine and noradrenaline from their stores in presynaptic nerve endings. However, the action on the synapse of the neurotransmitters released in this way is slight since they already undergo intracellular enzymatic degradation.

(4) The administration of biological precursors of serotonin, which can be converted to serotonin in the CNS, has no clear-cut antipsychotic effect in acute schizophrenic patients.

(5) In contrast to reserpine, chlorpromazine has neither a serotonin-like chemical structure nor does it release serotonin from nerve endings.

Despite its relatively fast and thorough rebuttal, the serotonin hypothesis of schizophrenia was fruitful in several respects. On the one hand it gave rise to the development of sensitive serotonin assay methods and proof that serotonin does occur in the brain (Carlsson, 1987), and on the other hand it served as the prototype for other simple and thus readily testable biochemical hypotheses of mental illnesses. Interest in serotonin has been reawakened in recent years in relation to the mechanism of action of some neuroleptics (Section 5.3.4); however, this development has nothing to do with the serotonin hypothesis of schizophrenia in its original version.

5.3.2   The transmethylation hypothesis of schizophrenia

Almost at the same time as the discovery of chlorpromazine and shortly before the publication of the serotonin hypothesis, Osmond and Smythies (1952) formulated the transmethylation hypothesis of schizophrenia, according to which the psychotic symptoms are an expression and consequence of abnormal biochemical processes in the brain: faulty methylation would cause

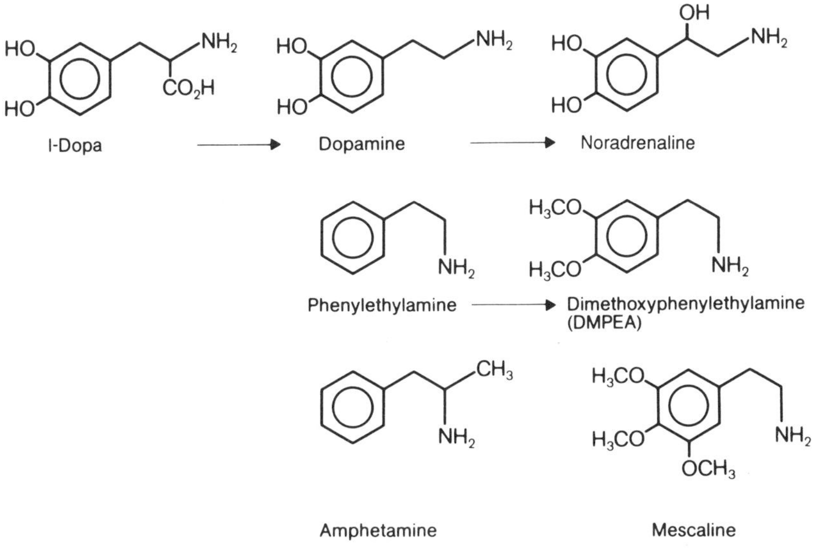

Figure 5.7. Abnormal methylation processes as a hypothetical cause of schizophrenia. The top line shows the physiologically normal conversion of L-dopa into the neurotransmitters dopamine and noradrenaline. L-Dopa, dopamine and noradrenaline (but also amphetamine and mescaline) contain the phenylethylamine skeleton (second line) which, according to the hypothesis, can be converted into hallucinogenic substances through the action of abnormal endogenous methylation processes. DMPEA was for some time regarded as being a possible hallucinogenic substance which can be formed by abnormal methylation (see text)

neurotransmitters to change into hallucinogenic compounds, e.g. tryptamine is converted to the hallucinogen dimethyltryptamine (DMT), serotonin becomes bufotenin and dopamine becomes mescaline (Fig. 5.7). Originally the hypothesis was based, above all, on the striking structural similarity between a number of endogenous substances and hallucinogens, whilst in the years that followed further findings were collected which also lent a certain empirical credibility to the transmethylation hypothesis:

- A methylated dopamine analogue (3,4-dimethoxyphenylethylamine, DMPEA) could be detected in the urine of schizophrenic patients, being revealed as a pink spot on paper chromatograms.
- High doses of methionine, an amino acid, can lead to acute psychotic reactions in chronic schizophrenics. Methionine is a so-called methyl group donor, i.e., it can favour – normal and pathological – methylation reactions in the organism.
- There was a temporal relationship between the appearance of methylated indolamines (serotonin, tryptamine) in the urine of schizophrenics and acute deteriorations in the condition of these patients (Tanimukai *et al.*, 1970).

Despite these interesting indications, the transmethylation hypothesis of schizophrenia had to be rejected for a number of reasons: firstly, DMPEA can also be detected as a pink spot in the urine of non-schizophrenics and is, moreover, not hallucinogenic; secondly, it has never been possible to identify hallucinogenic methyl derivatives of biogenic amines in schizophrenic patients; thirdly, the symptom-enhancing effect of high doses of methionine in certain chronic schizophrenics can also be explained in that this amino acid impedes the uptake into the brain of precursors of biogenic amines and exerts other direct and indirect effects on the brain (see Smythies, 1979).

5.3.3   The dopamine hypothesis of schizophrenia

The serotonin and transmethylation hypotheses of schizophrenia were formulated at approximately the same time as the discovery of the first neuroleptics, but had no direct connection with the pharmacological effects of these drugs. The situation is different in the case of the dopamine hypothesis; all known neuroleptics have an inhibitory action on dopaminergic neurons even though they vary considerably in their other pharmacological effects, and this anti-dopaminergic effect is considered to be responsible for the 'antipsychotic' actions of neuroleptics.

At the time of the discovery of chlorpromazine, dopamine could not be directly assayed and its role as a neurotransmitter was unknown (Carlsson, 1987). Chlorpromazine exerts a large number of pharmacological effects (see p. 37), all of which can in principle be considered as explaining its clinical action. Thus, it was first assumed that the antipsychotic action of chlorpromazine and other neuroleptics depends directly on their cataleptic potency, i.e., their ability to induce catalepsy in animal experiments or extra-pyramidal symptoms in clinical use. This assumption lost credibility when thioridazine, a neuroleptic with weak extrapyramidal effects but good anti-psychotic activity, became available; the assumed connection was definitively refuted with the introduction of clozapine.

In the late 1950s it was found that patients with Parkinson's disease have a dopamine deficiency in the basal ganglia that can be treated with L-dopa, a biological precursor of dopamine. This and the simultaneously observed similarity between some symptoms of Parkinson's disease and the dyskinesias noted during neuroleptic treatment led to the assumption that the 'neuroleptic Parkinsonoid' of schizophrenic patients could be due to a disturbance of dopaminergic neurotransmission. The postulated mechanism of the disturbance and the position of dopamine as a neurotransmitter were further clarified in animal experiments. Carlsson and Lindquist (1963) found that chlorpromazine increased the turnover of dopamine in mouse brain, whereas no corresponding effects arose after promethazine, a phenothiazine derivative without antipsychotic efficacy (p. 37). These authors interpreted the effect of chlorpromazine on dopamine turnover as being a consequence of a hypothetical blockage of dopamine neurotransmission through the action of the neuroleptic. It was assumed that presynaptic dopaminergic neurons tend to compensate for the blockade of postsynaptic receptors through increased dopamine synthesis and release in order to restore the functional balance disturbed by the antagonist.

Chlorpromazine and other neuroleptics were thus recognized as dopamine antagonists, and the next step was to clarify whether and to what extent the anti-dopamine action of various neuroleptics is related to their antipsychotic efficacy. In so-called receptor binding studies it was demonstrated that the affinities of various neuroleptics for dopamine receptors in the brain are highly correlated with their antipsychotic potencies (Creese et al., 1976), which again supported the dopamine hypothesis of neuroleptic action. However, a close correlation could be shown only with the dopamine D-2 receptor, whereas affinities for the D-1 receptor showed hardly any correlation with the strength of antipsychotic action (Seeman, 1980).

Despite some necessary refinement in later years, the dopamine hypothesis even in its original version ('neuroleptics act via blockade of postsynaptic dopamine receptors') can still explain many pharmacological and clinical observations, such as:

– In Parkinson patients treated with L-dopa or dopamine agonists, hallucinations and other psychosis-like states occur occasionally and may be interpreted in the sense of dopaminergic overstimulation.
– Large doses of amphetamine can provoke a toxic syndrome ('amphetamine psychosis') in healthy subjects that shows certain similarities to schizophrenic psychoses. By inducing massive catecholamine release from presynaptic sites, amphetamine produces a temporary excess supply of dopamine and noradrenaline in synapses.

– Even in small doses, amphetamine can exacerbate psychotic activity in schizophrenic patients, and similar symptom provocation also arises with other dopaminergic substances.

Further observations were published later which also pointed to the action of neuroleptics via dopaminergic mechanisms: alpha-methyl-*para*-tyrosine (AMPT), which inhibits the synthesis of dopamine and noradrenaline from their biological precursors (and thus also inhibits dopaminergic neurotransmission), augments the antipsychotic efficacy of neuroleptics. The toxic psychosis which arises in healthy subjects after large and repeated amphetamine doses can be antagonized by neuroleptics but not by noradrenaline antagonists. Schizophrenic patients with low DBH levels (DBH = dopamine beta-hydroxylase, an enzyme involved in the conversion of dopamine to noradrenaline) in whom intensified dopamine activity in the brain may therefore be assumed to occur, respond to neuroleptics better than schizophrenics with high DBH levels (Sternberg *et al.*, 1982).

Other empirical findings could not, however, be unequivocally incorporated into the dopamine hypothesis:

(1) The blockade of dopamine receptors is an immediate effect of neuroleptics that can be detected even after a single dose, whereas their therapeutic action becomes apparent only after several days or weeks of treatment.

(2) Dopaminergic agonists such as bromocriptine and apomorphine, which act directly on postsynaptic receptors (Table 5.2), do not provoke a psychosis-like state in healthy subjects.

(3) Some schizophrenics respond to amphetamine administration not with a deterioration but with an improvement in their state (Angrist *et al.*, 1982; van Kammen *et al.*, 1982).

(4) As shown by numerous individual studies, there is no convincing evidence for an elevated dopamine content or hypersensitivity of dopamine receptors in the brain of schizophrenic patients: breakdown products of dopamine and noradrenaline are elevated neither in the urine nor in the blood nor in the cerebrospinal fluid of schizophrenic patients. In some patients with chronic schizophrenia there is even evidence of dopamine hypofunction (Karoum *et al.*, 1987).

Despite these unexplained or contradictory findings, the dopamine hypothesis still represents the best developed theoretical basis on which to explain many biochemical, animal experimental, human pharmacological, and clinical results (McKenna, 1987). Criticism is often directed at the over-emphasis on one individual neurotransmitter, i.e., disregard for the fact that the transmitter systems in the CNS work in close mutual interdependence (Fritze, 1992), and also at the tendency to create a pathophysiological theory of schizophrenia from a model to explain the actions of neuroleptics. A possible criticism from the viewpoint of drug research is that the dopamine hypothesis is a rather retrograde theory which has so far not led to any basically novel antipsychotic medicaments (Crow, 1987).

5.3.4   Further development of the dopamine hypothesis

Davis (1974) proposed an early reformulation of the dopamine hypothesis in the form of a two-factor theory, which is particularly interesting from the clinical standpoint. This takes into account the fact that, although neuroleptics exert a dopamine antagonistic effect from the very first moment, their antipsychotic action generally only becomes evident after weeks or months. It may therefore be assumed that schizophrenic disorders have their origin in defects other than dopaminergic overstimulation, although this is involved as a second factor and augments the psychotic process. This second factor responds to treatment with neuroleptics so that the disorder becomes attenuated and, ultimately, intrinsic repair processes succeed in bringing about a complete cure of the disorder in some cases. The two-factor theory does not clarify the nature of the structural, biochemical, psychological or other factors which lie at the origin of the pathological process.

Another hypothesis that can resolve some contradictions of the dopamine hypothesis was developed by Crow (1982) and involves a division of schizophrenias into two types: 'Type I corresponds to acute schizophrenia or schizophreniform disorder in which one observes more positive symptoms of hallucinations and delusions with a good prognosis and excellent response to neuroleptics . . . Type II represents chronic schizophrenia with affective flattening, poverty of speech and loss of drive, the so-called negative symptoms of schizophrenia. Type II patients respond less well to neuroleptics . . .' (Snyder, 1982). Type I patients would thus fit into the dopamine hypothesis of schizophrenia, whereas a pathophysiological basis other than dopaminergic hyperactivity must be assumed for type II patients. However, Snyder (1982) emphasized that 'one should be cautious about drawing such a distinction [between different types of schizophrenia] solely on the basis of drug response'.

Newer variants of the dopamine hypothesis have mostly been derived from the profile of actions of the 'atypical' neuroleptic clozapine (p. 24) and seek to relate pharmacological findings to the unusual clinical actions of this product; at the same time one hopes to use clozapine as a basis for obtaining neuroleptics which are safer and even more effective. If the major clinical and pharmacological effects of clozapine are compared, the following picture is obtained:

Clinical features	*Effects in animals (selection)*
• Marked antipsychotic efficacy, even in some patients refractory to other treatment	• Inhibition of motor activity and conditioned avoidance
• Action on negative symptoms	• Relatively strong binding to (dopamine) D_1 receptors

- Beneficial effects on mood and well-being
- No extrapyramidal side effects

- Anticholinergic side effects, marked sedation at start of therapy

- Blockade of (serotonin) 5-HT$_2$ receptors
- No catalepsy, no marked antagonism of apomorphine
- Anticholinergic effects, sedation

It is not known which pharmacological effects are responsible for which aspects of the clinical action of clozapine, but there are two main and possibly complementary hypotheses today, namely the so-called 5-HT$_2$:D$_2$ hypothesis and the D$_1$:D$_2$ equilibrium hypothesis. According to the first one, the beneficial actions of clozapine are the result of simultaneous blockade of (serotonin) 5-HT$_2$ and (dopamine) D$_2$ receptors (Meltzer, 1989), whereas according to the other hypothesis, the clinical effects of clozapine and particularly the absence of extrapyramidal side effects are associated with the balanced action of clozapine on dopamine D$_1$ and D$_2$ receptors (Markstein, 1994). Both hypotheses have given rise to dozens of studies (see review by Deutsch *et al.*, 1991), but it is still not known which of these two or any other hypotheses, such as that of frontal dopaminergic underactivity with compensatory mesolimbic hyperactivity (Davis *et al.*, 1991), is closer to the truth. Good use can be made of both hypotheses from the viewpoint of pharmaceutical research, i.e., in the development of specific preparations (combined D$_2$/5-HT$_2$ antagonists or D$_1$/D$_2$ antagonists, e.g., risperidone), although experience shows that it will take several years before any of the said pharmacological concepts (and thus a specific mechanistic hypothesis) can be confirmed or refuted.

5.4 HYPOTHESES REGARDING THE MODE OF ACTION OF ANTIDEPRESSANTS

After the discovery of medicaments with antidepressant activity in the late 1950s, an intensive search was undertaken for pharmacological models which would provide an understanding of the therapeutic effects observed and at the same time assist in the development of other, still more effective and specific antidepressants. In traditional pharmacological tests, the prototype imipramine was characterized by sedative, antihistaminic and anticholinergic effects and thus did not differ fundamentally from other medicaments with no antidepressant activity, e.g. antihistamines. The following observations then led to a further step forward in the development of hypotheses:

- The behavioural syndrome induced in mice and rats by reserpine (sedation, catalepsy, ptosis) can be reversed by imipramine.
- The effect of noradrenaline on various organs is potentiated by imipramine.
- Imipramine inhibits the reuptake of previously released noradrenaline in isolated tissues.

All these findings suggested that imipramine augments the action of nor-adrenaline ('*amine potentiation*'), or is able to correct a state brought about through noradrenaline deficiency. Once it became known that reserpine, which had been used to treat hypertension, triggered depression in some patients and that it also released the neurotransmitters noradrenaline, dopamine and serotonin from their protected presynaptic stores and thus exposed them to inactivation by intracellular enzymes, then the first hypotheses were developed concerning the relationship between depressive syndromes and disturbances in the metabolism of these neurotransmitters: the catecholamine and serotonin hypotheses of depression.

5.4.1   The catecholamine hypothesis of depression

This was formulated in 1965 by J. Schildkraut and states that 'some, if not all, depressions are the consequence of an absolute or relative deficiency of cate-cholamines, particularly norepinephrine, at functionally important adrenergic receptor sites in the brain' (Schildkraut, 1965, p. 509). The material brought forward in support of this hypothesis was impressive (Table 5.3) since it covered both clinical and multifarious pharmacological findings. The antidepressant effect of imipramine and of the MAO inhibitors was attributed to the fact that these medicaments bring about an increased supply of functionally available catecholamines at the synapse:

- Imipramine prevents the reuptake (and hence the inactivation) of previously released noradrenaline from the synaptic cleft into the presynaptic nerve ending.
- MAO inhibitors prevent the breakdown of the released and functionally available catecholamines by the enzyme monoamine oxidase present in the extracellular space (within the cells, monoamines are protected by the vesi-cles, cf. Fig. 5.4).

The catecholamine hypothesis brought several pharmacological findings to-gether in an illuminating relationship, but contradicted a number of clinical observations (Section 5.4.3). The serotonin hypothesis, which constitutes a similar overall approach, was formulated at about the same time.

5.4.2   The serotonin hypothesis of depression

This states that some or all depressions are due to a lack of serotonin in certain parts of the brain stem (Coppen, 1967). Numerous pharmacological and biochemical findings support this hypothesis:

- The antidepressant imipramine inhibits not only the reuptake of catechola-mines into presynaptic nerve endings but also inhibits serotonin reuptake.
- MAO inhibitors inhibit serotonin inactivation in the extracellular compart-ment, just as they inhibit catecholamine inactivation.

Table 5.3. The catecholamine hypothesis of depression

Substance	Effect on mood in man	Effect on behaviour in animals	Effect on catecholamines in the brain (at the synapse)
Reserpine	Sedation, in some patients depression	Sedation, catalepsy, hypothermia	Reduction (intracellular release, hence more rapid degradation and inactivation)
Amphetamine	Stimulation, mood improvement	Stimulation	Release of noradrenaline (and dopamine) and inhibition of reuptake
MAO inhibitors	Antidepressant effect	Stimulation, prevents sedation after reserpine	Increase (prevention of degradation after release into the synaptic cleft)
Imipramine	Antidepressant effect	Prevents sedation after reserpine, potentiates effect of amphetamine	Increase (prevention of reuptake from the synaptic cleft)
DOPA (precursor of dopamine and noradrenaline)	Antidepressant effect in individual cases	Prevents sedation after reserpine	Increase (through greater supply of noradrenaline precursors)

- Reserpine, which can trigger depressions, releases not only catecholamines but also serotonin from the presynaptic stores.
- Serotonin and its metabolites are reduced in the cerebrospinal fluid of some depressive patients, which suggests reduced serotoninergic activity in the brain of these individuals.
- Serotonin precursors (L-tryptophan, 5-hydroxytryptophan) have an anti-depressant action in some cases, whereas a reduction in the blood tryptophan level in remitted depressed patients can provoke a clear relapse (Delgado *et al.*, 1990).

This list clearly shows that some pharmacological and clinical–pharmacological findings can be interpreted both in favour of the catecholamine hypothesis and in the sense of the serotonin hypothesis. In clinical as well as in biochemical terms, depression does not represent a single uniform disease since evidence has been found of catecholaminergic hypofunction in a proportion of depressive patients, while others have features of serotoninergic hypofunction. However, a reliable relationship between biochemical substrates and the various clinical courses or states has not yet been found (Schatzberg *et al.*, 1982). Consequently, the previous hope that subgroups of depression could be defined on the basis of biochemical features and be used to predict optimal drug treatment (Maas, 1975; Asberg *et al.*, 1976) has not yet been fulfilled.

Numerous new antidepressants have been synthesized, developed and, in some cases, marketed on the basis of the serotonin hypothesis over the last 15 years. These are the so-called selective serotonin reuptake inhibitors (SSRIs) such as fluoxetine, paroxetine, fluvoxamine and sertraline. There are only minor differences between their clinical profiles and they are similarly effective as conventional antidepressants, but have the great advantage of being less toxic than the latter and of not inducing anticholinergically mediated side effects. In the opinion of some authors, SSRIs come closer to the 'ideal antidepressant' than any previous products (Warrington, 1992), and from the scientific point of view represent an example of mechanistic, hypothesis-driven research and development in psychopharmacology.

5.4.3   Extensions of the monoamine hypotheses of depression

As with the dopamine theory of schizophrenia, the monoamine hypotheses of depression have been developed emphasizing one or more aspects of the actions of clinically effective drugs in pharmacological tests. However, whereas dopamine antagonism seems to be a common element of action of all neuroleptics, antidepressants differ much more greatly with regard to their pharmacological spectrum of activities, and a common 'core of action' has not so far been found. This can be interpreted in various ways: firstly, one could assume that the actual mechanism of action of antidepressants is still unknown since the pharmacological models used capture only epiphenomena of the actions relevant to the clinical effect. Another conclusion would be to critically interrogate the over-emphasis on individual transmitter systems as postulated bases for depressions.

Since the various transmitter systems in the brain are directly and indirectly linked together, purely catecholaminergically or purely serotoninergically based depressions are unlikely. Furthermore, the majority of antidepressants known today have multiple effects, especially after repeated administration, and thus affect a number of transmitter systems simultaneously. This fact is taken into account by more recent hypotheses of depression in that a balance between several transmitter systems is postulated as a prerequisite for mental health, whereas affective psychoses are believed to be a reflection of an imbalance (review by Fritze *et al.*, 1992). In an older catecholaminergic–cholinergic equilibrium model postulated by Janowsky *et al.* (1972), depression corresponds to cholinergic overactivity, whereas mania corresponds to catecholaminergic overactivity. Another, more complex model was proposed by Siever and Davis (1985) whereas authors like Murphy *et al.* (1986) seemed to cast general doubt on the possibility of a uniform hypothesis of the mechanism of antidepressant action. Brown and Gershon (1993) recalled the importance of the neurotransmitter dopamine for the development of depression in the elderly, with the major features of loss of drive and, in psychopathological terms, some similarity with Parkinson's disease.

However, neither the older nor the more recent monoamine hypotheses explain why the therapeutic effect of antidepressant drugs only sets in after several days or weeks, unlike their known pharmacological actions. Although some authors consider that the late onset of antidepressant action is a function of pharmacokinetics and so seek to achieve high blood levels of the drugs as quickly as possible by appropriate administration techniques (e.g. Pollock *et al.*, 1986), others search for effects of antidepressants which arise after relatively prolonged application of the substance, the timing of which fits in better with clinically observed actions.

Thus, experimental studies in animals have shown that the number and sensitivity of monoaminergic receptors change under chronic treatment with antidepressants: the number of beta-adrenergic receptors (a subgroup of the noradrenergic receptors) drops in the rat brain after the animals have been treated for a few weeks with tricyclic antidepressants, and there is also a drop in the sensitivity of other pre- and postsynaptic noradrenergic receptors following the repeated intake of such medication. Sulser *et al.* (1978) proposed a revised catecholamine hypothesis on the basis of these findings, according to which depression is not due to catecholaminergic subfunction but to hypersensitivity of the appropriate receptors in certain areas of the brain. According to this hypothesis, when there is an oversupply of noradrenaline – such as in a chronic stress situation – no downregulation occurs in the depressed patient, i.e., no decrease in receptor sensitivity and thus no easing of the stress situation from the 'inside'. Treatment with antidepressants and the resulting massive catecholamine oversupply at the synapses will in the end lead to downregulation, the decrease in receptor sensitivity with the possibility that the patient can cope better with the situation.

This concludes our brief summary of hypotheses relating to the mode of action of antidepressants. In much the same way as with neuroleptics, the question with antidepressants is which of the numerous pharmacological actions observed are responsible for the therapeutic effect of these drugs. As already noted, it has been particularly difficult to understand the latency in the therapeutic action of antidepressants. Unlike the situation with neuroleptics, where a principle of action newer and better than that of clozapine has not been discovered since the early 1970s, some therapeutic advance in the antidepressant field has been made with the introduction of SSRIs, although our understanding of the mechanism of action of antidepressants has not grown substantially (see Leonard, 1993).

5.5 HYPOTHESES REGARDING THE MECHANISM OF ACTION OF TRANQUILLIZERS

The mechanism of action of benzodiazepines (BZDs) as typical tranquillizers has been largely clarified in the last 15 years and is now less controversial than that of neuroleptics and antidepressants. Since the pharmacology of BZDs has been dealt with in several recent reviews (Enna and Möhler, 1987; Haefely, 1991), we will be brief here.

The calming, relaxing action of tranquillizers is attributed to the ability of BZD molecules to reinforce the actions of the neurotransmitter GABA. The site of BZD action is the GABAergic synapse, the sensitivity of which is increased by BZD molecules. A given presynaptically released amount of GABA induces a stronger or a longer postsynaptic inhibition in the presence of BZD molecules. As a result of BZD supply, the activity in the nerve cells behind GABAergic neurons is reduced. In addition, activation of GABAergic interneurons can also inhibit the activity of the upstream neuron (so-called feedback or intercurrent inhibition). The particular localization of GABA neurons in practically all segments of the CNS is thought to be the reason why BZDs primarily inhibit an excessive, 'unphysiological' stimulation and why the inhibition cannot exceed a given degree.

Like other psychopharmaceuticals, BZDs act on receptors located in the cell membrane. The name *BZD receptors* has become fashionable for the receptors which react with BZDs, although other substances can interact with these BZD receptors as well. BZD receptors are stimulated by suitable molecules and, as in the case of tranquillizers, intensify the actions of GABA. However, it is also possible for BZD receptors to be occupied by molecules which inhibit or prevent the action of BZD and structurally similar compounds. Such substances, called BZD antagonists, are used in anaesthesiology and emergency medicine, primarily to terminate anaesthesia and to treat BZD overdosage. Other molecules which can occupy BZD receptors and which have actions opposite to those of BZDs are called *inverse agonists*: they are reported to induce severe feelings of anxiety in healthy subjects (Dorow *et al.*, 1983).

The *beta-receptor blockers* used as anxiolytics in some indications act not through the CNS but via peripheral mechanisms; they will be briefly discussed in Chapter 8. The non-BZD-like tranquillizer *buspirone* and its derivatives gepirone and ipsapirone have both dopamine (D_2)-antagonistic and serotoninergic effects. The specific action of these compounds on 5-HT_{1A} receptors, i.e., a subgroup of serotoninergic receptors, is considered to be responsible for their anxiolytic effects. By stimulating presynaptic 5-HT receptors, there is thought to be a reduction of serotonin turnover in parts of the limbic system. However, this hypothetical mechanism of action is not without its critics (Palfreyman and Kehne, 1991) and does not explain why, in contrast to the anxiolytic effects of benzodiazepines, the clinical action of buspirone develops only after two or three weeks. It is also still unclear whether another group of serotoninergic substances, the so-called 5-HT_3 antagonists, have clinically useful anxiolytic actions in humans; in any event, these substances have shown marked anxiolytic effects in various animal models (Costall *et al.*, 1990).

5.6 COMMENTS

The past 40 years have seen a remarkable upswing in psychopharmacology, especially in its fundamental scientific disciplines of neurobiochemistry, neuroendocrinology and neurophysiology, which has led to a plethora of experimental results in almost all areas. Hypotheses concerning the mechanisms of action of neuroleptics, antidepressants, etc. have been formulated, refined and partially or entirely rejected, and much the same has happened with the pathophysiological hypotheses of schizophrenia, depression, etc. We do not yet have a coherent and generally acknowledged theory for any of these illnesses even though great advances have been made in areas of pathophysiology, diagnosis and pharmacotherapeutic possibilities.

Two major, interconnected reasons can be named for the comparatively slow theoretical progress in psychopharmacology: the multifactorial origin and structure of mental disorders on the one hand and the complexity and restricted accessibility of the most likely site of the pathological process, the human brain, on the other hand. Animal models of mental disorders only ever represent a fraction and possibly an irrelevant fraction of the processes which occur in mentally ill humans. Neurophysiological, neurobiochemical and other experiments are reductionist by design, and the possibilities for studying electrical, chemical and other processes inside the human brain directly and in relation to mental processes are still quite limited.

In an earlier edition of this book (1989, p. 130 f.) we critically discussed the conventional approaches of biological psychiatry, i.e., studies of neurotransmitters and their metabolites in blood, urine and cerebrospinal fluid, biochemical analyses of postmortem tissues, and the experimental administration of substances which selectively promote or inhibit parts of neuro-

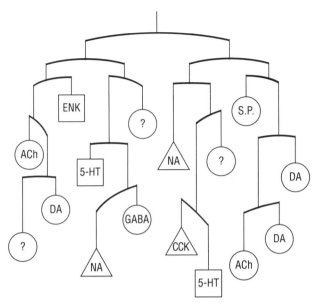

Figure 5.8.   Equilibrium model of neurotransmitters. This model, drawn by analogy to Calder's mobiles, should illustrate the complexity of the mutual influence of several neurotransmitter systems. This view is rather distant from the simple dopamine, catecholamine and serotonin hypotheses in their original versions (concept and realization: J. M. Vigouret)

transmission; a revision of this topic does not seem necessary here. In contrast, the introduction of procedures such as PET (positron emission tomography) and magnetic resonance spectroscopy (MRS) has brought a clear advance. Depending on the type of study, significant features can be studied in relation to the course of regional and total brain metabolism, the synthesis and concentrations of neurotransmitters, and the binding and release of agonists and antagonists at CNS binding sites and receptors in healthy and mentally ill subjects. PET and MRS have fundamental limitations with regard to their resolution capacity in time and space, but both procedures have already proved to be fruitful in several areas of study (dopamine hypothesis of schizophrenia, glucose turnover in the brain of dementia patients, etc.).

   Finally, a figure is presented to remind us visually of the complexity of neuronal circuitry and particularly the mutual dependency of the neurotransmitter systems: the mobile as presented to the art world by Calder in the 1950s (Fig. 5.8). If one part of the system is moved, the whole of it swings into movement and only after many attempts can the new equilibrium in which it will swing be predicted.

CHAPTER 6

Clinical research in psychopharmacology

Clinical research involves sick persons and aims ultimately at improving existing treatments and discovering new and better ones. Questions of diagnosis and classification of diseases as well as parts of basic medical research also come under the heading of clinical research insofar as they concern the study of causes and mechanisms of diseases and their symptoms in humans. In psychiatry, clinical research in the sense of therapy research includes pharmacotherapeutic and non-pharmacological therapeutic approaches. The following chapter deals exclusively with drug treatments.

As the following section shows, clinical research may imply that patients are treated with possibly ineffective or still inadequately tested drugs and procedures from which they may actually draw no direct benefit and which may even be superfluous to their individual curative process. Is clinical research therefore compatible with the duty of the doctor to put the well-being of patients in first place and especially not to expose them to any harm? Is it permissible to deny patients a proven (although not always optimally effective or tolerable) treatment in order to test a new and possibly better but also possible inferior treatment?

Clearly there is a conflict of purposes in clinical research, which has been and still is evaluated differently at different times and under different circumstances. Opinion today is that a patient should, whenever possible, be the master of his own fate and not be delivered defenceless to the doctor – an opinion which has been reflected in laws and guidelines.

6.1 PROTECTING THE PATIENT

Medical activity is covered, on the one hand, by national civil and criminal law and, on the other hand, by what are known as medical ethics. These are standards of behaviour which govern the doctor's dealings with his patients and by which every doctor should feel himself bound. The Hippocratic oath is part of the medical code of ethics which has been further extended over the past 30 years, particularly in view of clinical research. The 18th World

Doctors' Conference (1964) passed the Declaration of Helsinki, containing recommendations intended to guide physicians engaged in biomedical research on human subjects. This Declaration was revised in 1975 (Tokyo Revision of the Declaration of Helsinki) and covers many points which are also of importance in the present context (see box).

Consequences for clinical–psychopharmacological research arise above all out of the following requirements:

(1) Evaluation of the trial protocol by an independent board (§I.2).
(2) Duty of information *vis-à-vis* the patient (§I.9).
(3) Consent of the patient or his legal representative to participate in a trial.
(4) Ensurance of the best therapeutic method (§II.3).

In university clinics and other hospitals engaged in research, ethics committees (also called Institutional Review Boards = IRBs) have been formed over the last 20 years which monitor clinical research activities from scientific, legal, ethical and social viewpoints. All protocols relating to clinical trials have to be submitted to these committees, which are generally made up of one or several doctors, a lawyer, and a representative of the nursing staff, and often also include a social worker and/or priest. This composition forces clinical researchers to set out their intentions in such a way as to be clear enough for a lay person to understand and to assess whether the unpleasantness and risks involved for the patient are in reasonable relationship to the possible benefit of the planned trial.

The duty of information and the requirement to seek the consent of the patient or his legal representative can be difficult to carry out in practice. How can one adequately explain a drug study to a suspicious, paranoid schizophrenic with fears of poisoning, fears which extend to drugs also? How can a severely depressive patient, clinging in desperation to the doctor and nursing staff in the fear of being abandoned, be prevented from agreeing to a trial, the significance of which he cannot understand anyway? What use is the 'informed consent' obtained from a demented patient who cannot remember or only dimly recall the information given to him? As can be seen from paragraph II.5, for cases of this nature the Declaration of Helsinki allows a certain relaxation of the duty of information, although this must be substantiated in the trial protocol and be approved by the ethics committee. (In this context see Schafer, 1982, who takes a strict view in this matter, and Brewin, 1982, who adopts a more moderate approach somewhat closer to clinical reality.) On no account, however, does the informed consent by the patient or by his representative imply any reduction in the medical, moral or legal responsibility of the doctor conducting the trial.

Extracts from the Declaration of Helsinki (Tokyo Revision 1975)

I. *Basic principles* (summary)

Biomedical research involving human subjects must conform to generally accepted scientific principles (I.1); a detailed plan of the experiment should be set out in a written experimental protocol which is to be approved by an independent committee (I.2).

A clinically experienced doctor should always supervise medical experiments in human subjects (I.3); the importance of the objective must be in proportion to the inherent risk to the subject (I.4). Concern for the interests of the subject must always prevail over the interests of science and society (I.5).

The privacy of the research subject must be respected and the impact of the study on the physical and mental integrity and on the personality of the subject are to be minimized (I.6).

Each potential subject must be adequately informed of the aims, methods, anticipated benefits and potential hazards of the study and the discomfort it may entail. The right to abstain from participation or to withdraw at any time must be ensured. The doctor should then obtain the subject's freely-given informed consent, preferably in writing (I.9). Should the subject be in a dependent relationship to the doctor, the informed consent should be obtained by a doctor who is not engaged in the investigation (I.10).

Where physical or mental incapacity makes it impossible to obtain informed consent, or in the case of minors, permission is to be obtained from the responsible relative in accordance with national legislation (I.11).

II. *Medical research combined with professional care* (quotation)

1. In the treatment of the sick person, the doctor must be free to use a new diagnostic and therapeutic measure, if in his or her judgement it offers hope of saving life, reestablishing health or alleviating suffering.

2. The potential benefits, hazards and discomfort of a new method should be weighed against the advantages of the best current diagnostic and therapeutic methods.

3. In any medical study, every patient – including those of a control group, if any – should be assured of the best proven diagnostic and therapeutic method.

4. The refusal of the patient to participate in a study must never interfere with the doctor–patient relationship.

5. If the doctor considers it essential not to obtain informed consent, the specific reasons for this proposal should be stated in the experimental protocol for transmission to the independent committee.

6. The doctor can combine medical research with professional care, the objective being the acquisition of new medical knowledge, only to the extent that medical research is justified by its potential diagnostic or therapeutic value for the patient.

Much is now expected of the development work preceding a clinical trial, as a consequence of the requirement that each patient should obtain the best treatment currently available. If animal experiments and trials in healthy volunteers provide results which convince the responsible doctor of the potential advantages of an experimental drug, he is then justified in using the new, clinically still largely unknown substance – although the decision as to what can be regarded as a convincing indication of possible superiority is often a matter of opinion. A practical consequence of Paragraph II.3 of the Declaration of Helsinki, therefore, is the need to test new preparations, both in animal experiments and possibly in healthy volunteers, in such a way that any advantages are clearly apparent at every stage.

In common with any other medical code of ethics the Declaration of Helsinki cannot provide absolute protection for the individual patient. What it does prevent are clinical trials which are, in the opinion of the public (or its representatives), unnecessary, unconsidered, and unacceptable for the patient in question. Above all, however, it compels clinical researchers to examine the purpose and necessity of each step of any planned investigation.

From the many areas of clinical–psychopharmaceutical research, we have selected three which deal with the improvement of existing treatments or the development of new treatments. These are predictor research (Section 6.2), studies of pharmacokinetic–pharmacodynamic relationships (Section 6.3) and the testing of new drugs (Section 6.4). Some special questions, mainly methodological, will be discussed in Section 6.5.

6.2 PREDICTOR RESEARCH IN PSYCHOPHARMACOLOGY

As discussed in Chapter 1, none of the psychopharmaceuticals known today has an exclusively beneficial action. Neuroleptics often induce severe side effects, antidepressants are therapeutically ineffective in about one-third of patients, and the other classes of psychopharmaceuticals have various types of drawbacks also. The ability to estimate, preferably before the start of treatment, how an individual patient will respond to the planned drug would therefore be desirable. In other words, does the patient present features, or predictors, which normally allow therapeutic success to be expected, or are particular risks such as side effects to be expected in his/her particular case?

The question of potential predictors of therapeutic effects does not arise with the same urgency for neuroleptics, antidepressants, tranquillizers, etc. since the disorders treated with these drugs differ in severity and since the drugs themselves differ greatly in their efficacies and side effects. If the number of publications reflects the importance of the problem being studied, then the prediction of success of therapy constitutes a central problem mainly in the case of antidepressants (which is not surprising in view of the failure rate of about one-third); there are far fewer studies of this kind published regarding the other classes of psychopharmaceuticals.

With regard to the possible predictors of therapeutic drug effects, distinction must be made between features recorded in the usual clinical and psychiatric examinations, such as age, sex, diagnosis and anamnestic data, and test results which require special, e.g. biochemical or electrophysiological, examinations. Distinction also has to be made between features which are normally determined before the start of drug therapy (status, case history, special examinations) and observation made only after the onset of therapy and which may predict the further course of treatment. In the first case one usually speaks of primary predictors, and in the second case of secondary predictors (see Fig. 6.1).

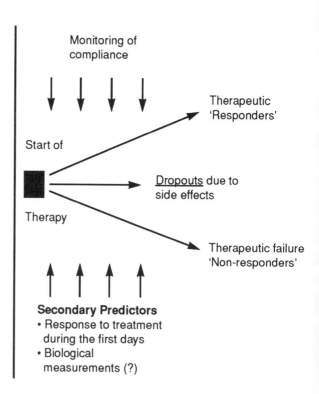

Figure 6.1. Primary and secondary predictors of therapeutic success

6.2.1   Demographic, anamnestic and clinical features

Studies in depressed patients

As long ago as 1976, Bielski and Friedel discussed the following possible predictors of the antidepressant actions of imipramine and amitriptyline on the basis of 40 placebo-controlled trials which they considered to be methodologically acceptable:

- demographic features such as age, sex, education, socioeconomic class;
- personality features such as neuroticism, hypochondria, hysterical traits;
- case history features such as prior mental illnesses and illnesses in the family;
- features of the course of the current illness;
- special symptoms and syndromes;
- biochemical predictors.

A few features (weight loss, insomnia, psychomotor inhibition, higher socioeconomic class) proved to be reproducible predictors of a positive effect of medication, but Bielski and Friedel stressed that even these features were based only on a few studies and that caution is required in using them as predictive criteria in practice. They identified the following features as *negative predictors* of antidepressant actions significantly superior to those of placebo:

- neurotic, hypochondriac or hysterical personality traits;
- several prior depressive episodes;
- depressive delusions.

As the authors noted, the predictors of therapeutic success of imipramine and amitriptyline correspond overall to the features of endogenous depression, whereas patients who did not respond to antidepressants better than to placebo were mainly to be classified as neurotic depressives. This is no great surprise since Kuhn (1957) had already emphasized in his first report on the antidepressant action of imipramine that patients with endogenous depressions, especially those with vital-depressive features, showed the best therapeutic response. This observation was subsequently confirmed by several authors, although, as Raskin (1968) had commented in an early review article, there were also reports indicating otherwise. In his view, the contradictions between different studies were due to the unclear and controversial differentiation between endogenous, reactive and neurotic depressions. Nevertheless, there is some evidence according to Raskin that tricyclic antidepressants such as imipramine and amitriptyline are more suitable for severe [sic!] depressions whereas monoamine oxidase (MAO) inhibitors are more suitable for neurotic depressions with hysterical overtones and accentuated anxiety.

In a more recent analysis (Joyce and Paykel, 1989), the following features and their relationship with the therapeutic action of antidepressants were identified:

- *Personality:* Patients with neurotic, hypochondriac and histrionic (theatrical) traits respond less well to tricyclic compounds.
- *Age:* Older depressives respond rather poorly to antidepressants (albeit 'age' might be statistically confounded with 'chronicity').
- *Chronicity:* The risk of becoming chronic increases (and the chance of a therapeutic success decreases) with every new episode of depression.
- *Life events and events during the episode of depression:* The results of various studies on this question are contradictory.
- *Form of depression:* Patients with depressive delusions respond less well to antidepressants.

In all, Joyce and Paykel consider that patients 'with a good premorbid personality, an insidious onset of depression, psychomotor retardation and an intermediate level of severity and endogeneity but without psychotic features' (1989, p. 95) may respond best to tricyclic antidepressants, although these drugs can also be prescribed with the expectation of therapeutic benefits in patients not matching this profile.

The results of a large multicentre study sponsored by the NIMH (US National Institute of Mental Health) in 239 ambulatory patients with 'major depressive disorder' (Sotsky *et al.*, 1991) are in line with the findings reported by Joyce and Paykel: imipramine, the only antidepressant used in this trial, was particularly effective in patients with moderately severe endogenous depression who were predominantly suffering from disruption of work but showed only low cognitive dysfunction. In a recent review, Woggon (1993) confirmed the prognostic factors proposed by Joyce and Paykel, but specified that the two aspects of 'severity' and 'endogenicity' of depressions are not independent of each other: severe depressions tend to be classed as endogenous and experience shows that they respond less well to placebo, so that in trials comparing antidepressants and placebo, clearer differences in favour of the active medication are obtained than in trials with patients having milder depression and tending to be classed as neurotic.

Studies in schizophrenics

With regard to the drug treatment of schizophrenias, Schied (1983, p. 264) came to the conclusion 'that there are no empirically confirmed and testable criteria allowing reliable predictions of therapeutic success before the start of treatment with neuroleptics'. This statement partially contradicts the experience of other authors: it is well established that women generally respond to neuroleptics better than men, and also require smaller doses on average (Woggon, 1992). In addition, a particularly rapid and beneficial action of neuroleptics can be expected when the current psychiatric symptoms have been present for only a short time (McEvoy et al., 1991b; Lieberman et al., 1993).

A study by Honigfeld and Patin (1989) concerning the identification of potential predictors of a beneficial response to clozapine (Clozaril®) is of practical interest. As noted in Chapter 1, clozapine is therapeutically superior to other neuroleptics but induces potentially fatal changes of white blood cell counts more frequently than other products. If predictors could be found for therapeutic success or failure with clozapine, the number of patients unnecessarily exposed to the risk of side effects could be reduced further. In a sample of 126 patients treated with clozapine, the authors examined a total of 46 features for their prognostic relevance, including six diagnostic, eight relating to case history and many symptomatic criteria, but found only a single predictor that could be considered responsible for a significant part of the therapeutic success. It was consistently clear that, as with other neuroleptics, patients with paranoid symptoms showed the best improvements with clozapine.

6.2.2   Biological predictors

Studies in depressed patients

The biological test and possible predictor most discussed for years in the field of depression research is the *dexamethasone suppression test (DST)*, an endocrinological stimulation test that is easy to perform. After the administration of a small dose of dexamethasone (a synthetic glucocorticoid) in the evening there is a decrease in the concentration of the hormone cortisol in the blood of healthy subjects, reaching very low values and normally remaining suppressed for at least 24 hours. This inhibitory action of dexamethasone on cortisol is frequently absent in patients with depressions, so that Carroll et al. (1981) developed the concept that the DST could be used as a biological test in the diagnosis of depression. Many other authors have subsequently confirmed the frequent occurrence of abnormal DST findings in depressed patients.

The utility of a diagnostic test is, among other things, determined by its sensitivity and its specificity. By sensitivity is meant the percentage of patients with a diagnosed disease who have abnormal values in the test in question. In a test which is 100% sensitive, all patients show abnormal values. Specificity expresses how many of the subjects with abnormal test results actually suffer from the disease in question; a test with 100% specificity would therefore respond only to individuals with the disease in question. The sensitivity of the DST with regard to depressions (major depressive disorders) is estimated to be 30–70%, and 50–60% in cases of severe illnesses requiring hospitalization; the figures for specificity of the test lie between 70% and 90% depending on the study (Braddock, 1986; APA Task Force, 1987). The DST thus often supplies false negative results, and false positive results occur in the presence of various physical illnesses, weight loss, alcohol consumption and the consumption of various drugs, as well as in the elderly and in dementia.

Despite its lack of diagnostic sensitivity and specificity, studies have been undertaken to determine if the DST can be of use as a predictor of success of antidepressant treatment in general or as a predictor of the efficacy of specific antidepressants. These are two questions that have led to entirely different answers in various clinical studies. Braddock (1986) discussed a number of these studies and warned against drawing far-reaching conclusions about treatment prediction on the basis of what are usually small numbers of patients. In his opinion, neither the success of antidepressant treatment in general nor the suitability of specific drugs for subgroups of depressives can be predicted on the basis of DST findings. Regardless of this overall negative evaluation, it is of interest to consider in more detail one of the methodologically better studies on the prediction of therapeutic results by means of the DST.

Unlike other authors, Beckmann *et al.* (1984) did not design their investigation as a retrospective study but as a prospective one; i.e., they treated 43 patients under double-blind conditions according to the following scheme:

– Of 23 patients with initially abnormal DST findings (DST+), 13 received the antidepressant nomifensine (which has a primarily noradrenergic action) and 10 received amitriptyline (with noradrenergic and anticholinergic actions).
– Of 20 patients with normal DST findings (DST–), 10 received nomifensine and 10 amitriptyline.

Both products have similar degrees of serotoninergic actions. Based on theoretical considerations, the authors predicted that DST+ patients would respond positively to amitriptyline and would not show favourable responses to nomifensine, whereas DST– patients would tend to have a better therapeutic response to nomifensine. However, the results summarized in Fig. 6.2 reveal the following:

(1) At the end of four weeks of treatment, all four groups showed a marked decrease in their symptoms as expressed by the Hamilton Depression Rating Scale (the improvements were much less marked in the self-evaluations by the patients).
(2) In all, the therapeutic results with amitriptyline were better than those with nomifensine, especially early in the treatment: the difference was statistically significant on treatment days 5 and 10, and was still detectable as a trend at the end of the study.
(3) As predicted, the lowest Hamilton scale scores, i.e., the best therapeutic results on average, were obtained in DST+ patients with amitriptyline and by DST– patients with nomifensine, but the differences between the four groups were not very great when the baseline values are taken into account.

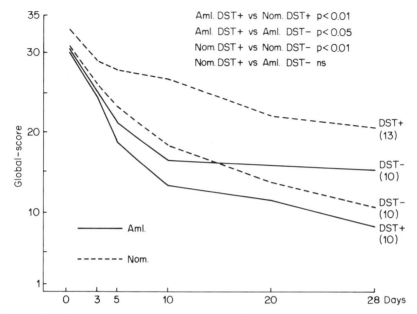

Figure 6.2. Dexamethasone suppression test (DST) and responses to various antidepressants. The figure shows the decrease in the total Hamilton Depression Rating Scale scores (as a measure for the severity of depression) in four groups:

DST+, dashed line: patients with abnormal DST findings, treated with nomifensine; $n = 13$;
DST–, continuous line: patients with normal DST findings treated with amitriptyline; $n = 10$;
DST–, dashed line: patients with normal DST findings, treated with nomifensine; $n = 10$;
DST+, continuous line: patients with abnormal DST findings, treated with amitryptiline; $n = 10$.
Above right: level of significance of some pair comparisons
(From Beckmann *et al.*, 1984, with permission)

In the discussion of their results, the authors pointed out that abnormal DST findings occur more often in severe endogenous depression; these patients then respond better to an anticholinergic antidepressant such as amitriptyline. According to Beckmann *et al.*, patients with normal DST findings, in contrast, suffer more from mild depressions and respond well to a primarily noradrenergic product such as nomifensine, and in these cases more anticholinergic side effects occur with amitriptyline and this could have an adverse effect on the therapeutic outcome.

As mentioned, the study by Beckmann *et al.* is one of the few prospective trials of the prognostic significance of the DST for the pharmacotherapy of depressions. However, it must be said that many authors have cast doubt on the utility of the DST as a predictor of antidepressant therapy (Emrich *et al.*, 1987; Steardo *et al.*, 1987) and that even the study of Beckmann *et al.* only partially confirmed the original hypothesis. A study by Rihmer *et al.* (1985)

with the two antidepressants maprotiline (predominantly noradrenergic) and amitriptyline (noradrenergic and anticholinergic) even provided the opposite result, namely a better response of DST+ patients to maprotiline. Thus, after a critical evaluation of 17 clinical drug studies, a Task Force of the American Psychiatric Association (APA, 1987) came to the conclusion that the DST can make no significant contribution to the short-term prognosis of antidepressant therapy (APA Task Force, p. 1257). Since the success rate with antidepressant drug therapies in both DST+ and DST– patients is approximately 70%, the Task Force sees no reason to withhold antidepressant treatment from patients with normal DST findings. Accordingly, the DST can be considered neither as a reliable predictor of the success of antidepressant treatments in general nor as an aid in selecting specific antidepressants (with regard to the second point, see also Modai et al., 1986; Emrich et al., 1987).

Another biological test, the TRH–TSH reaction, has been described by Langer et al. (1986) as a possible predictor of drug therapy in depressions as well as in schizophrenia and schizoaffective psychosis. However, not enough data are available with this procedure to allow an estimation of its sensitivity and specificity (assumed to be low). We cannot discuss here some other possible biological predictors (metabolites of noradrenaline and serotonin in the cerebrospinal fluid (CSF) and blood, [^{3}H]imipramine binding to platelets) which have attracted great attention over many years. They are presented in review papers by Cowdry and Goodwin (1981, with good critical comments on predictor research in general) and by Bunney et al. (1986, including a differentiation between state, trait and vulnerability markers).

Like other authors before her, Woggon (1992) came to the conclusion that there are at present no reliable and practically useful biological predictors which allow the therapeutic result of antidepressant treatment to be forecast.

Studies in schizophrenic patients

According to a study by Sternberg et al. (1982), patients with low dopamine beta-hydroxylase levels in the CSF respond better to neuroleptics than schizophrenics with high CSF levels of this enzyme, which is required for the conversion of dopamine to noradrenaline. To our knowledge, however, this relationship, which is also of theoretical interest, has never been confirmed and is not mentioned in more recent reviews. As Lieberman et al. (1993) and several other groups before them have established, chronic schizophrenic patients with enlarged cerebral ventricles and other structural deviations in the brain often have an unsatisfactory therapeutic response to neuroleptics. However, the relationship is not close enough to justify withholding drug therapy from patients with these features.

In contrast, a number of studies show the relevance of *secondary predictors* in evaluating the prospects of neuroleptic treatment. Thus, the success or failure of a neuroleptic drug can be estimated after a few days of treatment on the basis of the changes observed at that time. According to Woggon (1992), two-thirds to three-quarters of the overall changes in symptoms achieved in the end can be detected by the 10th day of treatment. Neuroleptic therapy which is insufficiently active or which is poorly tolerated could thus be rapidly corrected or withdrawn on the basis of secondary predictors.

6.2.3   Neurophysiological predictors

Apart from some biological indicators, so-called REM latency has attracted interest as a neurophysiological marker in the diagnosis of depressions. REM latency designates the time interval between the onset of sleep and the first appearance of a REM period in polygraphic sleep recordings (Chapter 4). In healthy subjects the REM latency is generally 40–80 minutes, depending on age, but in depressive patients it is often shorter and occasionally lasts for only a few minutes (Kupfer *et al.*, 1978). However, short REM latencies can also occur in non-depressed subjects, particularly in the elderly, and long REM latencies can occur in depressives, so that the sensitivity and specificity of this feature in the diagnosis of depressions is classed as low (Berger *et al.*, 1982; Rush *et al.*, 1983).

In a preliminary study, Gillin *et al.* (1978) observed that depressed patients responding favourably to an antidepressant drug showed a greater reduction in REM sleep as a direct response to the drug than those who later proved to be therapeutic failures. Another study in a larger number of patients showed that depressive patients who reacted to an antidepressant with a relatively marked prolongation of their previously shortened REM latencies showed better therapeutic effects than patients with a weak reaction of REM sleep to the product (Kupfer *et al.*, 1981). As in the case of the DST, it was therefore hoped that the therapeutic success of antidepressants could be predicted on the basis of this objective marker. Further studies, including one by Rush *et al.* (1983), rapidly dashed this hope. Prolongation of REM latency after certain antidepressant drugs is a pharmacological effect that also arises after single doses (p. 109) and has no direct connection with the therapeutic efficacy of these products (see Spiegel, 1984b).

6.2.4   Thoughts on predictor research

The paragraphs above provide a mainly negative result: the lack of practically usable and reliable primary predictors of therapeutic responses in psychiatric drug therapy despite hundreds of clinical and experimental studies, some of them very extensive. What factors are responsible for this globally disappointing result?

In the case of antidepressant therapy, the lack of uniform diagnosis is repeatedly noted as a source of error in clinical trials, together with the fact that patients enter studies at individually different phases of their illness and after various prior treatments so that they also have different therapeutic prospects. The difficulty in defining unequivocal criteria of treatment success is also stressed: is it complete freedom from symptoms, is it a 50% reduction in symptoms compared to baseline, or some other feature that is more difficult to quantify, such as social reintegration or improved 'quality of life'? The importance of all these sources of error is indisputable, but it seems that too little attention has been paid to another factor, namely the tendency to premature publication of the results of retrospective analyses, which may have been derived from small numbers of patients, without confirming them in prospective studies. Considerations in this regard include the following:

About 60–80% of treated patients respond to antidepressants within four weeks with a clinically relevant improvement. Depending on the study, 20–40% of patients also show an improvement with placebo (see Chapter 1). Therefore, in each clinical trial there will not only be true therapeutic failures but also many patients with spontaneous improvements, regardless of the therapeutic measures applied. From this it can be deduced that statements regarding predictors of therapeutic effects must be statistically supported, i.e., be based on studies with very large populations and preferably placebo-controlled studies, in order to avoid erroneous conclusions based on spontaneous improvement only. However, studies of this size can hardly be performed in single centres in a reasonable time; if the study is then distributed among several trial sites, differences in patient selection, classification and treatment cannot be avoided even with the best coordination, which makes further enlargement of the sample population necessary (see p. 176 f.).

Another problem is the choice of criteria of therapeutic success. 'Rating scales' (see Section 6.5.6) are normally used to evaluate the results of treatment, but they provide multidimensional measurements which often do not fully agree with the global evaluation of therapeutic success. If predictors of successful treatment are in question, it is advantageous to use only one criterion of success, e.g. the global evaluation 'unimproved–slightly improved–clearly improved–fully remitted' and to relate it to the possible predictor variables. If several criteria of success are used in parallel, the relationships with predictor variables will usually vary and the interpretation of the study becomes uncertain.

The number of potential predictor variables represents the next difficulty: if a study is started without a specific hypothesis, then basically all features of the patients (social, psychological, biological) can be considered as possible predictors so that dozens or hundreds of statistical comparisons have to be made between successfully and unsuccessfully treated cases. According to the rules of probability, some of these comparisons will lead to significant differences by chance alone, so that features which may be completely irrelevant are identified as 'predictor variables'. This mistake, which is known as type I error in statistics, can be avoided if the search for predictors is either hypothesis-guided or if the potential predictors obtained retrospectively from a large number of statistical comparisons as described above are checked for their validity in a second, independent sample (Goldberg, 1987). This second step, also called cross-validation, is hardly ever taken and in this sense many of the numerous contradictory reports on predictor variables can be considered as unsuccessful attempts to validate supposed predictors.

Finally reference should be made to another, probably underestimated problem in predictor research and in clinical research in general, i.e., that of treatment compliance, the obeying of therapeutic instructions (see Section 6.3). It goes without saying that the search for predictors of the success of medical treatment must fail if some of the examined patients do not take the prescribed drugs regularly or not at all!

6.3 STUDIES OF PHARMACOKINETIC–PHARMACODYNAMIC RELATIONSHIPS
Pierre Baumann and René Spiegel

6.3.1 The questions examined

This section deals with the question of whether there is a quantitatively detectable and interpretable correlation between the dose of an administered drug or the concentration of the drug or its metabolites measured in the blood or plasma ('blood or plasma level') and the therapeutic or side effects observed. Studies relating to questions of this type are called PK–PD (pharmacokinetic–pharmacodynamic) studies.

PK–PD studies are of interest for both practical and theoretical reasons. The treating doctor would be best served if there were a linear correlation between the administered dose of a drug and its therapeutic or side effects; in this case he need not worry about plasma levels, metabolites and PK–PD relationships but could prescribe uniform doses of the drug based, for example, on the body weight of his patients. However, this is not the rule in practice: the optimal dose of the same drug varies from patient to patient even if body weight is taken into account, and the plasma concentrations after one and the same dose may vary by a factor of 10 to 30 or more between different patients. In view of these great differences, the question arises as to whether the clinical effects of a drug are related more to plasma levels rather than to the administered doses. If this were the case, then both underdosage and overdosage of a drug could be detected from the plasma levels and a treatment could be withdrawn if it is clinically ineffective or leads to unacceptable side effects despite the maintenance of what is considered to be the optimal drug plasma level. PK–PD studies of this type are also known as *'therapeutic plasma level monitoring'* and can be useful in the following situations (Baumann, 1992a):

(1) In the case of drugs with a narrow therapeutic safety margin. This is typical for certain tricyclic antidepressants (Preskorn *et al.*, 1993) and some neuroleptics (Balant-Gorgia *et al.*, 1993), and is a situation where there is only a relatively narrow dosage range available due to the risk of toxic side effects.

(2) In the case of patients not responding to a dose known to be normally effective. In this situation the determination of plasma levels can reveal evidence that the patient metabolizes the drug particularly rapidly and thus presents lower plasma levels so that a higher dose is required.

(3) In the case of impaired liver or kidney function. In this situation the usual dosages could lead to intoxication since drugs are broken down and excreted more slowly than normal. By determining plasma levels, the dose can be adjusted to a level that is still tolerated well.

(4) In the case of the co-administration of several drugs which mutually affect (usually inhibit) each other's degradation and excretion. Here also, the measurement of plasma levels offers a possible means of avoiding overdosage or underdosage and thus of achieving an optimal therapeutic effect.

(5) By far the most frequent use of therapeutic plasma level monitoring concerns *compliance checking*, especially with neuroleptics and antidepressants. If it is true that, depending on the indication, 30–60% of all patients do not comply with their physician's instructions (Garfield, 1982), then plasma level monitoring would be very useful both for practical and for research purposes.

In terms of theoretical and applied research there is great interest in the PK–PD correlations of psychopharmaceuticals since drugs may differ greatly in their spectrum of action depending on whether they are tested *in vitro* ('in the test-tube', e.g. in receptor preparations or in single cells) or in the living organism (*in vivo*), where they must first reach their site of action and are repeatedly exposed to metabolic enzymes. The metabolites formed in this way may have a spectrum of action very different from the parent substance: for example, the antidepressant chlorimipramine is a selective serotonin reuptake inhibitor, but its metabolite desmethyl-chlorimipramine is a selective noradrenaline reuptake inhibitor (Baumann, 1992b). Consequently, a mixed serotoninergic–noradrenergic action of chlorimipramine is to be expected *in vivo*, and thus also when used clinically. Extreme cases of this type are the *prodrugs*, which have no pharmacological effects in themselves but give rise to degradation products which are the true drugs. An example of a prodrug is clorazepate, which is metabolized in the intestine to the active anxiolytic substance desmethyl-diazepam.

6.3.2 Basic pharmacokinetic terms and models

The most important areas of pharmacokinetic study are absorption (uptake of a drug from the digestive tract), distribution (compartmentalization in the body), metabolism (conversion or breakdown, especially in the liver) and elimination (excretion). They are summarized by the abbreviation *ADME*.

The time elapsed from ingestion of a drug to the achievement of its peak concentration (C_{max}) in the blood or plasma is called t_{max}. The elimination half-life ($t^{1/2}$) is the interval between t_{max} and the time at which the remaining concentration amounts to only 50% of the previously achieved C_{max}. In the case of drugs which produce their desired effect after just a single dose, such as hypnotics, the pharmacokinetic properties which are relevant differ from those of drugs which have to be taken repeatedly over a longer time, such as neuroleptics and antidepressants. Thus, assuming that the pharmacokinetic features coincide in time with the pharmacodynamic properties, a hypnotic should have a short t_{max} and a short $t_{1/2}$, i.e., a fast onset of action and a fast decline. In the case of neuroleptics and antidepressants, t_{max} is less important and $t_{1/2}$ should be 12 or more hours so that not more than one or two doses are required each day. Typical $t_{1/2}$ values for antidepressants are 12–50 hours; it takes about 4–5 half-lives to reach a stable concentration or 'steady state' (C_{ss}) after repeated administration (Fig. 6.3). Therapeutic plasma level monitoring, e.g. for compliance control, is sensible only under steady-state conditions.

As the central pharmacokinetic parameter for repeatedly administered drugs and as shown in the following formula, C_{ss} is dependent on several factors:

$$C_{ss} = \frac{f*D}{CL*\tau} = \frac{AUC_{ss\tau}}{\tau}$$

where D stands for the single dose administered, f for bioavailability, CL for clearance (a measure of elimination) and Υ for the time interval between two administrations. According to this formula, the steady-state concentration increases with increasing dose and with increasing bioavailability of a substance, and decreases with increasing clearance and increasing interval between administrations.

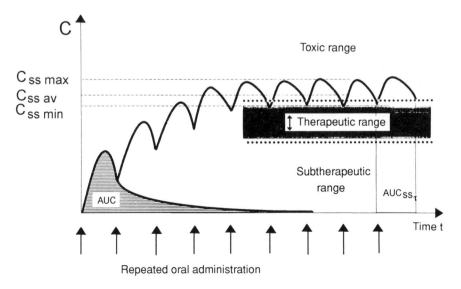

Figure 6.3.   Plasma concentration curve of a drug after single and repeated administration

Fig. 6.3 also shows the so-called *therapeutic range* of a compound, i.e., the steady-state concentrations at which experience shows the probability of a response to therapy is greatest but the risk of side effects is still low or at least tolerable. If the C_{ss} falls within the subtherapeutic range, there is a great likelihood that the desired therapeutic effect cannot be achieved with the selected dose. In the case illustrated here, the selected dose is certainly favourable for therapeutic success but the C_{ss} is relatively high, so that there is some risk of side effects.

Correlations with liver enzyme activities

Not all the factors which determine the fate of a drug in the body in the ADME sense can be considered in detail here, as there have been considerable advances in recent years in explaining both the metabolism of psychopharmaceuticals and the role of the enzymes responsible for this metabolism.

Certain enzymes of the cytochrome P-450 family perform the oxidative degradation of drugs, whereby different enzymes designated as CYPD6, CYP1A2 and CYP3A4 differ in their substrate activities. These activities, i.e. their abilities to metabolize exogenous substances ('xenobiotics'), vary from person to person and also vary at different times in the same person. The differences are due to genetic factors as well as environmental influences, for example the concomitant ingestion of other substances. Thus, it is known that by inducing certain enzymes barbiturates can lead to the faster breakdown of neuroleptics and antidepressants. In contrast, antidepressants such as fluoxetine and fluvoxamine, acting by partially different mechanisms, inhibit the breakdown of other concomitantly administered antidepressants and neuroleptics. Such interactions are of clinical relevance since they alter the steady-state concentrations of the administered drugs and thereby attenuate or enhance their therapeutic effects, and can lead to intoxications in extreme cases. The purpose of plasma level assays here is to adjust the dose to suit the new situation.

6.3.3   Methodological aspects

In PK–PD studies, correlations are considered between parameters that are determined in very different ways and which, from the statistical viewpoint, do not exhibit the same data level, i.e., drug concentrations on the one hand and the various types of clinical action of these drugs on the other hand (Steimer *et al.*, 1993).

Analytical procedures

Drugs are mostly assayed in the plasma or serum, and the results are usually given as 'total concentrations'. For methodological reasons, but also due to lack of studies providing clear evidence of a correlation between the 'free' concentration of a drug and its clinical effects, the results presented and used in PK–PD studies are not free concentrations (corresponding to the fraction not bound to plasma proteins) but are, not quite correctly, total concentrations. The physiological significance of plasma protein binding depends in turn on several factors such as the volume of distribution of a drug: accordingly, this binding can promote or inhibit the transport and distribution of the drug (Hervé *et al.*, 1994).

The assay methods for antidepressants and neuroleptics must have a sensitivity limit in the lower nanogram (ng) range. In addition, these methods must give precise, accurate and reproducible results.

The procedures must be specific enough to distinguish between different metabolites of the studied compounds and between other drugs administered concomitantly. Drugs and their metabolites are therefore generally extracted and, if necessary, converted to more easily analysable derivatives before or after chromatographic separation, then are finally measured with sensitive detectors (Fig. 6.4). Gas chromatography (GC) and high-performance liquid chromatography (HPLC) are the methods of choice. In order to achieve high specificity, the apparatus can be coupled to a mass spectrometer (GC–MS, LC–MS). Capillary electrophoresis offers great promise for the future: in this case the solution with the drugs to be separated is applied to a glass capillary exposed to an electrical field. The substances are separated in the same way as in normal electrophoresis and their concentrations are finally measured with a detector. Immunological procedures such as radioimmunoassay (RIA) or the enzyme-multiplied immunotechnique (EMIT) are suitable for certain applications, although they are generally not specific enough for studies in which metabolites have to be determined as well as the original substances. However, since they are easier to automate, their significance in routine clinical applications is increasing. Lithium (see below) is today measured with flame

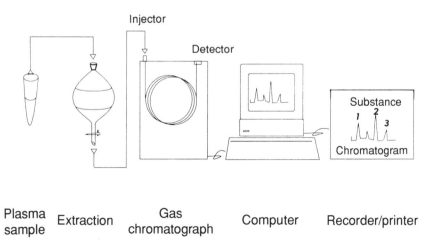

Figure 6.4. Diagram of a chromatographic assay method for psychopharmaceuticals

photometers or a system using ion-selective electrodes without prior extraction.

The requirements regarding quality control have increased in recent years in connection with the assay of drugs in body fluids. American and European boards have established regulations which have become known under the term 'Good Laboratory Practice' (GLP). GLP is designed to ensure that all laboratory analyses are performed as carefully as possible by correctly trained personnel in a suitably equipped laboratory, following detailed descriptions of the procedures and applying quality control tests. In laboratories, GLP is equivalent to Good Clinical Practice (GCP) in hospitals.

Clinical methods

With regard to clinical parameters, the possible sources of error in PK–PD studies are even more numerous than in the case of chemical assay methods. In order to create comparable conditions within individual studies and between several studies, the following criteria have to be checked or taken into consideration:

– patient characteristics such as age, sex, body weight and metabolic type (see Section 6.3.5);
– features of the disease such as precise diagnosis, duration and severity of illness, number and severity of previous episodes of illness, profile of symptoms;
– medication and additional drug treatment: doses, administration intervals, previous treatments now discontinued.

Even from this list it is clear that correlative studies between drug levels and clinical effects can only lead to unequivocal results when carried out with very homogeneous patient samples or, if they should be representative, in large but precisely described groups. Other problems on the clinical side that were also discussed in connection with predictor research include the number and choice of criteria of therapeutic success and especially the fact that placebo responders and patients with spontaneous remissions can blur the clinical results to an unknown degree.

Technical questions to be resolved with the aid of a detailed experimental protocol concern the timing of blood sampling and the timing of clinical evaluations.

6.3.4 Studies with antidepressants

Most PK–PD studies published in the last 25 years have been concerned with antidepressants, after Asberg *et al.* (1971) had reported on a curvilinear relationship between nortriptyline plasma levels and its therapeutic efficacy. Nortriptyline showed best effects at concentrations from 50 to 150 ng/ml, and its therapeutic action was less above and below this range. This study gave rise to the hope that a 'therapeutic window' could be defined for other products also.

Dozens of studies were subsequently carried out with amitriptyline, imipramine, desimipramine, maprotiline, doxepine and other antidepressants, but led to strikingly contradictory results (de Oliveira *et al.*, 1989a, 1989b; Preskorn *et al.*, 1993).

Preskorn (1989) incorporated the empirically discovered relationship between plasma levels of tricyclic antidepressants and their side effects into a scheme which defines the probability ranges for the appearance of a therapeutic effect or of side effects in relation to the measured plasma levels. On the basis of numerous case studies, it emerges that there are drug concentration ranges characteristic for certain side effects which are due to either noradrenergic or anticholinergic mechanisms. The picture shown in Fig. 6.5 is, for example, observed in patients treated with amitriptyline: the plasma levels correspond to the sum of concentrations of amitriptyline and its active metabolite nortriptyline and, when applied to the therapeutic situation, allow the use of this antidepressant to be evaluated in the sense of a benefit/risk assessment. However, clinical experience shows that certain patients respond to therapy only with plasma levels of about 750 ng/ml amitriptyline + nortriptyline, i.e., at a concentration which can trigger marked central side effects

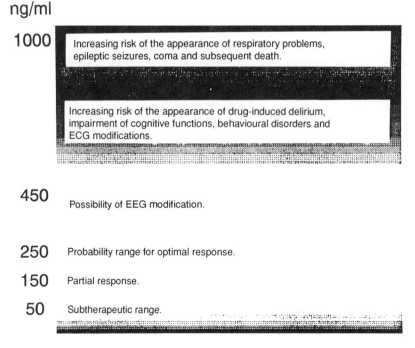

ng/ml

1000 Increasing risk of the appearance of respiratory problems, epileptic seizures, coma and subsequent death.

Increasing risk of the appearance of drug-induced delirium, impairment of cognitive functions, behavioural disorders and ECG modifications.

450 Possibility of EEG modification.

250 Probability range for optimal response.

150 Partial response.

50 Subtherapeutic range.

Figure 6.5. Correlation between plasma levels and clinical effects of tricyclic antidepressants (from Preskorn, 1989; see text).

such as memory disorders or even delirium in other patients. This is an indication that plasma level assays for psychopharmaceuticals must be seen only as one tool among others for optimization of therapy.

More recent antidepressants, i.e. some MAO inhibitors and selective serotonin reuptake inhibitors (SSRIs), differ from tricyclic drugs in their profile of pharmacological action. For example, SSRIs have little or no action on noradrenergic, adrenergic or cholinergic receptors. The relationship between plasma concentrations and side effects demonstrated in Fig. 6.5 therefore does not apply to these classes of drugs. On the other hand, a so-called 'serotonin syndrome' is observed with SSRIs, characterized by gastrointestinal upsets, agitation, shivering, fever and muscle cramps, and can have a fatal outcome in extreme cases. This syndrome is rare and has been observed almost exclusively in cases where the action of the SSRI on serotoninergic neurons has been enhanced further by MAO inhibitors or the similarly serotoninergic antidepressant chlorimipramine (Sternbach, 1991). A 'therapeutic range' of plasma levels has not yet been defined for any of the SSRIs, all of which show relatively little toxicity. With these more modern antidepressants, plasma level assays appear to have a more limited application, e.g. in relation to compliance problems or in the case of interactions with other drugs.

6.3.5   Lithium as an example

Lithium is used for the treatment of manias and for the prophylaxis of manic and depressive phases in bipolar affective psychosis (Chapter 1). With the same doses, the plasma lithium levels can vary by a factor of four in chronically treated patients. Since both the therapeutic effect and the side effects of lithium are closely correlated with plasma concentrations, regular controls of substance levels are now part of routine clinical monitoring.

Lithium has an elimination half-life of 10–30 hours. Since excretion occurs mainly via the kidneys, regular plasma level determinations are particularly indicated in elderly patients and those with renal insufficiency. Blood is normally obtained from patients 12 hours after the last dose. The plasma lithium level should then be between 0.5 and 0.8 mmol/l if the drug is used prophylactically. Even higher concentrations may be necessary in the treatment of mania unless lithium is combined with neuroleptics (Greil and van Calker, 1983).

As an example of a close correlation between pharmacokinetic and pharmacodynamic features, lithium is atypical in psychopharmacology since it is not metabolized (so that there is no problem of pharmacologically active degradation products) and since it can be assayed with very simple analytical methods. Nevertheless, even in the case of lithium it took years before a plasma concentration range that has proved to be well tolerated and effective in the great majority of patients was determined and agreed upon.

6.3.6 Neuroleptics

Empirical studies on the topic of 'therapeutic windows' of neuroleptics have led to variable and predominantly negative results (reviews by Berrios, 1982; Dahl, 1986). Simpson and Yadalam (1985) reported studies with the following substances: chlorpromazine, seven studies; thioridazine, five studies; thiothixene three studies; fluphenazine, four studies; butaperazine, three studies; haloperidol, 11 studies. For none of these neuroleptics could a reproducible correlation between plasma levels and therapeutic effect be found, which is surprising in view of the fact that representatives of various chemical classes with different metabolic behaviours were investigated. Thus 75 metabolites have been described for chlorpromazine, including many pharmacologically active ones, whereas haloperidol probably forms only one active metabolite. Since the therapeutic efficacy of neuroleptics can be described more clearly than that of antidepressants and is also confounded less with spontaneous improvements, it must be concluded that the correlation between plasma concentrations and clinical effects is actually quite loose with the said neuroleptics and not helpful in determining optimal doses. Simpson and Yadalam (1985) therefore recommend that, under normal conditions, the doses of neuroleptics be determined according to the state of the patient and not on the basis of supposed optimal plasma concentrations. Wirshing et al. (1995) list a number of circumstances, similar to the ones on pp 153/154 in which plasma level monitoring may be useful.

6.3.7 Other aspects

From a clinical point of view there is not the same urgency in the question of PK–PD correlations for *tranquillizers* and *hypnotics* since underdosage is simple to recognize and can be quickly corrected. The recognition of overdosage is more difficult, especially in elderly patients, since it often does not arise in the form of clearly manifest symptoms. In any case, the correlations between administered doses, the short-term and longer-term plasma levels achieved and the clinical effects are not at all straightforward with benzodiazepines (Greenblatt et al., 1987), so that no guidance for the dosage of these drugs can be obtained on the basis of isolated plasma level determinations. As in the case of neuroleptics, the individually correct dose of a benzodiazepine must be determined from clinical observations, additionally keeping in mind the problems of tolerance and dependency with these drugs (Chapter 1).

A partial explanation for the sometimes considerable individual differences in plasma concentrations (after the administration of the same doses) has been found in the form of a *genetic polymorphism* (Baumann, 1992c; Kalow, 1992): 5–10% of the continental European population has a genetically determined deficiency in their ability to metabolize substances like debrisoquine, spartein or dextromorphan. Since the metabolism of certain psychopharmaceuticals is dependent on the same enzymes as that of debrisoquine, etc., these 'poor metabolizers' rapidly achieve very high plasma concentrations of the drugs in question after usual doses.

A practical application of this knowledge is the *debrisoquine test*: patients with unexpected reactions to certain psychopharmaceuticals are given a test dose of debrisoquine and, where applicable, can be identified as abnormal metabolizers, so that the dose of their psychopharmaceutical can be corrected downwards. The debrisoquine test is also useful in clarifying unexpected drug interactions which are due to metabolic defects in some cases.

Here we leave these questions of PK–PD relationships, which were heavily concentrated on clinical aspects. In the clinical testing of new drugs as discussed in the following sections, substances have to be thoroughly investigated with regard to the relationships between administered doses, plasma levels of the substance and its metabolites, and the clinical effects.

6.4   CLINICAL INVESTIGATION OF NEW PSYCHOPHARMACEUTICALS

6.4.1   Introductory considerations

An important area of clinical research in psychiatry is the testing of new drugs to determine their therapeutic actions. Why are these studies necessary? Is it desirable at all to add further to the long list of psychopharmaceuticals with their often very similar properties of actions? This question should certainly be answered in the affirmative for several indications since there is a lack of:

- antipsychotic drugs which have no extrapyramidal effects and are generally well tolerated;
- anxiolytics with reliable action but not generally causing sedation and leading to dependency;
- drugs for the effective treatment of cognitive disorders occurring in the elderly (dementias).

How are these novel drugs discovered? If we consider the way in which the prototypes of psychopharmaceuticals used today were discovered (Chapter 2) the general answer would be: by the clinical study of the greatest possible number of substances exhibiting novel and previously unknown patterns of activity in preclinical experiments, and hoping for another lucky break. However, for various reasons, particularly legal and ethical, this approach in no longer practicable today. On the other hand there is no doubt that the rational development of drugs on the basis of scientific hypotheses also has only a slight chance of success and that no one has developed a formula for finding the psychopharmaceuticals of the future.

The search for new psychopharmaceuticals lies largely in the hands of pharmaceutical companies and is thus strongly influenced by economic interests. During the development of new compounds, these companies work closely with universities and other research institutes, and later with doctors and psychologists in clinics, hospitals and private practice. This cooperative work is supervised to different degrees by the state or regional authorities in different countries. The licensing of new drugs for general use after successful completion of clinical trials also falls within the competence of governmental authorities. Books by Burley and Binns (1985) and Mathieu (1994) give information on the corresponding regulations in Europe and the USA.

In the following pages we set out some typical problems and considerations related to clinical–psychopharmaceutical research, taking as our example a fictitious experimental preparation, the safety and efficacy of which is to be tested in man after the completion of the necessary pharmacological and toxicological tests in animals. More extensive discussions on questions of clinical drug testing in general can be found in a book by Glenny and Nelmes (1986) and, for psychopharmaceuticals in particular, in a chapter authored by Robinson and Prien (1995).

The research and development (R&D) work on our fictitious experimental substance is preceded by some basic considerations regarding the research area, the allocation of resources and scientific procedures that can be summarized by the terms research portfolio, strategy and tactics or methodology.

Within the context of developing the *research portfolio* of a pharmaceutical company, some of the questions which arise are:

- What are the urgent unsolved therapeutic problems in an area of medicine such as psychiatry? How many patients are affected in this way? What are the economic consequences?
- Is the company already present in this segment of the market? With which products? How are the company's products and those of its competitors developing? What changes can be forecast in the market in question?
- What are the prospects for resolving the remaining therapeutic problems? On what time scale? With how much resources?
- Do the company's R&D departments have experience in the therapeutic field in question? Are there links with other research groups?
- What effects will there be on the rest of the organization if the field considered to be of interest is further developed (or newly developed)?

Some of these questions are of a qualitative type and cannot be answered with precise figures, so that entrepreneurial decisions are required. Since decisions concerning the R&D portfolio will tie up personnel and financial resources for years, they are of highest relevance to a company as a whole. In order to limit the risk, most companies compile a portfolio of R&D projects which includes a mixture of long-term and short-term, rather conservative and rather high-risk R&D areas, and they also undertake regular reviews of their portfolio.

Research strategy includes questions of the following type:

- How is a specific objective within the R&D portfolio, e.g. the search for a neuroleptic lacking extrapyramidal effects as a possible way to improve the treatment of schizophrenia, to be partitioned and divided up so that individual working groups and researchers with their different methods can be sensibly integrated into the project?
- Which areas can be dealt with inside the company with its own know-how and which should be farmed out to external organizations such as university institutes?
- How many compounds from a given chemical class, with a given pharmacological profile and starting from a given hypothesis, should be developed and taken up to clinical testing?

Unlike the R&D portfolio, which forms part of business policy, questions of this type are usually discussed and decided not by the company top management but within the specialist divisions. Planning covers one to three years and is regularly checked.

The following topics form part of *research tactics* or *methodology* (in our case of clinical research):

- Outlining of the objectives and hypotheses for series of experiments and individual studies.
- Statistical planning of individual experiments and determination of the evaluation methods.
- Definition of the levels of assessment, evaluation criteria and measurement instruments.
- Selection of samples: definition of inclusion and exclusion criteria.
- Duration of treatment, dosage of the experimental product and of reference substances.

The choice of methods and possible methodological developments fall within the competence of the research groups and the individual researchers working on a project. The topics dealt with in the following paragraphs relate almost exclusively to this level.

6.4.2 The preclinical phase

Research on a new chemical compound from its first synthesis in the research chemist's laboratory to its first use in humans, called the preclinical phase, lasts for about three years on average. Among other things, the following work is carried out during this period:

(1) The compound is characterized in pharmacological experiments, i.e., is described quantitatively in numerous 'pharmacological models' in relation to its possible clinical use.

(2) Its mechanism of action is examined; i.e., an understanding is sought of how the actions encountered in various pharmacological models are produced.

(3) The compound is examined for toxic effects which would prevent further development.

(4) Manufacture of the compound is scaled up in a stepwise manner from the laboratory to industrial production since increasingly larger amounts of the active agent are required for the extensive pharmacological, toxicological and, finally, clinical studies.

(5) Pharmaceutical forms are developed which make it possible for the compound to be administered to humans, namely capsules, tablets, ampoules, etc., depending on the nature of the active ingredient and the planned method of use (see Padfield, 1985).

The methods used in *pharmacological testing* (Table 6.1) are partly based on the pathophysiological hypotheses presented in Chapter 5 (e.g. amphetamine antagonism by neuroleptics), partly on simple analogies with known drugs, and occasionally also on ethological considerations (Dixon, 1986). In the first case we speak of a rational or mechanistic approach since the test models used are based on a pathophysiological hypothesis. In the second case we speak of empirical or analogous procedures – some authors speak of correlation models (Schuurman *et al.*, 1992) – since the model is based not on any pathophysiological hypothesis but only on the experience that, for many compounds, there is a correlation between certain actions of a substance in the model and its clinical effects. Ethological approaches should rather be termed rational since they assume homology between experimental animals in the test situation and humans. Both approaches may include experiments on cell components, single cells, cell assemblies (cultures), isolated organs and, as in the ethological approach, in intact animals. It is also necessary to distinguish between studies related to the desired therapeutic effects of a drug (e.g. promotion of learning in the case of potential antidementia drugs) and the clarification of other effects belonging to the pharmacological profile of the compound and indicating potential side effects, e.g. studies involving the cardiovascular system.

Animal experiments are also used to show whether, and in what dosage, the compound is acutely toxic and whether repeated administration causes transient or permanent changes in function and structure (Table 6.2), whether it influences embryonic development in pregnant animals (teratogenesis), and whether it causes genetic changes (mutagenesis). On average, only one of several hundred newly synthesized compounds reach the clinical trial stage; the rest either fail to display any interesting biological activity during preclinical tests or the relationship between desirable and undesirable effects, such as the suspected presence of an antidepressant as opposed to a cardiotoxic effect, is too unfavourable to justify testing the substance in man.

Hypotheses as to the clinical application of a substance are formulated on the basis of results obtained in animal experiments. Such *pharmacological*

Table 6.1. Pharmacological characterization of potentially CNS-active substances (see Spiegelstein and Levy, 1982; Schuurman *et al.*, 1992; Geyer and Markou, 1995)

Behaviour	Effect on spontaneous, undisturbed behaviour: ethological trials Influence on conditioned behaviour: classical or operant conditioning
Neurophysiology	EEG recordings, evoked potentials in waking and sleeping animals; recordings from selected brain areas Single-cell recordings
Antagonisms	Neutralization of the effect of tetrabenazine: typical for conventional antidepressants Neutralization of the effect of amphetamine: typical for conventional neuroleptics
Binding studies	Binding of the substance to receptors for dopamine, noradrenaline, serotonin, etc.
Biochemistry	Action on neurotransmitter turnover
Vital functions	Effect on cardiovascular parameters, on respiration, digestive functions. Influence on water and electrolyte excretion

hypotheses can be either more or less specific. For a compound stemming from an already known chemical class, showing a profile of action during animal trials similar to that of established medicaments, the hypothesis may, for example, be formulated along these lines: 'In animal experiments the preparation XY has the profile of action of a classic antidepressant. It should be as effective as imipramine when given in a similar dosage range, but with fewer cardiovascular effects. Clinical testing should concentrate initially on patients with depression, in particular endogenous depression.' Such a precise hypothesis can be proposed when a compound is not very innovative, i.e., when its chemical structure is similar to that of known drugs, when it has been tested using long-established methods, and when its profile of action in animal experiments does not deviate to any major extent from that of already marketed drugs. In current jargon, such substances are called 'me-too' drugs.

A different situation arises when a substance possessing a 'high degree of innovation' is to be clinically tested. Such compounds would be derived from as yet relatively unknown chemical classes, would have shown a qualitatively

Table 6.2. Toxicological studies

Acute toxicity	Symptoms of poisoning after single oral and parenteral administration, estimation of the lethal dose in several animal species
Chronic toxicity	Administration over several weeks to several years: determination of NTEL (no toxic effect level) = highest still well-tolerated dose
Teratogenesis	Effects of the substance on the developing fetus, effects detrimental to the cells of propagation
Mutagenicity testing	Effect on genetic information Carcinogenic effects

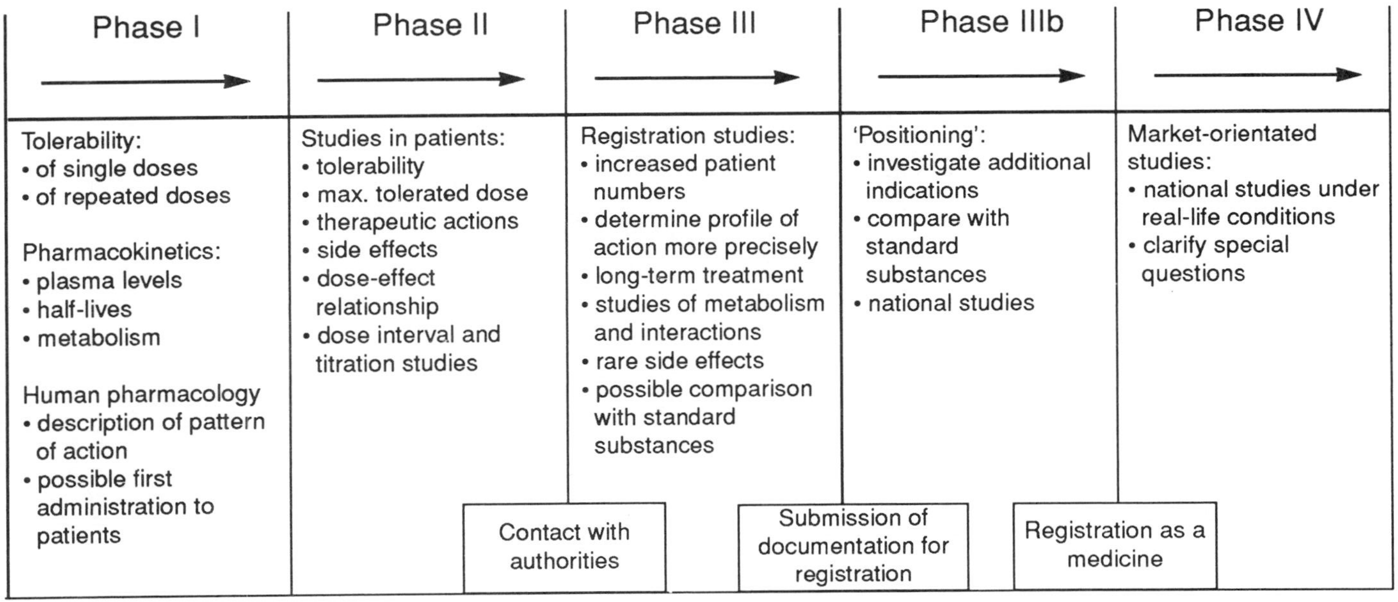

Phase I	Phase II	Phase III	Phase IIIb	Phase IV
Tolerability: • of single doses • of repeated doses Pharmacokinetics: • plasma levels • half-lives • metabolism Human pharmacology • description of pattern of action • possible first administration to patients	Studies in patients: • tolerability • max. tolerated dose • therapeutic actions • side effects • dose-effect relationship • dose interval and titration studies	Registration studies: • increased patient numbers • determine profile of action more precisely • long-term treatment • studies of metabolism and interactions • rare side effects • possible comparison with standard substances	'Positioning': • investigate additional indications • compare with standard substances • national studies	Market-orientated studies: • national studies under real-life conditions • clarify special questions

Contact with authorities

Submission of documentation for registration

Registration as a medicine

Figure 6.6. Phase division of the clinical testing of psychopharmaceuticals. Schematic diagram of the Food and Drug Administration guidelines (FDA Guidelines, 1977a,b) and the WHO guidelines derived therefrom (WHO Guidelines, 1985)

novel profile of action during animal experiments, or would have been tested using methods about which little was known to date. In circumstances such as these, the pharmacological hypothesis on which first clinical trials are based is less specific, and testing in man must be devised in such a way as also to reveal unexpected aspects of the substance and its action.

The clinical study of a new substance proceeds in several steps or phases (Fig. 6.6). The purpose of this subdivision is to minimize the risk to the participating subjects and patients at each point in time and to allow each individual part of the study to flow one from the other so that a maximum of information from one trial can be obtained for the following studies.

6.4.3 Phase I clinical trials: tolerability, pharmacokinetics, human pharmacology

Tolerability trials and pharmacokinetics

The testing of a new psychotropic substance in man always begins with investigations into its tolerability. These are normally conducted in healthy subjects who are informed about the aims and possible risks of a study and who then volunteer to participate in the trial, generally receiving some financial compensation (Rogers and Spector, 1986). Tolerability trials call for close medical supervision and readiness to deal with any emergencies, even though the first doses of the new substance to be tested in man, based as they are on the results of animal experiments, are so low that they generally have no effect at all. The dosage is increased gradually in order to keep the risk for the volunteers as low as possible. Tolerability trials can basically be run as open trials – i.e., without placebo control – until dosages are reached at which distinct effects become apparent. These are generally followed by placebo-controlled trials of several dosages found to have some effect in open trials.

After the first trials in normal subjects one may have some indication as to the nature and duration of the effect of a substance on the central nervous system. Although it is not normally feasible to include comprehensive psychological or psychophysiological testing during first tolerability trials, since medical aspects have to be paramount at this stage, it is possible to determine with considerable reliability any pronounced central actions of a substance as well as the approximate duration of such effects. Assuming that the substance is well tolerated, the next stage of a clinical investigation could thus be embarked on with the following newly acquired information: 'Dosages of from . . . to . . . mg of the substance have a sedating/stimulating/euphoria-inducing action; a central effect becomes apparent about . . . minutes after administration, attains its maximum effect . . . hours after administration and this action lasts for about . . . hours'. Further data will also be available as to the effects of the preparation on vital functions such as respiration and circulation, as well as on biochemical laboratory readings.

Within the context of initial tolerability testing, blood samples may be taken from the subjects at predetermined intervals of time. Tests are then conducted on them to determine if, when and in what concentrations the substance and its metabolites are detectable in the blood, when peak blood levels are reached and the way in which they decrease. These data make it possible to establish more precisely the intervals which should elapse between doses during later studies involving the repeated administration of the substance. They also permit a rough estimation of the absorption of a test substance after oral administration.

Phase I also includes safety testing with repeated administration of the new substance. Studies of this type can, depending on the product, be carried out in healthy subjects or in selected patients with an illness corresponding to one of the pharmacological hypotheses.

Human pharmacological investigations

If the new substance is well tolerated, it is either examined further in healthy subjects in order to gain additional insight into its profile of action or it is administered for the first time to patients who are mentally ill. The choice of the course of action taken depends on several factors, above all on the information derived from preclinical studies and from initial human tolerability trials.

Should the substance in question have little innovative character and be based on a specific pharmacological hypothesis, testing in patients ought to commence as early as possible. Animal experiments will have yielded the hypothetical profile of action and the presumed therapeutic indication, and a centrally active single dose in humans can already be estimated from the tolerability trials in healthy subjects. The risk of the first patients receiving either a totally inactive substance or inadequate doses of the new preparation is comparatively low, although it is never possible entirely to eliminate the possibility of negative surprises. In the case of compounds with little innovative character, early testing in patients is appropriate since 'me-too' preparations are expected to have clearly defined advantages as compared to already marketed drugs: lower dosages, longer duration of action per individual dose, a more favourable relationship between therapeutically desirable and undesirable effects. Should such advantages not be confirmed during therapeutic trials, the clinical testing of the substance can be discontinued quickly, at least for the originally proposed indication.

In the case of chemically and pharmacologically novel substances, great significance attaches to the studies of tolerability and, especially, of human pharmacology in healthy subjects. As discussed in Chapters 3 and 4, such studies give a guide to the following points:

– pattern of action in respect of subjective, performance, and electrophysiological parameters in comparison with known substances;

- onset of action, maximum effect, and duration of action following administration of a single dose;
- relationship between central and peripheral (side) effects.

These data are important in the planning of the clinical trials to follow, even though they do not permit any reliable forecast to be made of the therapeutic drug effects. Studies in patients can then commence with doses which have shown central activity; the dosage interval may be estimated more precisely and the doctors or scientists responsible for planning the therapeutic studies are not left entirely in the dark as regards the profile of action and side effects.

6.4.4 Phase II and III clinical studies: trials in patients

Should an experimental preparation have passed through the preclinical developmental phase as well as initial experiments in man, and shown central effects, but no prohibitive side effects, it is then possible to commence its testing in patients. The aim of *clinical–therapeutic trials* is to establish the suitability of a new substance for patients with a specific illness, or for a subgroup of such patients. This includes clarifying the effective and safe dosage range for single and repeated administration, defining the precise pattern of action, including side effects, under hospital and outpatient conditions, and, finally, the question as to whether the new substance possesses sufficient advantages over existing drugs to make its introduction on the market medically and commercially advisable.

In view of the numerous and interrelated questions that have to be answered in Phase II (Fig. 6.6), some authors (e.g. Möller, 1992) have proposed that a phase IIA and a phase IIB should be differentiated. According to this scheme, open, exploratory trials would be performed in small homogeneous groups of subjects, whereas controlled, i.e., comparative studies in larger groups of patients would be performed in phase IIB. We shall return to this question in Section 6.5.

The first steps in any therapeutic trial involve a job of translation: the results of the preceding experiments in animals and in healthy subjects have to be translated into clinical hypotheses. Patients suitable for inclusion in the trial must be defined exactly on the basis of diagnoses and target symptoms; possible reasons for their exclusion, contraindications, admissible or non-admissible concomitant medication, and additional therapeutic measures have to be stated. Decisions must be taken as to the initial doses of the experimental preparation to be given, the intervals to elapse between administrations and the steps by which the dosage should be increased. Agreement must be reached as to the conditions under which the patients are to be observed, the instruments to be used in this assessment and the persons by whom such assessments are to be made. Finally, a timetable must be set for all these activities and measures must be decided upon for any possible emergencies. The outcome of all these considerations is a written *study protocol* (Table

Table 6.3. Protocol of a clinical study

1. *Information regarding the experimental product*
   Chemistry, pharmacology, toxicology
   Results of previous studies in man

2. *Purpose of the study*
   Pharmacological hypothesis/hypotheses
   Questions that require answering

3. *Selection of patients*
   Age, sex, diagnoses, target symptoms
   Exclusion criteria, concomitant diseases, contraindications
   Permitted and unallowed concomitant medication

4. *Experimental design*
   Type of trial (open, double-blind), reference treatments, timetable for control
   examinations: clinical evaluation, psychometric tests, medical examinations

5. *Parameters investigated*
   Rating scales, test procedures
   Medical parameters, laboratory tests, special procedures

6. *Drugs and doses*
   Doses, methods of administration, administration intervals, dose increase,
   maximum dose, maximum duration of administration, information on placebo
   and/or reference products

7. *Documentation*
   Documentation of findings, presentation and evaluation of the results, reporting

8. *Response to emergency situations*
   In the event that the experimental product is ineffective, in the case of adverse
   events, information regarding antidote (if known)

9. *Statistical aspects*
   Estimation of the sample size
   Intended evaluation procedures

10. *Ethical considerations*
    Informing the patient
    Ethical committee

6.3) which is normally discussed with all the persons involved in the trial (see
Greenberg, 1982).

It is not always possible to adhere to all of the intended points laid down
in a study protocol, even when this is prepared thoroughly and on the basis
of extensive experience: patients becoming ill or having accidents, absence
of nursing staff due to illness, unforeseeable events inside and outside of the
clinic, and even lack of interest, suspicion of the trial or simple forgetfulness
on the part of nursing staff often cause even the most carefully planned
clinical trials to go awry. Clinical monitoring, i.e., regular supervision of
studies on behalf of the sponsoring company, is therefore of greatest
importance.

6.5 SPECIAL QUESTIONS IN THE CLINICAL TESTING OF PSYCHOPHARMACEUTICALS

6.5.1 Problems of patient selection

For reasons of safety, trial preparations in an early stage of clinical development must be tested under hospital conditions. However, neurotic, depressed and even schizophrenic patients are only hospitalized when they are very ill, when they endanger themselves or their surroundings and/or do not respond (or no longer respond) to available drugs. Most of the patients in hospitals are thus seriously ill and possibly resistant to therapy, and are not representative of the majority of persons taking tranquillizers, antidepressants and neuroleptics. If an experimental preparation were to be tested exclusively on such patients, a false impression of its efficacy or lack of efficacy can be obtained, and an interesting substance might perhaps be abandoned prematurely and unnecessarily.

Investigators are thus facing a dilemma: on the one hand every patient has the right to the best treatment available at any given time (Section 6.1) and should consequently not be treated with what might be an ineffective experimental compound; on the other hand new substances should, if possible, be tested in the type of patients for whom they would later be intended and not on an atypical, therapy-resistant minority. True, one could claim that a preparation representing a real advance would act on just those patients who had failed to respond to existing drugs; and yet this would be an unfair demand: resistance to therapy may be due to a variety of reasons (failure to adhere to instructions regarding therapy, inadequate absorption of the drug, particular sensitivity to certain side effects, incorrect diagnosis) and the development of a new preparation may even be justified when it exhibits properties such as a faster onset of action or superior tolerability, and not necessarily through efficacy in hitherto resistant patients. It is therefore essential for a trial preparation already in its early stages of testing also to be examined in newly admitted, as yet untreated patients. What could be a solution to these contradictory requirements?

There is no standard procedure covering all types of psychopharmaceuticals since the information derived from animal trials and experiments in healthy subjects, which precede the first clinical applications, is not always of the same significance and since the demands made of a medicament vary according to its indications. In the case of neuroleptics, where parts of the spectrum of activity can be characterized in animal experiments and where a rapid onset of therapeutic action is desired, the following procedure is frequently adopted.

The experimental compound is administered to schizophrenic patients with productive symptoms at a dose range derived from the initial tolerability studies in humans and any other Phase I human pharmacology trials. In this approach, newly ill, relapsed or even chronic patients can be treated if they have not previously received neuroleptics and in whom 'positive symptoms' such as unrest, hallucinations and delusions dominate the clinical picture. The dose of the experimental product is low to start with but is rapidly increased if the effect is inadequate. If no clear improvement occurs after a few days, the experimental product is withdrawn and a standard drug assumed to be best for the case in question is administered. On the basis of experience in the first few patients, the dose can be estimated better for the following cases so that the risk of ineffective treatment decreases steadily. In this manner, each individual patient will still receive effective treatment since he can be switched at any time to what should be the best standard drug for his particular need, if necessary after only two or three days.

Pilot studies of this nature generally cover not more than 10–20 patients each in several hospitals and provide information on the basic suitability of a test product as a neuroleptic. Restriction of the drug administration to 7–10 days in the event of inadequate efficacy (or two to three days in the very first patients) is therapeutically sensible since a neuroleptic must have a rapid onset of action.

Time limits of this kind are also logical since the efficacy of neuroleptic treatment can be quite reliably predicted on the basis of changes arising in the first few days of treatment (see p. 144: 'Secondary predictors') so that the continuation of a clearly ineffective treatment beyond this time would not be justified.

A similar procedure applies in the case of *antidepressants*. Here also, treatment must be restricted to a few weeks should the test compound fail to show any significant therapeutic effect. There is little risk of unjustifiably dropping an interesting substance on the basis of short-term trials of this nature since compounds not showing a therapeutic effect within two weeks would hardly be acceptable as an antidepressant today (see Quitkin *et al.*, 1984, for a different view on antidepressant trial duration).

The dilemma arising between medical and scientific requirements is less sharp in other indications (dementias, anxiety disorders, insomnia) since either there are still no convincingly effective and safe medicines available as alternatives (as in the case of dementia) or, as in the case of tranquillizers and hypnotics, the information gained from experiments in healthy subjects is more relevant (Chapter 3) and the patients participating in clinical trials are not so severely ill as in the case of hospitalized patients with schizophrenia and depression. The risk of causing or prolonging suffering with an inadequately effective experimental compound is thus smaller in these instances.

6.5.2   Drug effects, spontaneous course of the disease and historical comparisons

Psychiatric symptoms and illnesses follow a spontaneous course: sleep disorders and so-called vegetative symptoms frequently arise during times of greater stress and anxious anticipation and often disappear without any treatment. Depression can follow a cyclic course with remission into a normal state or shift into mania. The symptoms of schizophrenic psychoses are also subject to change which can occur within days, months or years and can include very different states. Precise knowledge of psychopathological developments in general, and of the earlier course undergone by the individual patient in particular, are consequently essential prerequisites if the effect of a therapeutic measure is to be correctly assessed in each individual case.

For example: should there be an improvement in the state of an endogenous depressive patient after two weeks' treatment with a new antidepressant, this would not necessarily point to a causal relationship between the medicament and the clinical change (because the patient might have improved spontaneously). A causal connection would, however, be more likely if it were known that the patient in question had already experienced several depressive phases of between 8 and 10 months' duration, none of which had shown any real response to medication, whereas the present phase had only begun two weeks prior to commencement of the trial substance and had then swiftly responded to the new preparation.

In this fictitious case, a current observation is compared with earlier observations – this is called a *historical comparison*: the patient is his own comparative subject. Let us assume that similar observations have been made in a total of 15 of 20 patients treated with a new antidepressant who have previously shown inadequate or no response to standard antidepressants. Would this enable one to conclude that the trial preparation has a pronounced antidepressant action? The answer is no, not with any certainty. There might have been decisive changes in the social environment of some of the patients at the time of the trial; in some of the other patients the symptoms of depression may have waned earlier than expected on unknown grounds, whereas in yet other patients the enthusiasm of the medical team in response to the initial results may have been the critical factor. This is of course a fictitious situation which merely serves to show that historical comparisons, such as those customarily conducted in early phases of psychopharmacological research, do not, in themselves, suffice as definite proof of therapeutic efficacy.

Consequently (and for other reasons also), many authors believe that open trials or trials with only historical controls are scientifically worthless in so-called Phase IIA; it is recommended that controlled comparative trials versus a standard product and/or placebo be performed even in the early developmental phases (Awad, 1993).

The term historical comparison is also used when a current result of treatment is compared with the 'natural history' of an illness. Assuming, for example, that according to reliable statistics a specific disease leads to death an average of six months after it first becomes manifest, then any treatment which is well tolerated and which lengthens the survival period by an average of three years will arouse interest. In such cases, the historical comparison can constitute a major portion of the clinical proof of action, based on the statistics covering the spontaneous course of the illness and in the light of the ethical difficulties involved in running untreated comparative groups. In psychiatry and in clinical psychopharmacology, however, where there are numerous and complex biological and social factors having an impact upon patients, historical comparisons are of lesser importance than in the case of purely somatic illnesses.

In order to distinguish spontaneously occurring from drug-induced changes, it would in principle be possible to treat one and the same patient alternately with a trial preparation and with placebo or a standard preparation, and then to compare the results of the individual treatment phases in a longitudinal study. However, such an 'intensive design' (Chassan, 1960; Huber, 1978) imposes prerequisites which are not usually fulfilled in psychiatry: firstly, the disorder being treated must respond rapidly to the medicament and reappear quickly after drug discontinuation so that each change can be related to the preparation being given at that particular time. Secondly, the symptoms or illness being treated must theoretically remain more or less unchanged over a long period of time to enable comparisons to be made between treatment periods. Neither of these prerequisites is generally fulfilled in the case of mental disorders. Finally, the third prerequisite, namely that the patient or his legal representative must agree to the entire procedure (Section 6.1), likely to present a problem.

6.5.3 Maintenance of constant conditions

A requirement which must be fulfilled in psychopharmacological trials, as in any scientific experiment, is that apart from the independent variables which are intentionally varied, other factors also capable of influencing the observed behaviour (the dependent variables) must be kept constant or must at least be controlled. Only in this way is it possible to distinguish between the effects of independent variables – in our case the trial substance – and more or less coincidental circumstances accompanying the study. However, in clinical trials it is barely possible to keep other independent variables constant.

– Every illness has its spontaneous course with symptomatic improvements, deteriorations, and general ups and downs which cannot always be linked to alterations in the patient's environment. The presumed effect of a trial substance must consequently be delimited from spontaneous alterations in the illness.
– The surroundings of a patient are another factor subject to variation: seasons and weather conditions change, family and other social factors tend to fluctuate or to alter abruptly (in hospital this can be due to changes in doctors and nursing staff and to the arrival of new and the departure of familiar fellow patients).
– The trial itself causes changes in the patient's environment, independent of the pharmacological action of the preparation. He receives new tablets or capsules, is the object of greater attention and closer scrutiny, he is examined more frequently and more thoroughly, his urine is collected and blood samples taken, and apparatus-based examinations are conducted. Particularly in the case of long-stay patients, such measures constitute massive encroachment on their familiar routine and affect the individual and his illness.

There can consequently be no question of keeping all possible influences constant during a clinical trial. All that can be kept constant are at best those factors which are involved on a short-term basis; however, a clinical trial is run over weeks and months and is consequently subject to different laws than is a short-term experiment.

All this leads to the need to perform clinical studies with new forms of treatment, e.g. with an experimental product, as 'controlled' trials in which a reference group of patients (control group) treated with a known effective medicine or, in some indications, with a placebo is included alongside the group of patients receiving the trial compound. This design is intended to allow the actions observed with the new compound to be differentiated from:

(a) changes which occur spontaneously or as a result of the experimental conditions; comparison with placebo is used for this delimitation;
(b) changes which typically occur with a therapy recognized as being effective; this comparison is made possible by using a standard reference product.

If feasible, comparisons between trial products, placebo and standard drugs should be performed 'blind'. However, this requirement cannot always be fulfilled (Section 6.5.5). The selection of reference groups can also lead to problems, as will be discussed briefly below.

6.5.4 Formation of comparative (control) groups; multicentre trials

Since every patient is a unique individual is it possible to create genuinely comparable groups of patients in a therapeutic trial? If we assume that factors such as age and sex of the patients, number and duration of earlier instances of hospitalization, duration of current illness, and success of earlier treatment certainly do not represent reliable predictors of the therapeutic effect but nevertheless can have a bearing on the treatment result, it would then be necessary for experimental and control groups to be exactly comparable in respect of 6–10 characteristics. Technically speaking, one would have to stratify the subjects on the basis of these characteristics and would thus arrive at a matrix with 50–100 cells which would have to be occupied in a balanced manner by the experimental and comparative groups. From this example it can be seen that the creation of entirely similar control groups is almost always an unattainable requirement – all the more so since one does not know in advance which factors will display a relevant relation to the result of the treatment (Netter, 1992).

In practice one consequently trusts to chance and aims at creating control groups which, *as a whole*, do not deviate systematically from the trial group, i.e., in which there are an equal number of men and women and in which the average age, the number and nature of earlier disorders, as well as additional factors, correspond as a whole to the characteristics of the trial group. Even under such simplified conditions it is often difficult to find sufficient numbers of patients in one and the same centre who correspond to all the criteria of the trial in question and who are also prepared to participate in a comparative study.

One solution to such sampling problems lies in dividing up the trial between several clinics, all working according to the same protocol. Depending on the field of application of the new substance *multicentre studies* of this nature are unavoidable and bring with them both advantages and disadvantages from the viewpoint of trial design. A major advantage lies in the fact that especially favourable or unfavourable conditions prevailing in a particular clinic, which could consequently bias the result of a trial, can be equalled out through the participation of several clinics, thus permitting a more representative picture to be formed of the drug being investigated. A distinct disadvantage of multi-centre studies lies in the heterogeneity of the trial conditions prevailing in different clinics. This can be reduced by suitable measures (initial joint discussion of the protocol with all participating investigators, so-called rater training, use of video tapes to demonstrate model cases, and perhaps even staff exchanges between the participating clinics), but cannot be entirely excluded (see Klimt, 1979; Möller, 1992).

Even when a comparative trial is organized on a multicentre basis and covers a large number of patients, it is frequently still not possible to achieve a complete balance between experimental and comparative groups. This is particularly so when the allocation of the trial and comparative preparations to the patients is conducted according to a random sequence. Thus, for example, it may emerge at the end of a study that the average duration of illness was significantly shorter in the control group than in the group of patients receiving the trial preparation – in which case the two groups will not have been comparable in respect of this criterion. Appropriate statistical methods are available to cope with such situations, which become all the more likely the greater the number of variables being considered (for examples, see Hsu, 1992). For example, uneven baseline values for individual variables can be transformed or brought into relationship with the modification encountered, and the influence of independent variables on the result of a trial can be estimated, and in part corrected, with the aid of the appropriate techniques (formation of blocks, covariance analyses) (for more details, see Schmidtke, 1992).

6.5.5 So-called blind trials: comparison with placebo and/or standard drugs

The form of study which leaves the individual patient uninformed as to the medicament administered to him is termed a single-blind trial; that in which the nursing staff and doctor or psychologist making the assessment are also ignorant as to the treatments given is known as a double-blind trial. Blind trials should prevent intended or unintended distortion of the results through prejudice, expectations or anxiety on the part of the participants. Blind trials are generally comparisons between two or more treatments which are used either by the same patients at different times or at the same time by different patients. In the first (rarer) case, we speak of a cross-over trial, and in the second case of a parallel group trial.

In blind trials it is possible to compare a product with placebo and/or with standard drugs for the indication in question. By *placebo* is meant a pharmacologically inactive galenic preparation, e.g. a capsule filled with corn starch, which may show pronounced effects under given circumstances and thereby can simulate a pharmacological effect. A considerable volume of literature is concerned with various aspects of placebo reactions: whether 'placebo responders' are characterized by specific personality features, which situations favour placebo responses, and how the placebo phenomenon can best be explained theoretically (reviews by Schindel, 1967; Shapiro, 1978; Netter, 1992).

In connection with clinical trials of new drugs, 'placebo effects' are primarily seen as distorting factors since they blend with the specific effects of the substance and make a reliable evaluation of the experimental product difficult. The use of placebos in clinical studies therefore does not have the purpose of keeping patients and other study participants in the dark but should make it possible to separate the true pharmacological actions of a substance from the non-specific effects governed by the situation: in placebo-controlled studies, the difference between the modifications arising with the experimental product and those arising with placebo is considered to be the specific drug effect.

The use of placebo and active reference drugs for controlled studies is not handled in the same way in all psychiatric indications: tranquillizers and hypnotics are usually compared with placebo since the treated diseases are mainly of a subjective nature, show great spontaneous variations and also are rarely so serious that a pharmacologically effective treatment has to be ensured for medical ethical reasons. The situation is different in trials with antidepressants and neuroleptics: severely depressed, possibly suicidal patients must not run the risk of being treated with blank product for a long time, and the same applies to acute schizophrenic patients. In such cases, an experimental substance which has shown some efficacy in open Phase I and IIa studies is compared with a standard drug for the same indication. The efficacy of the new product is then considered to be demonstrated if it proves to be superior to or at least equivalent to the standard drug.

Although this procedure seems ethically acceptable and scientifically plausible, objections have repeatedly been raised against the trend detectable in some countries to accept evidence of the efficacy of new psychopharmaceuticals solely on the basis of open Phase I and IIA studies and of non-placebo controlled Phase IIB and III studies (see Maier and Benkert, 1987). It is argued that the superiority or inferiority of an active substance, e.g. a trial preparation, relative to another form of treatment can be demonstrated only in studies with very large numbers of patients. However, if merely the equivalence of two substances is shown, there is the danger that new drugs which have no significant advantage or which are actually inferior will reach the market. It should therefore be a requirement, according to these authors, that the efficacy of new products be demonstrated whenever possible in placebo-controlled studies and that a product licence be issued only when superiority over previously available drugs has been demonstrated in at least one relevant area (efficacy, safety, efficacy in a subpopulation, etc.).

From a technical viewpoint, the double-blind comparison between a trial preparation and placebo and/or standard medicament in randomly selected groups of patients comparable in relevant criteria constitutes the ideal case of a controlled therapeutic trial: all the treatments have an equal chance to develop a therapeutic effect, any differences in the results of the trial groups being interpretable as being due to different pharmacological effects. In practice, however, a number of limitations apply also in the case of the double-blind principle and need to be handled in different ways, depending on the product and the objective of the trial.

As pointed out by Blackwell and Sternberg (1971), Brownell and Stunkard (1982) and more recent authors, psychopharmaceuticals can often be recognized from their side effects, so that experienced doctors and nurses as well as patients can rapidly find out whether an active substance or a placebo is being administered in a particular case. There is thus the threat of undesirable 'unblinding' of the trial which, depending on the circumstances, can be prevented by the use of independent evaluators (raters) not involved in the care of the patient. These additional raters are bound to make their evaluation of the action of a treatment only on the basis of psychological and psychopathological criteria; all the other data (laboratory values, results of physical examinations, observations made by the nursing staff and relatives) remain unavailable to them. By recording the rating interview one can also ensure that 'unblinding', e.g. by mentioning side effects, does not occur. (However, it must be taken into account that placebos can also cause 'side effects' and that an excessively complicated study design can produce more harm than good.)

In this connection we should mention some points affecting the atmosphere surrounding double-blind trials (Plutchik et al., 1969) and which can jeopardize their 'ecological validity':

- The doctor often feels his freedom of action to be restricted by the double-blind trial arrangement, particularly as regards the possibility of dosing a medicament according to clinical requirements.
- Double-blind trials can create an artificial situation: an experimental, affectively neutral relationship arises in place of a therapeutic one.
- When drugs with different time/activity characteristics are used, the double-blind trial can become very cumbersome, if not quite impossible.

As far as possible, all these points must be taken into account when planning a comparative trial (Hellman and Hellman, 1991). For example, the doctor must be given the opportunity to adjust the doses of the experimental and comparative treatments within a specified range and also to apply other suitable medical measures in individual cases. An affectively neutral, non-therapeutic relationship between treating physicians and patients can be prevented if the study-related interviews, tests, etc. are carried out by separate personnel with clearly defined roles. Finally, the comparison of medicaments with different time/ activity characteristics represents a technical problem which can almost always be solved – use of additional placebo capsules, so-called double-dummy techniques, are just examples of this. A further reservation raised by Plutchik and his co-workers in connection with double-blind trials cannot, however, be solved even with experimental perspicacity: some methods of treatment such as electroshock and psychotherapy cannot be compared in a really 'double-blind' manner with pharmacotherapy (Carroll *et al.*, 1994).

6.5.6 Assessment criteria

The therapeutic effects of psychopharmaceuticals are expressed as changes in well-being and behaviour. The clinical testing of new substances therefore involves the reliable determination of these modifications in a form that can subsequently undergo statistical analysis. Three basic types of methods are available for this purpose: questioning of the patients themselves (or other procedures to determine subjective effects), behavioural observations of various degrees of complexity, and test procedures for specific mental functions.

Questioning of patients

Whenever possible, the treated patients should be the first source of information about a drug effect. Depending on the nature of the psychiatric disorder, the questioning can certainly be difficult or even impossible, but nevertheless is essential in the case of depressive patients, neurotics and many schizophrenics. Only the patients themselves can give information on how they feel, their mood, anxieties, hopes, etc., and in addition many side effects of psychopharmaceuticals are exclusively of a subjective nature.

Scales of various types are available for the quantification of statements made by patients (see *ECDEU manual*, 1976; *CIPS handbook*, 1986). Methods used in German-speaking countries are the well-being scales BS and BS' (Table 6.4), Zung's Self-rating Depression Scale (SDS) (1965) and the procedures discussed in Chapter 3 (p. 54 ff.). Further methods are referenced in a book edited by Sartorius and Ban (1986). In addition, some rating scales (see below) also include items which have to be scored on the basis of the patient's own statements. With these instruments and open questioning of the patients, the essential subjective effects of a treatment can be determined.

Observation of behaviour

The behaviour of a patient under hospital conditions can be observed by nursing staff, doctors or observers specially engaged for this purpose. In particular, nursing staff who see patients in their own surroundings for days and weeks can reliably determine if and to what extent they engage in activities, whether they make contacts with other patients or tend to keep to themselves, and how they react to questions, requests and other contacts. These are all features which make it possible to evaluate and to some extent to quantify the need for nursing and the patient's social behaviour and mood, although it must also be borne in mind that personal likes and dislikes play a direct role even in apparently objective observations: difficult, quarrelsome, withdrawn patients are generally less favourably assessed, and contaminations may occur between various assessment levels. Moreover, times of observation and the conditions under which a patient is observed fluctuate from day to day. It is therefore possible to engage independent observers, uninvolved in the day-to-day nursing schedule, to rate the patients under conditions that are as standardized as possible and at predetermined times. In the case of outpatient treatment, the behaviour of the patients can be observed by relatives and other contact persons. Relatives are understandably often by no means neutral observers and therefore cannot always make reliable observations. In many instances it would also endanger the doctor–patient relationship if a system of communication were to be set up with the relatives behind the patient's back. Nevertheless, standardized behavioural observations in the habitual environment have great value in the case of children, for example, in the documentation of drug therapy of the hyperkinetic syndrome (Bachmann, 1976; Hechtman and Weiss, 1977; Whalen et al., 1979), and should also play an important role in the psychopharmacology of the elderly (see Chapter 7).

Psychological tests

So-called personality tests come less into consideration for the documentation of drug effects since they are intended to determine features that are stable in time and which are hardly relevant in the present context. Procedures for the measurement of performance (Chapter 3) are occasionally used in order to study adverse drug effects such as sedation after antidepressants and tranquillizers. As parameters of desirable therapeutic effects, these methods are relevant to the testing of substances which improve cognitive performance in patients with age-associated cognitive deficits (Crook et al., 1983; Coper et al., 1987a).

Rating scales

This expression designates evaluation scales which generally encompass several aspects (mood, social behaviour, unusual behaviours, psychopathological features) and which are also not uniform with regard to the sources of information (behavioural observation, patient interview, evaluation of third-party reports). In principle, rating scales should fulfil the same requirements as other psychological assessment and measurement methods (sensitivity, reliability, validity; see Wittenborn, 1972). Some of the best-known methods are listed in Table 6.4.

Table 6.4. A selection of well-known clinical evaluation methods (see van Riezen and Segal, 1988, for comprehensive documentation)

Self-rating scales
B–S   *Well-being Scale* (Befindlichkeits-Skala): von Zerssen *et al.* (1970).
B–S'   28 pairs of properties which are graded by the patient as present/absent/
       neither–nor. Encompasses a general drive-mood dimension
SDS   *Self-rating Depression Scale*: Zung, 1965.
       20 statements on mood and behaviour which are answered as always/
       frequently/sometimes/never or rarely. Encompasses depressivity in one
       dimension

Observation of behaviour
NOSIE *Nurses' Observation Scale for Inpatient Evaluation*: Honigfeld (1974).
       30 items that are answered as always/mostly/often/never. Assessment of
       everyday behaviour by the nursing staff; evaluation according to seven
       dimensions and a total score

Rating scales (composite evaluation scales)
BPRS   *Brief Psychiatric Rating Scale*: Overall and Gorham (1962).
       18 items that are graded on a seven-point scale from 'absent' to 'extremely
       marked'. Assessment based on observations and direct questioning of
       patients; evaluation according to five dimensions
AMDP   *Arbeitsgemeinschaft für Methodik und Dokumentation in der Psychiatrie*:
       Angst *et al.* (1969).
       Extensive documentation system which includes a list of characteristics
       which are evaluated on a five-point scale. Assessment based on observation
       and direct questioning
HDS   *Hamilton Depression Scale*: Hamilton (1960).
       17 items which are evaluated on three- to five-point scales. Assessment on
       the basis of observations and information given by the patient. Evaluation
       mostly as summed scores (methodologically dubious!)

Rating scales such as the BPRS (Brief Psychiatric Rating Scale) and the Hamilton Depression Scale offer the doctor or psychologist several practical advantages. He is reminded of the areas of behaviour to watch out for and what aspects he should cover in his interview with the patient. He obtains concrete instructions (which in some scales are quite specific) as to how to make his assessments and how to convert these to quantitative data. Finally, he is reminded of the importance of converting into a quantitative judgement clinical impressions obtained of the same patient at different times or of various patients at the same time. The statistical evaluation of clinical trials is greatly simplified by the use of standardized rating scales, since it can be performed on the basis of uniform quantitative data instead of individual verbal reports. Despite all the practical advantages inherent in standardized rating scales, one must not forget a few disadvantages:

– Some typical rating scales only cover pathologically orientated items and, in the event of clinical improvement, merely indicate reduction in pathology or, in the ideal case, normalization. What they do not record are positive, desirable forms of behaviour which are also present or which can supplant pathological characteristics in the course of therapy.

– The individual items are not independent of one another and for this reason it is most unlikely that one characteristic would change in isolation. However, by dividing up observed behaviours into several differently formulated questionnaire items, one may create the wrong impression of independence and equality of symptoms.

– Adding the scores of several items up to form sum scores can give misleading figures as estimates of the severity of an illness. Simply because the individual items are not independent and not equivalent, the greatest caution must be adopted when arriving at and interpreting such sum scores (see Immich *et al.*, 1971). Similar sums in different patients do not necessarily indicate comparable psychopathological conditions.

– Rating scales can flatten out the clinical situation. An event that would stand out as a dramatic situation in a case history may be levelled out when rating scales are used.

– Individual behaviour which is part of a sensible whole is artificially broken down and looked at in isolation, at a risk of becoming incomprehensible.

Despite these limitations, rating scales are today the preferred clinical recording instrument in most areas of psychopharmacology. In order to cancel out the disadvantages they are often combined with brief case histories or, occasionally, with symptom lists, which can be prepared individually for each patient.

CHAPTER 7

Drugs and memory

7.1 MODELS OF MEMORY AND PSYCHOPHARMACEUTICALS

In colloquial use the term 'memory' relates to an ability: one speaks of people having a good memory for names, events, faces, tunes, smells. What is meant is the ability to recall without difficulty names mentioned a long time ago, to describe in every significant detail some event in the past, to recognize a face seen years before. The powers of memory include active recollection (example: spontaneous recall of a name) and recognition (example: recognition of an individual face amongst many faces) as well as the recall of isolated incidents ('episodic' memory) and the reproduction of systematically learned material. We know from our everyday life that children are able to remember details about events which adults can barely remember, whilst old people's lapses of memory often provoke an indulgent smile – or sometimes even impatience and anger. Memories can be jogged. Events which have slipped our mind come to life again through the reminiscences of one who was also present; we remember and are quite unexpectedly able to contribute details of the event which we thought long forgotten. Re-reading a book which we read years before not only brings its content back to us again, it also conjures up moods and events which affected us and our surroundings at the time of first reading.

Whereas everyday routine provides repeated opportunities to observe and describe feats of memory, scientific psychology is attempting to quantify these phenomena, to elaborate general laws and work out models according to which it is possible to explain as many empirical phenomena as possible (historical account in Norman, 1969). Some of these memory models will briefly be mentioned.

The division of memory into a *short-term* and a *long-term store* takes into account the experience, also confirmed experimentally, that the recollection of events just past is not identical with the reproduction of occurrences going back further in time: that only a portion of what we remember for a short time is available on a long-term basis. The spatial and statical expression 'store' is used, although active processes may be assumed to exist which constantly rearrange the material acquired. According to the general view, the short-term store has a limited capacity whereas the long-term store is of unrestricted capacity. The dual-store model of memory is expanded by the assumption of *sensory registers*. These are understood to be sensory-specific stores with an extremely short retention time and are intended to explain certain phenomena on the borderline between perception and memory. The unnoticed overhearing of, and counting of, the chimes of a clock; the ability to allow one's thoughts to wander and yet subsequently still grasp words or entire sentences uttered by one's interlocutor; the seeing, but only subsequent realization of an object, a person or a printed word – these are a few examples. Attentiveness is critical for the further fate of a piece of information – where there is no attentiveness, the items in the sensory register decay after a few seconds, or else they are transferred into the short-term store. From here they can pass into the long-term store, provided they are repeated or rehearsed. Only material that is refreshed deliberately (by conscious practice) or spontaneously (because it recurs frequently or is important for the individual), enters the long-term store after it has been 'encoded' in a suitable manner.

Craik and Lockhart (1972) were able to show that the durability of storage in the long-term memory increases with increasing 'depth' of processing of the corresponding material. In experiments with incidental learning, it was found that words which had been classified by suitably instructed test subjects according to various criteria were remembered best when the subjects had paid attention to their actual meaning and not to other features (size of print, phonetic criteria). The so-called 'levels of processing' approach is attractive since it deals with unintentional, incidental learning as well as the rules of encoding as a prerequisite for storage in the long-term store. However, it does not lead to an extension of the storage models of memory.

From Tulving (1985) comes a differentiation of the contents in the long-term store, which are designated by the terms episodic, semantic and procedural. *Episodic memories* form the individual, autobiographic memory of events in our lives which have occurred at a specific time and in a specific place. *Semantic memory* refers to general knowledge, e.g. speech, understanding of terms, rules and connections, without the subject necessarily having been conscious of the occasions on which the corresponding memories were acquired. *Procedural memory* largely encompasses automatic, rather motor-type abilities and skills that are necessary in everyday life and which are applied without their details and rules necessarily being accessible to conscious reflection. As Parkin (1987) emphasizes, the differentiation between episodic, semantic and procedural parts of the long-term store is especially valuable in the study and evaluation of pathological memory disorders.

Newer models of memory are quite complex, which can be explained by the desire of their authors to include phenomena going beyond the traditional learning of meaningless syllables or word lists. In connection with psychopharmaceuticals there is the question of which model of memory should best be used to accommodate the experimental and clinical data available. As shown in the following sections, most cited studies have not been carried out on the basis of a uniform model of memory, but readily relate to the general temporal scheme of the learning and memory process presented in Chapter 3 (Fig. 3.2). It is therefore useful to distinguish between works in which the actions of substances on the acquisition, storage and retrieval processes were studied. The corresponding questions are:

- Can learning, i.e., the *acquisition* of new memory content, be positively or negatively influenced by drugs?
- Can the *storage* of memory material be affected by pharmacological agents?
- Can the *retrieval* of learned material be qualitatively or quantitatively modified by drugs?

The structure of this chapter follows again the classification of psychopharmaceuticals into neuroleptics, antidepressants, tranquillizers, etc. In addition, distinction is made between experiments in healthy subjects (if not already discussed in Chapter 3) and studies in patients taking the drug in question for therapeutic purposes. The last section of this chapter (7.6) deals with memory disorders in the elderly and the possibilities of treatment by pharmacological means. Alzheimer's disease stands at the centre here, and for some years has been researched particularly intensively.

This chapter concentrates on studies in humans, although it should be mentioned that animal experiments conducted in various species have over decades yielded a large amount of information on the subject of drugs and memory (reviews by Hunter *et al.*, 1977; Alpern and Jackson, 1978; Sanger *et al.*, 1992) and that the physiology and biochemistry of learning and memory processes represent vast fields of research in themselves (Squire, 1986; Thompson, 1986). Space does not allow us to discuss these aspects.

7.2   ACTIONS OF NEUROLEPTICS

7.2.1   Studies in healthy subjects

Although neuroleptics and notably those with initially highly sedating and sleep-inducing properties cause disturbances of attentiveness and performance in healthy subjects, there is no evidence that these medicines have a specific amnestic action (Chapter 3, Table 3.4). This experience obtained in single-dose experiments has been confirmed after the repeated administration of neuroleptics, e.g. as demonstrated by the following study by Liljequist *et al.* (1975).

Groups of 20 healthy subjects received the following treatment for two weeks:

- either the neuroleptic thioridazine at a dosage of 10 mg three times daily, rising to 20 mg three times daily in the second week;
- or the neuroleptic chlorpromazine at the same dosage.

Other groups of 20 subjects received sulpiride (a drug with mixed neuroleptic and antidepressant activities) or the tranquillizer bromazepam or placebo. After the two weeks of treatment, digit recall was tested as an indicator of short-term memory, and the learning of meaningless pairs of syllables was assessed. Neither of these test procedures revealed an action of the neuroleptics compared to placebo, so that the authors concluded that neither memory nor learning had been adversely affected by either of the two neuroleptics given at low doses. The result of the study is noteworthy in that 12 of 20 subjects given chlorpromazine and 10 of 20 subjects given thioridazine mentioned tiredness as a side effect and yet were able to solve the learning and memory tasks despite the sedation, which was considerable in some cases.

In another study in healthy subjects, single doses of 25 mg chlorpromazine also had no significant effect on learning and memory performance (Liljequist et al., 1978). However, since psychomotor performance tests also showed no impairment, the results of this and the previous experiment are not very relevant to a therapeutic situation in which doses 4–20 times larger are administered for some weeks. Mungas et al. (1990) administered single doses of 4 and 10 mg haloperidol to 49 healthy subjects and, 6 hours later, examined the effects of this large neuroleptic dose on verbal and spatial learning and memory performances. None of the parameters tested here was significantly altered, so that it could be concluded that typical neuroleptics over a broad range of doses have no influence on memory performances of healthy subjects.

7.2.2   Effects during therapeutic use

More recent clinically orientated textbooks of psychopharmacology (e.g. Baldessarini, 1985; Hinterhuber and Haring, 1992; Janicak et al., 1993) do not specifically address impairment of learning and memory functions during the therapeutic use of neuroleptics. Most authors consider that delirious states could occur principally in older patients with high doses of anticholinergic neuroleptics such as thioridazine and chlorpromazine, although there is no information on the incidence of such events. According to Davis and Casper (1978), the cognitive performance of schizophrenic patients usually improves during the course of neuroleptic treatment since the antipsychotic effect of these drugs more than compensates for their concomitant sedative action.

In a review article, Cassens et al. (1990) promote the view that the available literature contains no conclusive evidence of an adverse effect of neuroleptics on learning and memory functions of patients. On the other hand, the effects of anticholinergics, which are often administered together with neuroleptics, have been studied too little. In this connection a study by Perlick et al. (1986), which Cassens et al. did not cite, deserves to be mentioned: 17 hospitalized chronic schizophrenic patients aged 25–49 years (mean = 33 years) were studied to determine if there is a connection between performance in a battery of neuropsychological tests and the pharmacological actions of neuroleptics administered for some months. For this purpose, the plasma levels of the neuroleptics taken by these patients (five different products in individually adapted doses) were measured and recalculated as 'atropine equivalents' (as a measure of the anti-cholinergic action of the substances) and 'chlorpromazine equivalents' (as a measure of neuroleptic action). A significant negative correlation was found between the atropine equivalents and performance in the learning of a word list, suggesting a detrimental effect of the neuroleptics on certain learning per-formances. However, since all other correlations with learning and memory tasks were not significant, the authors concluded that the major memory func-tions in these patients had not been significantly affected by the administered neuroleptics. Nevertheless, in schizophrenic patients with disorders of attentive-ness and motivation, possible impairment by neuroleptics should be considered and the doses reduced whenever possible.

More recent studies, which will not be discussed in detail here, have to some extent provided contradictory results. Whereas Eitan *et al.* (1992) found that neuroleptics with anticholinergic activity, such as chlorpromazine and thioridazine, impair the short-term verbal memory of schizophrenic patients but that neuroleptics lacking anticholinergic action (haloperidol, trifluo-perazine) do not, Nigal *et al.* (1991) found that the performance of chronic schizophrenic patients as measured by a comprehensive battery of memory tests had deteriorated significantly four weeks after withdrawing combined neuroleptic and anticholinergic medication that had been given for some years. Cleghorn *et al.* (1990) showed that, depending on the test procedure used, the memory functions of schizophrenic patients either improved or remained unchanged during neuroleptic treatment. Finally, Goldberg *et al.* (1993) reported that 15 psychotic patients, including 13 schizophrenics, showed a marked clinical improvement after changing from conventional neuroleptics to the strongly anticholinergic clozapine, but that their perfor-mances in some memory tests tended to deteriorate.

Almost all the clinical studies mentioned here exhibit methodological de-fects with regard to the selection of patients, their allocation to the experi-mental and control groups, the separation of time effects and drug effects, and other relevant factors. However, in total they allow it to be concluded that neuroleptics at usual therapeutic doses have no pronounced effects on the learning and memory performances of schizophrenic patients and that any action of certain drugs on memory is of rather subordinate relevance com-pared to their other beneficial or adverse effects within the context of the therapy of schizophrenic psychoses.

7.3   EFFECTS OF ANTIDEPRESSANTS

7.3.1   Studies in healthy subjects

Antidepressants differ from one another in two areas of activity which may be of relevance to learning and memory: their varying degrees of sedative action and their anticholinergic effects. Impairment of memory as part of the general impairment of performance after using sedative products would not be surprising, and effects of this type would be classed as non-specific. On the other hand, impairment of learning and memory performance after using anticholinergically active antidepressants would be considered specific if it were not accompanied by general sedation. Several so-called conventional antidepressants have both sedative and anticholinergic activities, so that separation of specific and nonspecific effects on memory is hardly possible in this case.

The selection of experimental study results summarized in Table 3.5 of Chapter 3 reveals no evidence of specific effects of antidepressants on mnestic functions in healthy subjects: impairment of learning and memory performances are mainly found with sedating substances such as amitriptyline. In independent reviews, Deptula and Pomara (1990), Thompson (1991) and Curran (1992a) presented similar conclusions and stressed the close connection between general sedative activity and impairment of memory by some antidepressants in healthy subjects. It has occasionally been reported that the memory-impairing action of the antidepressant amitriptyline goes beyond what would be expected on the basis of its sedative action alone (Curran *et al.*, 1988); this is perhaps an expression of the central anticholinergic activity of amitriptyline. Such a view is supported by the observation that the drug's sedative action is subject to faster habituation than its effect on memory (Sakulsripong *et al.*, 1991).

It must be emphasized, however, that these results from studies in healthy subjects are mainly of theoretical interest, whereas the clinical relevance of any memory-impairing activities of antidepressant drugs can be estimated only in therapeutically orientated trials in patients.

7.3.2   Effects during therapeutic use

Older antidepressants such as imipramine and amitriptyline have peripheral and central anticholinergic effects, so that disturbances of attention and memory would be expected during the clinical use of these drugs. However, clinically orientated textbooks on psychopharmacology (see above) hardly mention any specific amnestic actions of antidepressants. States of confusion and delirium as side effects of some thymoleptics are known and often quoted; Hollister (1978) found these in 10–15% of cases, rising to 35% and more in patients aged over 40. States of confusion during treatment with antidepressants are mostly due to excessively high doses and disappear after withdrawing the drug or reducing the dose. Schatzberg *et al.* (1978) reported a symptom occasionally observed in patients receiving antidepressants, to which they gave the term *speech blockage*: patients had difficulty in finding the next logically following thought in a discussion or in expressing an idea in words. The appropriate word would occur to them after a pause of 1–3 seconds, but the unaccustomed interruptions in thought and speech processes often caused anxiety and worry. In the authors' views, speech blockage is more frequent in patients over 40 years old, and results from the central anticholinergic action of certain thymoleptics. The symptom disappeared completely when the dosage was reduced.

Branconnier *et al.* (1987) experimentally studied further the phenomenon of speech blockage after antidepressants. From a sample of 48 patients with major depressive disorders they formed three age groups: young (18–33 years), middle-aged (34–54 years) and elderly (55–78 years). After a medication-free period of one week with placebo, half the patients in each age group received the sedating and anticholinergic antidepressant amitriptyline as a single dose of 50 mg, and the other patients received the sedating but less anticholinergic product maprotiline. Two speech-orientated memory tests were applied about 3.5 hours after administration: the selective reminding paradigm of Buschke (1973) and the naming of words with a given initial letter (word fluency).

In both tests the elderly patients showed considerable impairment of performance after amitriptyline which, compared with the corresponding group given maprotiline, amounted to about 50% in the Buschke test and about 20% in the word fluency test. In the other patients, especially those of the middle-aged group, the differences between the compounds were small, so that the authors spoke of an age threshold effect: patients over 55–60 years are said to be particularly sensitive to the amnestic actions of an anticholinergic antidepressant such as amitriptyline. (It should be emphasized that this interpretation strictly applies only to single doses of 50 mg amitriptyline and patients previously treated with placebo for one week. However, in clinical practice it is usual to build up treatment with small or single doses in elderly patients.)

Complaints of memory disturbances or poor memory are common among depressed patients, especially if elderly, even though they cannot always be substantiated objectively, i.e., confirmed by use of memory tests (Weingartner and Silberman, 1982; O'Hara *et al.*, 1986). Memory disorders in depressed patients are seen as an expression of the 'altered motivation state' of these patients and thus generally regress as a depressive episode disappears. Antidepressants can therefore have direct and indirect actions on the memory of depressed patients: direct in the sense of a direct pharmacological action on learning and memory performance, and indirect as a result of the resolution of the depressive mood. Borrowing from Curran (1992a), this connection can be represented schematically as shown in Fig. 7.1.

Since antidepressants lead to the resolution of depressive phases on the one hand and may have sedative and anticholinergic actions on the other hand, the question of practical importance arises as to whether the use of specific compounds is associated with an improvement in depressive memory dysfunction or, in contrast, an additional deterioration. An older study by Sternberg and Jarvik (1976) provides a partial answer for the two classical antidepressants imipramine and amitriptyline.

The authors studied 26 patients with endogenous depression and 26 healthy subjects matched for age, sex and education (age data and sex distribution not

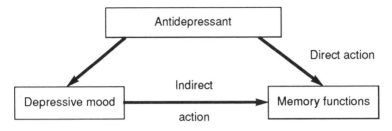

Figure 7.1. Direct (inhibitory) and indirect (facilitatory) effects of antidepressants on memory functions (Curran, 1992a)

reported). The patients were in hospital for the first time and had not yet received any antidepressants at the time of the first examination in the trial. The following tests were performed on the patients and subjects:

– learning of 15 weakly associated pairs of words;
– recognition of 15 drawings of familiar objects among 30 drawings;
– association of three portraits with three fictitious descriptions of people.

The test results before the start of drug therapy are presented in Figure 7.2. It is clear that the depressed patients were inferior to the healthy subjects in learning word pairs and in linking portraits with imaginary descriptions of people (left half of Fig. 7.2) but that the differences between the two groups were significantly reduced when the tests were repeated 3 hours later. The authors interpret this as evidence that immediate memory but not the ability to retain learned material was disturbed in the depressed patients. The patients were then treated with antidepressants, either imipramine or amitriptyline, at doses of 150–300 mg per day. The therapeutic results were evaluated four weeks later on the basis of observations made by the nursing staff and the patients' self-ratings. These results were:

Cured	4 patients (Group A)
Considerably improved	8 patients (Group B)
Moderately improved	8 patients (Group C)
No noticeable improvement	6 patients

The tests were then repeated at this time with the 20 clinically improved patients as well as with some of the healthy volunteers in order to compensate for any training effect. The patients showed a highly significant improvement in performance in all tasks involving immediate recall after presentation as compared to the values recorded four weeks earlier. In contrast, their memory performance 3 hours after presentation (which even before the start of therapy did not differ much from that of the reference group) showed hardly any improvement. There was a quantitative correlation between the improvement in clinical state and the improvement in memory since memory was improved most markedly in groups A and B.

These results are noteworthy since they stem from an attempt to assess the memory disturbances often mentioned by depressed patients in an objective way – an attempt which was successful for immediate memory but not for memory performance 3 hours later. Another interesting point is the effect of the drug treatment: imipramine and amitriptyline led to clinical improvement in the majority of patients which, despite the known anticholinergic effects of both antidepressants, was accompanied four weeks later by an improvement in memory also.

The findings of this early study have now been supplemented and partially confirmed by results obtained with other antidepressants (see reviews by Deptula and Pomara, 1990; Thompson, 1991; Curran, 1992a). Two other studies from the 1980s should also be mentioned briefly here.

Glass *et al.* (1981) studied a group of 32 outpatients with moderately severe to severe 'primary depression', i.e., depression not attributable to other illnesses. At the start of the study the patients showed significantly weaker performance in a recognition task than a reference group of non-depressed subjects. Their performance then improved by about 38% during treatment

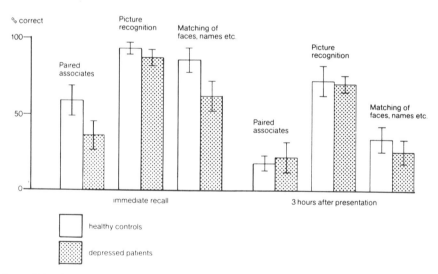

Figure 7.2. Learning and memory performance in depressive patients and in healthy controls. Three tasks yielded significant ($p < 0.05$ for recognition of drawings) and highly significant ($p < 0.001$ for learning of word pairs and association of personal details with the portraits of imaginary persons) differences between depressives and healthy subjects, when recall was tested immediately after presentation. Three hours later the differences between the two groups had disappeared, indicating impaired short-term memory (or anxiety about the experiment?), but not impairment of long-term memory in depressive patients (drawn after results given in Sternberg and Jarvik, 1976; $\bar{x} \pm$ s.d.)

with imipramine at 150 mg per day. Interestingly, the beneficial effect of the antidepressant on memory was obtained even though the clinical state of the patients as evaluated by rating scales had not changed significantly. Glass *et al.* interpreted their results as evidence that certain memory functions in depressed patients can improve independently of clinical status; on the other hand the study confirmed that, when administered at suitable dosages, antidepressants with anticholinergic activity do not lead to impairment of memory functions.

In a comparative study between the anticholinergic antidepressant amitriptyline and the non-anticholinergic selective serotinin reuptake inhibitor (SSRI) clovoxamine, Lamping *et al.* (1984) found a slight impairment of the patients in a word recognition test during amitriptyline treatment. Other learning and memory tests showed no differences between the two groups but to some extent reflected ceiling effects and were thus too simple for these subjects. It should also be noted that 11 of the original 21 patients given clovoxamine and seven of the 19 patients given amitriptyline dropped out during the course of treatment, mostly due to drug side effects, so that the generalizability of the study is greatly restricted.

There is evidence from various studies that depressed patients become accustomed after a few days or weeks to the sedative activity that is typical of some antidepressants. Consequently, massive impairment of attentiveness and memory as a result of antidepressant administration need not be expected in depressed patients under about 50 years of age. It remains to be seen whether this is also the case with the anticholinergic actions of drugs such as amitriptyline or imipramine; if the central anticholinergic effect of these products behaves in the same way as the peripheral one, then some mild impairment of memory functions not consistently detectable with psychological tests may be expected even after prolonged use (Meyers *et al.*, 1991). This present uncertainty should lead to corresponding caution in prescribing these drugs, especially in elderly patients, and may give cause to change to products lacking anticholinergic activity.

Lithium

A considerable number of clinical studies have been concerned with the question of whether lithium, which normally has to be administered for months or years, leads to detectable cognitive disturbance, particularly impairment of memory. The starting point for these studies was the observation that a proportion of patients treated with lithium complained of being mentally slower, less attentive and also more forgetful than they used to be.

In healthy subjects, lithium leads to slight psychomotor slowing which is also accompanied by a subjective feeling of impaired performance and learning capacity (Judd *et al.*, 1987), and which can last for several weeks.

Greil and Van Calker (1983) came to the conclusion in a review that the actions of lithium on cognitive functions, including memory, of patients on continuous treatment are slight – a view which also cannot be contradicted on the basis of more recent studies (Engelsmann *et al.*, 1988; Joffe *et al.*, 1988). However, a critical comment is that these are mostly 'empirical studies' which do not allow definitive conclusions. Measurements obtained before starting lithium treatment are presented in only a few cases; in addition, practically all the studies lack a control group not treated with lithium, with the consequence that a definitive evaluation of the observed effects is not possible. The opinion that lithium does not lead to serious cognitive impairments is primarily based on so-called clinical experience and on comparison of test results in lithium-treated patients with more or less reliable standard values in the corresponding tests.

Observations over 10 years and more have at any rate provided the comforting finding that, even after long-term treatment, lithium patients do not show memory disorders going beyond the expected age-related changes (Engelsmann *et al.*, 1988).

7.4 EFFECTS OF TRANQUILLIZERS

Tranquillizers and hypnotics of the benzodiazepine type (diazepam, oxazepam, lorazepam, nitrazepam, flurazepam and some newer substances) must represent the class of psychoactive drugs most studied in man. All benzodiazepine derivatives have dose-dependent sedative, myorelaxant and memory-impairing activities, and the question arose early on as to whether the effect on memory is part of the general sedative action or should be considered as a specific action of these drugs. If it is a specific effect, it would therefore arise even with low and possibly subtherapeutic doses, but if it is a non-specific effect it could at least be avoided by careful individual dosage adjustment. Another question concerns the duration of the memory-impairing activity of benzodiazepines during therapeutic use: does this effect diminish after a few days in the same way as the sedation, or are learning and memory impairments to be expected even after weeks or months of chronic administration?

7.4.1 Studies in healthy subjects

The fact that a single administration of benzodiazepine derivatives could have marked amnestic effects was first recognized in anaesthesiology, where these drugs are used to relax and sedate patients prior to surgery. It was found that after surgery and on waking from anaesthesia, patients had generally forgotten all events occurring between the benzodiazepine premedication and the operation. George and Dundee (1977) reported on a systematic study of this phenomenon.

The authors gave various *benzodiazepines* intravenously to groups of between 10 and 20 female patients immediately before they underwent minor surgery, in order to achieve preoperative sedation. The drugs used were diazepam (10 and 20 mg), flunitrazepam (1 and 2 mg) and lorazepam (4 mg). After injection of the medicament, each patient was shown 10 pictures at fixed intervals, the content of which they had to name, whilst the nurse showing the pictures simultaneously noted the degree of sleepiness. Later, 6 hours after the operation, when the patients had recovered, they were asked which pictures they remembered (free recall) and were subsequently shown 20 pictures from which those previously shown had to be selected (recognition). The experiment yielded the following results. (1) Some amnesia occurred after all three medicaments, although there were pronounced differences between the three preparations with regard to the time of onset of action, peak effect and duration of action. For example: the amnestic effect of diazepam occurred as soon as 1 minute after injection, but had abated completely 60 minutes later. (2) There was a close relationship between the extent of the memory impairment for a specific picture and the degree of sleepiness recorded by the nurse at the time when this picture had been presented. (3) No patient suffered total amnesia for the entire period of the investigation and recognition performance was always superior to free recall.

This clinical experiment, which has since been confirmed by many similar studies, permits the following interpretation: intravenous (as well as high-dose oral) doses of benzodiazepines cause pronounced sleepiness and eventually induce sleep. Despite the marked sedation, the patients were able to perceive and correctly name pictures shown to them before anaesthesia but later, after the effect of the substance has disappeared, had only a limited ability to remember the pictures. Accordingly, when given before the acquisition phase, benzodiazepines impair the consolidation of new material, the transition from a short-term to a long-term store. The impairment concerns not only visually presented learning stimuli but also words and other materials (Lister, 1985). The action of benzodiazepines in the acquisition phase is dose-dependent (Ghoneim *et al.*, 1984a,b) and, as shown by the experiment of George and Dundee (1977), has a different duration with different compounds, i.e., is related to the biological half-life of the drug in question.

As these studies show, benzodiazepines can induce *anterograde amnesia*; i.e., they impair the new data acquisition or registration phase in the information processing scheme reported on p. 61. If this scheme is followed further to the right, the question arises as to whether, if administered after the registration phase, benzodiazepines can also affect the encoding process, i.e., the phase of further processing of new information and its linking with existing memory. This phenomenon, called *retrograde amnesia*, is not known for benzodiazepines according to all available study results (Curran, 1991): information acquired before administration of these drugs remains available even at a later date.

It must again be noted that the temporal relationships in the recording and processing of new information and their precise correlation with the administration and action of drugs are complex and that many results obtained in experiments performed under circumscribed laboratory conditions may be far removed from the realities of the clinical use of the tranquillizers. Despite these restrictions, a series of experiments performed by Hinrichs *et al.* (1984) are of interest since they describe a seemingly paradoxical *retrograde improvement* of memory (retrograde facilitation) after a tranquillizer. In these experiments, male and female students were treated with a rather high dose of diazepam (0.3 mg/kg) or placebo and had to learn word lists of various difficulties presented to them at various times before and after medication. The following observations were made:

(1) When diazepam was administered *after* learning the word lists, it promoted the later remembrance of the learned words; in the experiment performed by Hinrichs *et al.*, almost twice as many words were remembered correctly compared to placebo.
(2) Retrograde facilitation could be demonstrated only when diazepam was administered after learning the first word list and before learning a second word list. If a second list was not presented, there was no retrograde facilitation of learning.
(3) The word lists presented in the second phase, i.e., after administration of diazepam, were learned significantly less well, which thus demonstrated the known anterograde amnestic effect of benzodiazepine.

The authors interpreted these results in the sense of the so-called *interference hypothesis*: according to this, 'improved recall of predrug information is not the result of any direct facilitating effect of diazepam but is a consequence of reduced learning of information presented after the drug takes effect. The reduced learning (of the later material) causes less interference with and therefore less forgetting of the material learned before the drug becomes effective' (Hinrichs *et al.*, 1984, p. 161). This interpretation explains the seemingly paradoxical improvement of memory performance after high doses of diazepam (see Fig. 7.3) and also agrees with the interpretation of similar experiments performed with alcohol (Parker *et al.*, 1981; Mueller *et al.*, 1983).

It emerges clearly from the foregoing that benzodiazepines can lead to anterograde but not retrograde amnesia, but that the question of specificity of action has not been answered. Curran (1991) referred to some of the methodological difficulties encountered in attempts to separate the general sedative action from the possibly specific amnestic action of a substance, but nevertheless came to the conclusion on the basis of her own work and numerous studies by other authors that the amnestic activity of benzodiazepines cannot be completely explained by their sedative effects (see also Kirk *et al.*, 1990). In addition, it has been established that different types of learning and memory performances are not affected in the same way by benzodiazepines: episodic memory is affected more than semantic memory, and voluntary cognitive processes more than automatic processes, whereas the learning of skills and procedures is hardly affected by benzodiazepines. On the other hand,

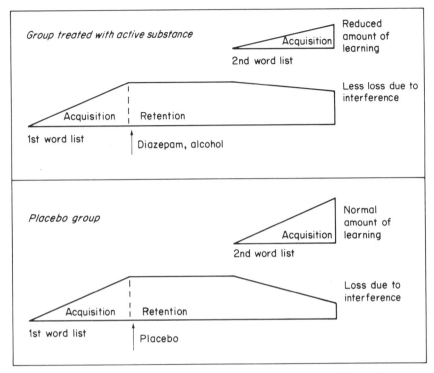

Figure 7.3. Protection of learned material against interference. Schematic representation of the interference hypothesis: the first word list is learned equally well by the subjects of the substance and placebo groups, and consolidation and retention are equal after the administration of active substance and placebo (arrows). Differences arise in the phase in which a second word list has to be learned: after administration of the active substance, the second list is learned less well (anterograde amnesia) but the first word list is retained better (retrograde facilitation) since, according to the hypothesis, the substance effect protects it against interference by the second list

different benzodiazepine derivatives seem to differ in their relative amnestic potencies, and the fact that time–effect relationships differ greatly from one substance to another complicates the experimental comparison of several aspects of their activity. After weighing up this and other points of view, King (1992) came to the conclusion that the amnestic action of benzodiazepines could be primarily explained by their effects on attentiveness and on rehearsal ability; however, it is not possible to attribute this entirely to the general sedative action of these drugs.

7.4.2   Effects during therapeutic use

On the basis of an analysis of the available literature, Taylor and Tinklenberg (1987) established that, like their general sedative effects, the amnestic activity of benzodiazepines undergoes rapid habituation after repeated administration. In the case of tranquillizers, this statement is based almost exclusively on clinical impressions and on studies in healthy subjects; only some benzodiazepine hypnotics have been examined in a significant number of controlled trials with relevant patients.

Tranquillizers

One of the few controlled clinical studies with tranquillizers (Lucki *et al.*, 1986) shows that, even with years of administration of benzodiazepines in medium to large doses, each additional individual dose can lead to mild anterograde amnesia. Although habituation to the sedative effects of benzodiazepines develops in various areas of performance, this is apparently not the case with regard to memory performance.

Golombok *et al.* (1988) performed a retrospective study that is of interest in this context: in long-term consumers of benzodiazepines (more than one year), they revealed a negative correlation between the cumulative dose of medicine over one year and the performance in some attention and learning tests. The higher the cumulative tranquillizer dose, the poorer the performance. On the other hand, Curran (1992b) established in a study of long-term benzodiazepine consumers (seven months to 28 years!) that an individually adjusted normal daily dose had no detectable influence on most aspects of performance, including learning and memory tests. The only exception was a two-stage word pair associations test, in which enhanced 'proactive interference' was seen after taking tranquillizers.

After analysing various studies, Curran came to the conclusion 'that the repeated use of benzodiazepines over weeks does not lead to tolerance of episodic memory impairments' (1991, p. 6), whereas King, in a review article published almost at the same time, took the view that with regard to habituation the amnestic action of benzodiazepines lies between the general sedative action (rapid habituation) and the anxiolytic action (no habituation) (1992, p. 84).

Hypnotics

In contrast to tranquillizers, benzodiazepine hypnotics also appear, even after prolonged use, to lead to clearly detectable impairment of memory on the following day. This is illustrated by the following observations:

A study by Linnoila and Viukari (1976) involving 20 patients in a psychogeriatric unit receiving 25 mg thioridazine, 10 mg nitrazepam or placebo in the evening as a hypnotic for a period of two weeks each, found both active substances to have an approximately equal sleep-promoting effect; however, although nitrazepam produced more frequent and severe impairment in the patients the following morning, Whereas performance in a simple memory test after nitrazepam dropped in 12 of 20 cases and was improved in two cases, thioridazine was found to cause slight impairment in eight cases and improvement in four cases.

Nitrazepam is a benzodiazepine derivative with a rather long plasma half-life, and patients in a psychogeriatric ward may not be representative of the majority of long-term consumers of hypnotics. It is all the more striking that an amnestic effect on the morning after an evening dose could also be detected in healthy subjects and in young and middle-aged insomniacs given midazolam and triazolam, two benzodiazepines with short or very short plasma half-lives (Bixler *et al.*, 1991; Borbély *et al.*, 1988; Weingartner *et al.*, 1992). There has been controversy for some years regarding whether some benzodiazepines may, perhaps as a result of particularly high affinity for specific benzodiazepine subreceptors, be able to induce greater disturbances of memory than others, or whether the pharmacokinetic features of the individual products are responsible for the specific effects (Ghoneim and Mewaldt, 1990). In any event, complete disappearance of the amnestic effect of benzodiazepine hypnotics after repeated administration cannot be expected, and impairment of memory can occur particularly in elderly insomniacs even after presumably small doses (Pomara *et al.*, 1989).

7.4.3 Commentary

A number of questions arising in connection with the administration of benzodiazepines still remain unanswered: why do products with a short plasma half-life have prolonged effects on memory whereas other benzodiazepines which form long-lived and pharmacologically active metabolites do not exhibit the corresponding effects? Why can the sedative–hypnotic actions of benzodiazepines be abolished with benzodiazepine antagonists but the amnestic effects of these drugs are at least partially resistant to antagonists (Ghoneim, 1992)? What are the consequences of benzodiazepines' actions on memory when the patient is receiving concomitant psychotherapy, i.e., has to learn new behaviours and cognitive patterns? Despite extensive research during the last 30 years, our knowledge in this area of psychopharmacology remains patchy and ought to be improved by further systematic studies, if feasible under real-life conditions.

7.5 EFFECTS OF PSYCHOSTIMULANTS AND NOOTROPICS

Whereas impairment of learning and memory functions may occur after the use of neuroleptics, of sedative and anticholinergic antidepressants, tranquillizers and hypnotics, an improvement in memory is rather to be expected after the use of medicines which increase performance and attentiveness, such as psychostimulants and perhaps also nootropics. As will be seen below, however, this expectation is not fulfilled in all cases.

7.5.1 Studies in healthy subjects

In an often quoted early study, Hurst *et al.* (1969) investigated whether the psychostimulant *d*-amphetamine promoted pair-association learning in the immediate or longer term. To this purpose, four groups of 17–18 students each received the following treatments under double-blind conditions:

	1st day of experiment	*1 week later*
Group 1	Placebo	Placebo
Group 2	Placebo	*d*-Amphetamine
Group 3	*d*-Amphetamine	Placebo
Group 4	*d*-Amphetamine	*d*-Amphetamine

The oral dosage of amphetamine given was 14 mg per 70 kg body weight; i.e., it was individually adjusted. The task involved was the learning off by heart of 12 lists each consisting of 14 pairs of words (paired associate learning) of differing degrees of difficulty. The experiments were conducted in the evenings and the learning tests were carried out between 80 and 175 minutes after administration of the medicaments.

Results: there were no significant differences between the groups receiving placebo on the first day of the experiment (groups 1 and 2) and the others which had been treated with amphetamine (groups 3 and 4), although acquisition in the case of the more difficult word lists (containing word pairs with a low association value) was somewhat improved after amphetamine. A distinct effect was, however, noticeable on the second day of the experiment, i.e., one week later. Here groups 3 and 4, which had received amphetamine on the first day, performed better: whereas their performance on the first day of the experiment had been only insignificantly better than it was in the subjects receiving placebo, they were, in the long-term, able to retain more word pairs. According to the authors' interpretation (Hurst *et al.*, 1969, p. 316), 'This finding is the opposite of what would be expected if amphetamines had no true learning effect, but acted instead to increase the performance potential at a given level of learning.'

This interpretation must, however, be countered with the following consideration: 14 mg per 70 kg body weight is a rather high amphetamine dose which, when given in the evening, would undoubtedly have led to sleep onset disorders. It is thus not unlikely that subjects, unable to sleep, relived the preceding experiment, in so doing intentionally or unintentionally rehearsing the word pairs, even if they did not know that the task would be repeated the following week. What is taken to be the favourable effect of amphetamine on long-term memory could therefore be a consequence of the waking effect of the preparation. An experiment involving methylphenidate and published by Kupietz *et al.* (1980) is more conclusive in this regard.

Nine healthy volunteers were given the task of learning to read Chinese characters (a form of paired associate learning), two different teaching methods being used. At each test session two lists of 12 words each were learned: one list with the aid of an easier, the other using a harder method. On each day of the experiment the two sessions took place 5 hours apart: one under the influence of 5 mg or 10 mg methylphenidate, the other using a placebo in both cases. The experiment lasted two days. Learning conditions, sequence of the administrations and doses were balanced. In the case of both teaching methods, performance was better under the influence of the active substance, although the difference was only significant in the case of the 5 mg dose and only for the harder method. In contrast to the study by Hurst *et al.* (1969) no attempt was made to show whether the improvement in learning success with methylphenidate was of any duration.

From the two experiments it can be seen that psychostimulants such as *d*-amphetamine and methylphenidate provide a slight *enhancement of acquisition performance* if administered before the registration phase (point 1 in the scheme of p. 61).

The study by Hurst *et al.* (1969) also examined whether the subjects who received *d*-amphetamine on the second day (groups 2 and 4) could reproduce better a list of word pairs learned one week previously and/or could then relearn it faster than those given placebo on the second day of the experiment (groups 1 and 3). However, reproduction was not improved after the psychostimulant, so that an effect of the substance on retrieval or reproduction (point 4 in the scheme on p. 61) was not detected. On the other hand, a slight but not statistically significant improvement in relearning was found, i.e., partial confirmation of the *effect on acquisition performance* seen in groups 3 and 4 on the first day of the experiment.

As mentioned above, the beneficial action of psychostimulants on learning and memory performance can be seen as a consequence of the improved attentiveness on this medication. On the other hand, no improvement in memory was found in healthy subjects given nootropics (see p. 74 f.).

A phenomenon which has attracted much interest for some years in relation to psychostimulants is known as *state-dependent learning (SDL)*. In SDL, which can be considered a special case of context-dependent learning and memory, the question is whether any material learned under specific conditions (e.g. under the influence of a drug) can be recalled under other conditions just as well as under the original conditions. SDL is discussed extensively in reviews by Overton (1968) and by Weingartner (1978), although the best-known experiments were performed with alcohol and nicotine rather than psychostimulants.

Goodwin *et al.* (1969) gave the following treatments to four groups of 12 students each on two successive days:

	Day 1	Day 2	
Group 1	Alcohol	Placebo	Dissociated
Group 2	Alcohol	Alcohol	conditions
Group 3	Placebo	Alcohol	Congruent
Group 4	Placebo	Placebo	conditions

The alcohol was presented in the form of a single dose of vodka which led to blood levels of between 0.8 and 1.4% alcohol. Forty minutes after the subjects had consumed the vodka or placebo beverages they were confronted with several learning and memory tests. These were carried out again the following day, under congruent treatment conditions in two groups (given the same beverage as on the previous day) and under dissociated conditions in the other two groups.

Results: on the first day of the experiment learning performance in groups 1 and 2, both of which had received alcohol, was significantly worse in two test tasks (an avoidance learning task, learning short sentences off by heart) and there was no difference in two other tests. On the second day of the experiment the volunteers in group 1, participating under dissociated conditions, learned a new avoidance task more quickly than the other subjects, whilst making more mistakes in learning short sentences off by heart. The authors interpreted these results in the context of state-dependent learning (the dissociated state facilitates learning of new arrangements in avoidance learning whilst impairing recall of learned verbal combinations) – an interpretation which is not entirely convincing in view of the non-uniform findings in the four tests used and the only just significant results in two tasks.

The second experiment to be described here may be of practical importance to smokers (Peters and McGee, 1982): four groups each composed of 14 habitual smokers received one of the following four combinations of treatments on two successive days: H–H; H–L; L–L; L–H (H = cigarette with high (1.4 mg) nicotine content; L = cigarette with low (0.2 mg) nicotine content). After the subjects had smoked the appropriate cigarettes on the first day they were shown a list of 15 words which they subsequently had to write down from memory. Memory performance (immediate recall) was similar for all four groups. On the second day the same list of words had to be reproduced after the appropriate cigarette had been smoked. Whilst there were no differences in groups H–H and L–L, performance in group L–H was slightly, and that in group H–L clearly and statistically significantly, diminished. Words which had been learned under the effect of a normal cigarette were thus less well reproduced after the low nicotine cigarette had been smoked. The difference from the H–H and L–L groups was over 30%!

In their experiment with *d*-amphetamine discussed on p. 200 f., Hurst *et al.* (1969) also analysed the findings with regard to the SDL phenomenon, but found no evidence that the two groups of subjects working under dissociated conditions on the second day of the experiment (groups 2 and 3) had worse performance than the other two groups. As these and other examples (see Spiegel 1989, p. 177 ff.) show, the experimental evidence for the occurrence and relevance of SDL after the use of psychostimulants is inconclusive.

7.5.2   Effects during therapeutic use

The acquisition and retention of new memory material is promoted by psychostimulants in hyperactive children (ADHD, see p. 22). Since the behavioural disorders of these children are assumed to be based on impaired attentiveness, the beneficial action of amphetamine and similar drugs on learning and memory may be seen as an indirect effect in the sense stated by Curran (1992a), i.e., a consequence of the improved attentiveness following the use of psychostimulants.

Psychostimulants are administered chronically in the therapy of ADHD. This raises the question of the possible consequences of state-dependent learning: in ADHD children given methylphenidate and similar drugs, is there a risk that the newly acquired and desirable behaviour patterns, scholastic knowledge and practical skills will no longer be available to them after withdrawal of their medication? Two older controlled trials can be examined with regard to this question.

Aman and Sprague (1974) treated 18 hyperactive children, having an average age of 8, in one of three different ways: 0.2 mg/kg d-amphetamine, 0.5–1.0 mg/kg methylphenidate, or placebo, 75 minutes in each case before commencement of the tests. All the subjects received all the treatments at 48-hour intervals. Functions tested were the recognition of pictures, the association of pictures and numbers (paired associates) and the learning off by heart of a path through a maze. The questions studied were whether the acquisition and retention of learned material was influenced by the two stimulants and whether performance was inferior under dissociated drug conditions than under congruent conditions. The answer to all three questions was a negative one since neither acquisition nor retention was improved after the stimulants and since there were no signs of a drop in performance under dissociated drug conditions.

Swanson and Kinsbourne (1976) conducted an experiment involving 48 children with a mean age of 10.5 years; they included 32 ADHD children and a control group of 16 children without ADHD. In the course of this experiment 10–20 mg methylphenidate or placebo were given on two successive days, the design of the trial (2 × 2) corresponding to that frequently used in connection with state-dependent learning. During the test the children were given the task of relating 48 animal pictures with four names of towns (paired associates). In each case the tests commenced 60 minutes after intake of the medicaments. Results were as follows:

(1) In the case of the hyperactive children there was a pronounced and statistically significant improvement in performance after methylphenidate on both the first and second day of the experiment: the number of errors until correct arrangement of pictures and towns was reduced on average by 25% on the first day and by 35–40% on the second day, as compared to placebo.
(2) In the case of the normal children, the reverse trend was apparent, i.e., they tended to learn relate the pictures and names less well after the psychostimulant.
(3) Under congruent drug conditions, the learning performance of the hyperactive children was significantly better on the second day than under

dissociated conditions – a result which may be interpreted in the sense of state-dependent learning.

(4) In the case of the normal children there was no significant difference in learning performance between congruent and dissociated drug conditions.

Here two experiments which were similar in respect of patient selection, nature and dose of the medicament and test method, whilst differing as to sample size and experimental design, led to opposite results. In the experiment by Aman and Sprague no significant effect was observed even in the acquisition phase after the psychostimulants, whereas Swanson and Kinsbourne found clear improvements in learning performance of the ADHD children after methylphenidate. State-dependent learning was only encountered in the second study, in which improvements in learning performance had also been observed with the stimulant. In the commentary on their study, Aman and Sprague postulated that, when given in doses which do not lead to pronounced alterations in consciousness, psychopharmaceuticals do not cause any dissociated state and consequently cannot give rise to state-dependent learning. Similarly, Swanson and Kinsbourne pointed out that state-dependent learning could only be observed when a significant pharmacological effect – be it positive or negative – occurred in the acquisition and reacquisition phase. The studies listed in Section 7.5.1, as well as a further experiment using methylphenidate (10 mg b.i.d. for two days) in hyperactive children (Steinhausen and Kreuzer, 1981), do conform with this generalization and yet one cannot understand why virtually the same doses of methylphenidate had no effect on learning in ADHD children when given by Aman and Sprague, whilst clearly promoting learning and relearning and leading to state-dependent learning in the study published by Swanson and Kinsbourne.

What practical consequences can emerge out of these results? In contrast to the experimental situation wherein individual performances are investigated in isolation from an everyday context, an individual does not normally learn in isolation, but by linking new material personally and biographically and, when important material or experiences are involved, by rehearsing these consciously or unconsciously. These are all factors which are thought to act against state-dependent learning (see Overton, 1968). However, the question still to be answered is the extent to which experiences acquired in the course of treatment with a psychopharmaceutical can be transferred to a subsequent, medicament-free condition.

7.6 DRUGS FOR THE TREATMENT OF DEMENTIA

7.6.1 Changes in cognitive functions in the elderly

Some decrease in memory performances with advancing age is considered to be 'normal'. Older people are thought of as being forgetful: they repeat the same story over and over again, keep asking the same question, mislay things they use every day, go out and forget what they wanted to do. These lapses are not isolated but are part of a change which occurs in the sensory, motor and cognitive faculties of people as they age: accuracy and speed of sensory perception and of voluntary motor activity diminish, and attentiveness, interests and motivation change during the course of life. Many of these functions are directly or indirectly associated with learning and memory processes, and the manner in which an individual copes with the changes in cognitive faculties that come with old age will also co-determine learning and memory performance.

However, ageing is not related to a general decline in intellectual abilities. There are losses in those areas which are directly dependent on intact sensory abilities, and it is also known that older persons tend to encounter difficulties when called upon to perform cognitive and other tests under pressure of time. The subjective significance of a task and familiarity with the test conditions are further factors which assume greater importance in older persons than in the young. It should be noted here that so-called cross-sectional studies demonstrate greater age-related changes in the cognitive sphere than longitudinal studies. In cross-sectional studies, subjects from different age groups are compared with each other at a given point in time, whereas in longitudinal studies the same population is studied repeatedly over a number of years or decades in order to document the actual effect of ageing (Schaie, 1983). Cross-sectional studies, which have produced most of the data and generalizations on ageing and memory, involve the risk that differences between different generations of subjects will be interpreted as effects of age (so-called cohort effects).

In a still relevant review of 'ageing and memory', Craik (1977) collated a large number of empirical studies and related them to a uniform model of memory processes. This involves three stages (sensory register, primary memory, secondary memory) and shows the following changes with age:

- *Sensory register:* Visual traces (icons) decay more rapidly with advancing age, and the same is true for the content of the (acoustic) echo memory. Age-related losses are particularly pronounced in situations calling for divided attention.
- *Primary memory:* The short-term retention of sequences of numbers, word lists, etc. is considered to reflect primary memory. The effects of age on primary memory are slight and can only be detected if the retentive capacity of this memory store is exceeded.
- *Secondary memory:* This faculty, also known as long-term memory (not to be confused with old memory), shows marked age-related losses (discussed extensively by Fleischmann, 1989). Craik and other authors attribute this decline in performance directly to the fact that older persons organize newly acquired information less efficiently and carry out more superficial encoding. There are no indications that material once acquired is lost more rapidly or that memory traces disintegrate faster in advanced age, and yet

older people are not as good as young people at effectively using the cue information when stored material is retrieved.

Over and above memory performance, the typical changes in cognitive functions occurring in advanced age can be summarized as follows (Craik and Salthouse, 1992):

- With age, the performance of the sensory organs and the speed of reactions decrease, especially in unaccustomed situations. Motor responses are also slower.
- Areas of performance which depend on experience and verbal functions show less marked or no decrease.
- Interindividual variation increases with increasing age in practically all cognitive areas examined, so that mean values are less representative of older groups than of younger ones, and the normal range is broader in older populations than in young subjects.
- Mental performance in older age depends on education and previous activities, and is additionally affected by the general state of health of the individual.

7.6.2 The dementia syndrome and Alzheimer's disease

When an elderly, physically sprightly person shows a generalized deterioration in cognitive functions which prevents him pursuing his usual activities in familiar surroundings, there is then the suspicion of incipient or possibly already advanced dementia. The term dementia signifies a 'global deterioration in all aspects of mental functioning, including memory, general intellect,

Table 7.1. DSM-III-R criteria for dementia[a]

A. Demonstrable impairment of short-term and long-term memory.
B. At least one of the following:
(1) Impairment in abstract thinking
(2) Impaired judgement
(3) Other disturbances of higher cortical function: aphasia, apraxia, agnosia, constructive apraxia
(4) Personality changes
C. The disturbance in A and B significantly interferes with work or usual social activities or relationships with others.
D. The disorders do not occur exclusively during the course of clouded consciousness (delirium).
E. Either (1) or (2):
(1) The case history, current status or laboratory data provide evidence of aetiologically related organic factors.
(2) The disorder is not attributable to non-organic mental illness, e.g. depression.

[a] See text.

emotional attributes and distinctive features of personality' (Roth, 1980). The term dementia has replaced older expressions such as chronic 'psycho-organic syndrome' (POS) or 'organic brain syndrome' (OBS). A diagnosis of dementia presumes the presence of several features according to DSM-III-R (APA, 1987) (Table 7.1) and DSM-IV (APA, 1994) which, in contrast to previous usage of the term, include neither the progression nor the irreversibility of the syndrome.

Dementias are very common in the very old: about 5% of all persons over 65 years and about 20% of all those aged 80 years are to be classed as demented (Henderson, 1986). According to Jorm *et al.* (1987), the number of dementias in the over 65s doubles for every five years or so of life. The DSM-III-R clinically divides dementias according to severity, which can be characterized as follows:

- *Mild dementia*: Although work or social activities are significantly impaired, the capacity for independent living remains, with adequate personal hygiene and relatively intact judgement.
- *Moderate dementia*: Independent living is hazardous, and some degree of supervision is necessary.
- *Severe dementia*: Activities of daily living are so impaired that continual supervision is required, e.g. unable to maintain minimal personal hygiene; largely incoherent or mute.

Assessment in methods which determine several fundamental mental functions (attention, orientation, memory, speech, understanding of speech, psychomotor functions) in a simple, practical way are recommended for the rough estimation of the severity of dementia. The best-known method is the Mini Mental Status (MMS, Folstein *et al.*, 1975), which allows the grading of dementia on a 30-point scale on the basis of a 5–10-minute examination. Other, rather more involved procedures include the Dementia Rating Scale of Mattis (1976) and the so-called Alzheimer Disease Assessment Scale (ADAS) of Rosen *et al.* (1984). Neuropsychological techniques are applied for a more precise description of the mental functions which are still retained and those which are impaired (Lezak, 1983; Weintraub and Mesulam, 1986).

A dementia syndrome may be caused by various underlying diseases which can be detected or excluded by extensive medical, neurological and psychiatric examinations (Fig. 7.4). The most common cause of dementia is Alzheimer's disease, but physical illnesses, endocrine disorders, dietary deficiencies and drug overdosage may also cause or aggravate dementia (see Kiloh, 1986; Mahendra, 1987).

Alzheimer's disease is a chronic, progressive and degenerative brain disease with a still not fully explained pathogenesis. It is macroscopically characterized by atrophy of the cerebral cortex which, at least in advanced stages, can be detected by computer-assisted tomography or magnetic resonance imaging (MRI). Plaques, neurofibrillary modifications (tangles), neuron loss and other abnormalities are observed as characteristic microscopic features

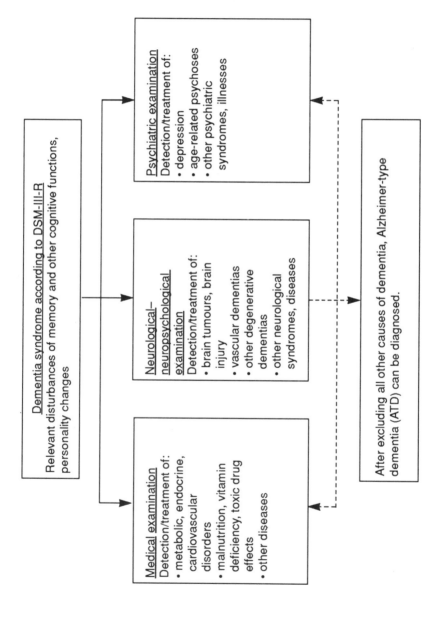

Figure 7.4. Transition from a syndrome diagnosis (dementia) to nosological diagnosis (Alzheimer-type dementia)

(Katzman, 1986). There is as yet no specific clinical, biochemical or neurological test for a diagnosis of Alzheimer's disease in the living patient, so that the diagnosis can strictly be made only by postmortem examination of the brain. As there is about 80–90% agreement between the clinical and postmortem diagnosis, most authors follow the advice of McKhann *et al.* (1984) and speak only of 'probable Alzheimer's disease' clinically, i.e., while the patient is alive. The terms DAT (dementia of the Alzheimer type) or ATD (Alzheimer-type dementia) are also often used.

Since plaques and in particular neurofibrillary tangles are quantitatively correlated with the severity of DAT, molecular biological and biochemical research has been directed over the past 10 years to the composition and possible genesis of these two neuropathological features of Alzheimer's disease (Murphy, 1992). The precursors and the intermediate steps leading to the material from which the plaques are mainly formed (so-called beta-amyloid) have been clarified, and some genetic factors which promote the excessive formation of beta-amyloid are also known (Rosenberg, 1993). Advances have been made in understanding the structure of the tangles and the pathway of their formation (Goedert *et al.*, 1992). On the other hand, however, there is fundamental uncertainty about the role of beta-amyloid and its precursors under normal and pathological conditions (Regland and Gottfries, 1992), so that prognoses regarding a causally orientated therapy of Alzheimer's disease vary greatly (Rossor, 1993).

7.6.3   The acetylcholine hypothesis of DAT

Some short-term advance in the drug therapy of DAT can be expected from the knowledge that the brains of DAT patients exhibit not only increased numbers of plaques and tangles but also marked disturbances of chemical neurotransmission. The noradrenergic, serotoninergic and other transmitter systems are affected, but the dysfunction is most pronounced in the cholinergic system (Bowen and Davison, 1986; Perry, 1987). This opens up the possibility of acting specifically on the appropriate neurotransmitter systems and in this way contributing to a functional improvement that should be expressed as a reduction in symptoms.

The *acetylcholine hypothesis of DAT*, sometimes also called the cholinergic hypothesis, has for years been the most popular mechanistic theory of Alzheimer's disease (Bartus *et al.*, 1982; Holttum and Gershon, 1992). It is based on data from extensive and in some cases old experimental, clinical, biochemical and neuropharmacological work demonstrating a close relationship between cholinergic neurotransmission and some mnestic functions.

1. *Experimental findings*: Cholinergic antagonists ('anticholinergics') such as as atropine and scopolamine cause dose-dependent disturbances of information intake and processing in healthy subjects, expressed as anterograde

amnesia (Petersen, 1977; Preston *et al.*, 1988). Practically all the actions of anticholinergics can be abolished by substances that increase acetylcholine supply to the synapses and thus restore cholinergic neurotransmission (Karczmar, 1979), so that the amnestic effects of scopolamine are also reversed (Mohs *et al.*, 1981; Preston *et al.*, 1989). Some authors have discussed the question of whether the actions of anticholinergics on memory functions are specific and thus whether they differ in nature and degree from the effects of benzodiazepines for example (Weingartner, 1985; Curran *et al.*, 1991). Also controversial is whether the activities of anticholinergics on learning and memory can be eliminated only by compounds with cholinergic action or also by compounds with other mechanisms of action. Finally, it has been contested whether the memory disturbances arising after scopolamine and similar substances are comparable to the cognitive losses observed in DAT patients, and thus whether the 'scopolamine syndrome' in healthy subjects is an appropriate experimental model for Alzheimer's disease (Holttum and Gershon, 1992). Despite all the limitations, the study of cognitive impairments which become apparent after scopolamine and similar drugs is of interest and supports a close connection between intact cerebral cholinergic processes and the ability to process and retain new information.

2. *Clinical biochemical data*: Bowen *et al.* and Davies and Maloney reported as long ago as 1976 that there is a marked decrease in indicators of cholinergic activity (so-called cholinergic markers) in the brains of patients who died while suffering from Alzheimer's disease. In the hippocampus (a brain structure essential, among others, for memory functions) and cerebral cortical areas there is a massive reduction in those enzymes required both for the formation and the breakdown of acetylcholine. The 'cholinergic deficit' in the brains of Alzheimer's patients has been confirmed in many studies, has been correlated with the degree of cognitive decline (Perry *et al.*, 1978), and has been delimited precisely in terms of cerebral anatomy (Price *et al.*, 1986), although always with evidence that not only the cholinergic but also other neurotransmitter pathways are severely disturbed and that the cholinergic deficit is probably a consequence of other disturbances (e.g. Harrison, 1986). This latter view has gained further support from new insights into the origin of plaques and tangles (Lamour, 1994). Nevertheless, further study of the cholinergic deficit in DAT as a possible site of action of substitutive therapy, especially in the early stage of the disease, is considered sensible (Gray *et al.*, 1989).

3. *Neuropharmacological data*: Since the postsynaptic elements of cholinergic neurotransmission in DAT appear to be less severely affected than the presynaptic side (the postsynaptic receptors are perhaps even hypersensitive; see Sunderland *et al.*, 1987), there are several possible approaches for substitutive cholinergic treatment of the disease:

– Increasing the supply of the biological precursors of acetylcholine, i.e., of lecithin or choline; this is analogous to the treatment of Parkinson's disease with L-dopa as a precursor of dopamine. This approach, tested in dozens of studies, has had no measurable effect at all on cognitive functions in DAT patients (review by Becker and Giacobini, 1988).

– Stimulation of postsynaptic cholinergic receptors by so-called cholinomimetics, i.e., compounds which can take over the function of acetylcholine at the synapse. Here also there is analogy with the treatment of Parkinson's disease with man-made dopaminomimetics such as bromocriptine (Poewe and Gerstenbrand, 1992). A conclusive appraisal of this approach cannot be given, but pilot studies with the muscarinic agonist RS 86 produced positive results in some individual cases only (Spiegel, 1991).

– Use of presynaptically active antagonists, i.e., substances which in theory, should produce increased synthesis in and release of acetylcholine from the presynaptic cholinergic neurons. This approach seems to have been left practically untested at present.

– Inhibition of the enzyme which breaks down the neurotransmitter acetylcholine (acetylcholinesterase, AChE) by so-called AChE inhibitors, which is analogous to the use of MAO inhibitors as antidepressants (Chapter 5). Known AChE inhibitors are physostigmine and tacrine.

After a long period of therapeutic studies with mostly negative results (see Becker and Giacobini, 1988), this last approach has attracted a new following thanks to a study by Summers *et al.* (1986). These authors described their spectacular therapeutic success with the AChE inhibitor tacrine in a group of 17 patients, some of whom had quite advanced DAT. The response to tacrine lasted for many months in some cases and allowed the patients to lead a socially integrated and satisfactory life. The study itself was subsequently criticized for methodological shortcomings and its thoroughly positive results could be confirmed only partially in larger and better controlled trials (Davis *et al.*, 1992; Farlow *et al.*, 1992). However, it had two important consequences with regard to therapeutic advance:

– Firstly, a pharmaceutical company took over the further development and clinical testing of tacrine, and after a period of five years was able to obtain a product licence (brand name Cognex®) from the American health authorities in 1993 and, subsequently, in other countries.

– Secondly, several pharmaceutical companies started searching for more effective and better-tolerated cholinergic substances. As we now know, tacrine acts to a clinically detectable degree only in a minority of DAT patients, and in addition is hepatotoxic in many cases at therapeutically active doses (Knapp *et al.*, 1994), so that much is left to be desired in relation to efficacy and safety. At present about 10 other cholinergic compounds, including AChE inhibitors with chemical structures unlike that of tacrine, are undergoing clinical testing and more precise information on the therapeutic potential of this pharmacological approach will therefore be available soon. There is particular interest in the question of whether AChE inhibitors and other cholinergic substances can have a beneficial effect on the course of DAT beyond their theoretically expected symptomatic effect, and thus whether a slowing of the generally progressive course of DAT can be expected (Lamy, 1994).

CHAPTER 8

Psychopharmaceuticals and the treatment of mental disorders

8.1 INTRODUCTION

In Chapter 1 of this book, psychopharmaceuticals were introduced as medicines which have a primarily symptomatic action but which are problematical
in several respects. Neuroleptics can cause serious side effects, antidepressants often exert their therapeutic effects only after a delay of weeks and in
many cases have unpleasant side effects. With tranquillizers, hypnotics and, in
particular, psychostimulants, there are problems with habituation and the
development of dependency, and nootropics have mostly not fulfilled the
therapeutic hopes placed in them. It is therefore not surprising that psychopharmaceuticals do not enjoy a very high reputation amongst many doctors
and the general public (see box), and have been given names such as 'chemical strait-jackets' for neuroleptics (Szasz, 1957) or 'chemical blinkers for the
mind' for tranquillizers. Elomaa (1993) even poses the question of whether
the long-term use of conventional neuroleptics to be considered a crime
against humanity.

A visit to a psychiatric hospital is also rarely suited to dispelling reserva-
tions about psychopharmaceuticals. Many of the patients wander around like
robots, their movements lack natural animation, their expressions are rigid,
they seem apathetic, cut off from their surroundings, stiff and sometimes
additionally handicapped by motor disorders. An encounter with a relative or
friend suffering from a mental illness and being treated with psychopharmaceuticals can be shocking and confusing, and the layperson is often not in a
position to evaluate whether the signs which they see and hear are expressions
of the illness being treated or effects of the administered medicines.

On the other hand, older nurses and doctors who lived through the period
before 1953/54 and then saw the introduction of modern psychopharmaceuticals can confirm the unprecedented therapeutic advances which these medicines have provided: how much suffering, anxiety and waste of human life
have been eliminated inside and outside of psychiatric hospitals. Relief and
sometimes elation, together with new therapeutic optimism, can also be detected in the early publications on the discovery of neuroleptics and antidepressants (see Chapter 2).

In the following paragraphs we will attempt to determine more precisely
the value and position of psychopharmaceuticals in the treatment of mental

---

The negative image of psychopharmaceuticals: a summary

(1) In hospitals, psychopharmaceuticals, especially neuroleptics, are used as a disciplinary measure: patients are forcibly subdued by means of medication. Medication is often used as a form of punishment for rebelliousness.

(2) Psychopharmaceuticals are employed for brainwashing: under the influence of psychopharmaceuticals the patients become indifferent, lose their own will, and adapt themselves to circumstances in an environment which is itself sick.

(3) Psychopharmaceuticals encourage 'revolving door' psychiatry: patients are often sent home as being 'cured' too soon and swiftly return to the clinic. As time goes by, they cease to believe in a cure and in themselves.

(4) Many doctors prescribe psychopharmaceuticals in order to get rid of difficult patients and so that they do not have to become more involved in the problems of their patients.

(5) For doctors and patients, psychopharmaceuticals are often the simplest way out of a difficult situation: they suppress a few acute symptoms, but do not lead to a permanent solution of the basic underlying problems.

---

disorders. This will be done on the basis of a literature survey referring, with few exceptions, to comparative studies between two or more forms of therapy. Historically, the following tendencies can be detected in this area of comparative therapeutic research:

– In the 1960s and early 1970s, the studies often related to the question of whether and in which particular therapeutic indications psychopharmaceuticals show superiority over placebo.
– At about the same time, studies were performed to determine whether psychopharmaceuticals or specific psychotherapeutic procedures produced better results in the treatment of mental disorders, especially schizophrenia and depression.
– In the last 15 years, interest has been primarily directed to the question of how psychopharmaceuticals and non-drug procedures relate to one another and how they can best be combined.

Problems of optimal dosage and duration of drug treatment for mental disorders have also been addressed in numerous controlled studies and are presented separately below for neuroleptics, antidepressants, tranquillizers and psychostimulants. This division again makes sense since the disorders treated and the therapeutic approaches used differ in significant features and since the empirical studies carried out in the individual indications show major qualitative and quantitative differences.

8.2 NEUROLEPTICS AND THE TREATMENT OF SCHIZOPHRENIA

8.2.1 Proof of efficacy

The efficacy of neuroleptics for the symptomatic treatment of schizophrenic psychoses is not disputed: a tranquillizing, emotion-subduing and anti-hallucinatory effect can be clearly seen in the majority of patients and has been confirmed in a large number of comparative studies versus placebo. According to a compilation by Davis and Casper (1978), even before 1969 there had been 66 comparative studies versus placebo performed in the USA with chlorpromazine, 18 with trifluoperazine, 15 with fluphenazine, 10 with triflupromazine, nine with haloperidol and seven with thioridazine: a vast majority of these studies demonstrated the superiority of the active product over placebo. The therapeutic effect of the neuroleptics arose in 60–75% of patients during the first six weeks of treatment, although later improvements were also observed. The symptoms most perceptibly improved by the use of neuroleptics were:

- psychotic thought disorder, paranoid ideation;
- hallucinations;
- mannerisms;
- autism;
- general slowness or motor hyperactivity;
- withdrawal, hostility;
- affective blunting and indifference.

According to a formulation of Heinrich (1976, p. 27), 'psychotic syndromes which are characterized by a lively emotional mobility, wealth of symptoms, active confrontation with one's own disease and with one's surroundings, react from experience appreciably better to neuroleptic drug therapy than do those syndromes which are, as it were, burnt out, torpid, lacking in symptoms, and emotionally frozen'. The prospects for patients with schizophrenia simplex and with schizophrenic defect or residual syndromes are less favourable than for patients having catatonic and paranoid-hallucinatory schizophrenias (Crow, 1982).

In connection with the introduction of newer, so-called 'atypical' neuroleptics, the question arises as to whether and to what degree these drugs have a beneficial effect not only on the positive (or productive) symptoms of schizophrenia but also on the negative part of the schizophrenic syndrome (apathy, social withdrawal, emotional blunting, impoverishment of thought and speech). Möller (1993a) emphasizes that so-called *negative symptoms* are observed at various stages of schizophrenic psychosis and are therefore to be evaluated differentially also. Depending on the type and stage of psychosis, they occur in association with positive symptoms or are isolated, and they also respond in a differential way to neuroleptics. One can speak of a particularly marked or even a specific effect of a neuroleptic on negative symptoms only when a preparation acts on apathy, social withdrawal, etc. after the acute positive symptoms have faded, but especially in patients with schizophrenic defect or chronic deficit state. This type of effect has been convincingly obtained so far only with the atypical neuroleptic clozapine, which is also used successfully in cases of so-called therapy resistance (Farmer and Blewett, 1993).

8.2.2   Questions of dosage and duration of treatment

There may be considerable differences between the lowest and the highest recommended doses for neuroleptics (see Table 1.2 in Chapter 1). The major reasons for the wide dosage range are the weight and age of the patients, their general physical health, and the type and severity of the mental disorders. Baldessarini emphasized (1985, p. 48) that 'there have been very few systematic investigations of dose–effect relationships, or comparisons of specific types of agents, in large numbers of psychotic patients diagnosed by reliable methods'. The published doses for neuroleptics should therefore be seen only as rough guidelines and the dosage must be tailor-made individually on the basis of the symptoms to be treated and tolerability.

Two dose–effect studies with haloperidol allow a statement to be made regarding adequate doses, at least for this neuroleptic: a double-blind comparison between daily doses of 10, 30 and 80 mg haloperidol in 87 recently hospitalized patients with schizophrenia revealed no advantage of the two higher doses over the dose of 10 mg per day (Rifkin et al., 1991), and a study by McEvoy et al. (1991a) in 106 patients with schizophrenia and schizoaffective psychoses showed that an increase in dose above an individually optimal level (mostly less than 10 mg per day in this study) produced no additional therapeutic effect but rather an increase in side effects, especially extrapyramidal symptoms.

Despite the clear trend to lower doses seen in newer works, some authors such as Schied (1983, p. 279 ff.) warn against experimenting with inadequate doses *at the beginning of a treatment*: especially in younger, physically healthy patients it is important to achieve a rapid antipsychotic action that is also clearly perceptible to the patient. (For questions of so-called 'high-dose' antipsychotic medication see Thomson, 1994.)

Dosage during long-term treatments

Baldessarini and Davis (1980) attempted to clarify, on the basis of studies published by other authors, whether there exists a significant relationship between maintenance dosages administered and risk of relapse in the case of chronic schizophrenics. Correlations calculated for 23 controlled studies showed no relationship between the chronically administered doses of neuroleptics and risk of relapse within a wide range. Based on this negative result, the authors ruled that the maintenance dosage for each individual patient should be kept as low as possible in order to prevent neuroleptics from causing undesirable delayed effects.

In a more recent paper, Kane and Lieberman (1987) critically discussed the possibility of dose reduction during long-term treatments. From several controlled studies it clearly emerged that the reduction of an originally administered neuroleptic dose and the risk of relapse are closely correlated. On the other hand, patients on lower neuroleptic doses were described as less emotionally withdrawn, livelier, more relaxed and less sluggish. Since these patients also showed fewer signs of incipient tardive dyskinesias, Kane and Lieberman drew the following conclusion: 'Dosage reduction can lead to a diminution in adverse effects and improvement in some subjective and objective measures of well-being; however, the risk of psychotic exacerbation increases, and patients must be observed carefully with a readiness to increase medication when necessary and usually on a temporary basis' (Kane and Lieberman, 1987, p. 1107).

In a pilot study with long-term chronic schizophrenic patients, Van Putten *et al.* (1993) showed that it is possible to decrease the neuroleptic dose even in so-called therapy-resistant patients, and were able to reduce the mean haloperidol dose from 62 mg to 17 mg daily. Two of the original 13 patients responded adversely to the dosage reduction, which was undertaken over a mean period of 32 weeks, but the others showed either no change in their condition or even an improvement ($n = 6$). In parallel with the dosage reduction, which was accomplished in a department with a high staffing level, there was a marked reduction in extrapyramidal symptoms.

Duration of treatment and compliance

In discussions of the necessary and sensible duration of treatment of schizophrenic patients with neuroleptics, two tendencies compete: on the one hand the desire to keep each patient in hospital for as short a time as possible and to keep exposure to potentially harmful neuroleptics as short as possible, and on the other hand the endeavour to avoid relapses and symptomatic deteriorations as far as possible.

According to Heinrich (1976), the hospital treatment of productive schizophrenic psychoses usually lasts about six weeks, sometimes less in the case of catatonic syndromes, and two to four months with schizophrenia simplex. Discharge from the hospital is striven for as early as possible so that the patient is not allowed to become used to the protective atmosphere in hospital for too long and so that the family and other social contacts are not unnecessarily hindered. On the other hand, patients may only be discharged when their state has stabilized to the extent that they are capable of coping with the stresses which will unavoidably occur on return into their usual environment. Each patient must be thoroughly prepared for his discharge: he must be made clearly to understand that he has to take his medication in the prescribed manner and he must learn to recognize signs of deterioration in his state as being possible premonitions of a psychotic episode. Inner unrest, sleep disturbances, a dejected or irritable mood lasting over some period of time, prolonged tiredness and disturbed concentration are warning signs which should quickly bring the patient to the doctor's surgery (Herz and Melville, 1980; Jolley *et al.*, 1989), although psychotic episodes may occur without identifiable prodromal symptoms (Malla and Norman, 1994).

Experience has shown that a large percentage of patients take the neuroleptics prescribed for them either irregularly or not at all (Fitzgerald, 1976). Precise figures are unknown, but doubtless very high and many relapses and readmissions to hospital are attributed in schizophrenics to 'noncompliance', i.e., to the failure to observe therapeutic instructions. Revolving door psychiatry would thus seem to be partly due to the patient's rejection of treatment. One possible remedy is to prescribe notoriously unreliable patients *depot neuroleptics*, i.e., injectable galenic formulations of neuroleptics which are released over a period of weeks from the muscle tissue and which then exert their therapeutic action. The most frequent cause of the failure to take medication as instructed – the unsatisfactory tolerability of conventional neuroleptics arising particularly with high doses – is, however, not eliminated by this procedure. Neuroleptics frequently lead to motor and vegetative disturbances (Chapter 1): tremor, stiffness, palpitations, outbreaks of sweating, impotence, dizziness, and the typical feeling of neuroleptic constraint are all phenomena which remind the discharged patient that he is actually still sick and which may cause him to discontinue the orally administered medication on his own initiative.

The intramuscular administration of neuroleptics acting for weeks prevents this independent action and improves compliance; on the other hand, only highly potent neuroleptics such as fluphenazine, flupenthixol and haloperidol are suitable for depot administration and it is precisely these medicines which more frequently lead to extrapyramidal symptoms and dysphoric mood (van Putten *et al.*, 1984).

8.2.3   Discontinuation trials with neuroleptics

The question of the optimal duration of neuroleptic treatment of schizophrenic patients has been investigated in so-called discontinuation trials: depending on the study, the medicine that had been administered for months or years abruptly or gradually withdrawn and, in the better-controlled studies, replaced by placebo. According to Gardos and Cole (1978) and Woggon (1979), who discussed the older literature, the mean relapse rate in schizophrenic patients six weeks after neuroleptic discontinuation is approximately

50%. Observations for two years show that chronic schizophrenic patients who had been switched to placebo experienced a relevant deterioration of their state 2.5–3 times more frequently than those patients who continued to take their original neuroleptic. Studies in which depot neuroleptics were discontinued confirm these figures (Odejide and Aderounmu, 1982; Wistedt et al., 1982).

Woggon (1979) emphasized that the risk of relapse in discontinuation trials depends on many non-pharmacological, often poorly controllable factors, and she specifically named the expectations of the patients, doctors and nurses, other environmental factors, the duration of hospitalization and prior treatment, and the time interval since the last acute psychotic episode. On the basis of an analysis of 14 more recent discontinuation trials, Kane and Lieberman (1987) found that the relapse rate varied greatly from study to study: depending on the trial, relapse rates of 30–86% with clustering around 60–70% have been reported in the first 12 months after placebo substitution. According to Kane and Lieberman, this scatter is a result of the different inclusion criteria applied and the different definitions of 'relapse'. They therefore proposed that a quantifiable increase in symptoms be used as the dependent variable instead of the relapse rate in future studies of this type.

More important in practice than percentages would be an answer to the question of whether the relapse or exacerbation tendencies of individual patients can be estimated on the basis of specific features even before the planned withdrawal of neuroleptics. Unfortunately, the answer is largely negative. According to present knowledge there are no reliable clinical features that speak for or against the maintenance of neuroleptic therapy in individual cases (Möller, 1992). An experimental study by J.A. Lieberman et al. (1987) certainly suggests that patients at risk of relapse can be differentiated with some degree of probability from those not at risk by means of an intravenous test dose of the psychostimulant methylphenidate, but provocation tests of this type will probably not become widely used for ethical and practical reasons. Placebo-substitution experiments (e.g. Crow et al., 1986) also provide no relapse-risk predictors of practical relevance.

Consequently, in most cases the recommendation remains that the neuroleptic treatment of schizophrenic patients should be continued for at least 12 months after the termination of the acute state, and then, if this concerns the first psychotic episode and productive symptoms are no longer detectable, to gradually reduce and eventually discontinue the neuroleptic (Kissling, 1991). Monthly check-ups by psychiatrists are necessary after this withdrawal of medication in order to recognize an impending relapse and to prevent it with initially low doses of neuroleptics. In patients with frequent relapses, continuous treatment with neuroleptics is preferred and efforts should then be directed at finding the minimum dose that is still effective (Schooler, 1991). Other factors which are also decisive in individual cases include patient relationship with the treating doctor, the attitude of the patient and relatives to the side effects of neuroleptics and to the possibility of renewed hospitalization, and finally easy access to outpatient and inpatient psychiatric services (see Schöny and Rittmannsberger, 1992).

Many authors consider that long-term neuroleptic therapy should not be given to chronic schizophrenic patients with so-called negative symptoms since these states may have a neurobiochemical basis different from that in acute states with florid symptoms (Crow, 1980, 1982). The long-term administration of dopamine receptor blockers with their known side effects would not be justified in states which are presumably not attributable to dopamine hyperactivity.

8.2.4 Drug therapy and psychotherapy of schizophrenia

The introduction of neuroleptics represented such a decisive advance in the treatment of schizophrenia that the endeavours made in the 1940s and 1950s concerning individual psychotherapy of schizophrenic patients were largely pushed into the background. Whereas older textbooks of psychiatry refer respectfully to the psychoanalytically orientated attempts at therapy for schizophrenics undertaken by Rosen and Benedetti, they generally qualify their remarks by adding that the results of these often heroic efforts were quantitatively modest and that the wider application of such methods is out of the question on practical grounds. Over a period of 10 years a qualified therapist could only treat some 40–60 schizophrenics (Müller, 1972).

Studies before 1968: comparisons between psychotherapy and drug treatment

A literature review (May, 1968) has shown that neuroleptics represent considerably more effective treatment for acute forms of schizophrenia than do various types of psychotherapy:

Neuroleptics versus psychotherapy (two comparative studies): Both studies covered large, statistically equivalent groups of patients with productive symptoms; one study compared group psychotherapy and neuroleptics, the other analytically orientated individual therapy and neuroleptics. The results were similar inasmuch as both trials showed the drug therapy to be markedly superior in almost all clinically relevant characteristics and symptoms.

Neuroleptics versus combined neuroleptic therapy and psychotherapy (five studies): Here too, the results were clearly in favour of drug therapy since there were virtually no relevant differences between patients receiving neuroleptics alone and those treated with neuroleptics plus psychotherapy. Three of the five studies involved group therapy, the other two individual psychotherapy, and neither of these forms of treatment augmented the effect of the simultaneously administered neuroleptics to any demonstrable extent.

Psychotherapy versus combined psychotherapy and drug therapy (two studies): In both studies the patients received analytically orientated individual therapies with the result that the effect of the combined therapies was appreciably superior to that of psychotherapy alone. It was found in both studies that the administration of drugs had no unfavourable effect on the course of, or the results of, the psychotherapy which had been going on for up to two years.

The conclusion which May reached on the basis of this analysis was quite clear: '. . . if one were faced with the hypothetical choice of using one and only one form of treatment in addition to the usual hospital care, the objective evidence would indicate that, for the average *hospitalized* schizophrenic patient, drug therapy would at present, generally speaking and on the average, be the treatment of choice over other physical and non-physical forms of treatment' (May, 1968, pp. 1170–1171). Interestingly enough, this statement also holds true for so-called environmental therapies, i.e., for occupational therapy, group activities, preparation for a profession, therapeutic community models, patient self-government, and other hospital-run programmes. In the opinion of May, eight additional controlled trials clearly showed the superiority of neuroleptic therapy as compared to such measures which, whilst somewhat increasing its prospects of success, come nowhere near to taking the place of drug therapy.

Two long-term studies from the 1970s

May's survey related almost exclusively to studies with hospitalized patients who, as experience shows, have quite variable outcomes: some of these patients will stay in the protected environment of a clinic for a long time, or even permanently, whereas the majority of schizophrenics can be discharged and will perhaps never return to the hospital again.

One aspect which is of great importance in the long term, namely a reduction in the relapse risk *after the subsidence of an acute schizophrenic episode*, forms the subject of two comprehensive studies involving schizophrenic patients who had been discharged from hospital.

In a study conducted by Hogarty and Goldberg (1973), a sample of 374 schizophrenic patients, who had been discharged after showing marked improvement and had been adjusted to ambulatory treatment with a neuroleptic for two months, was divided into four different treatment groups: chlorpromazine plus psychotherapy; placebo plus psychotherapy; chlorpromazine alone; placebo alone.

The psychotherapy consisted in regular individual sessions dealing with the patient's family as well as social and professional problems, the number of relapses during the following 12 months being taken as the criterion of therapeutic success. These were as follows for:

– chlorpromazine plus psychotherapy: 26% relapse;
– chlorpromazine without psychotherapy: 33% relapse;

– placebo plus psychotherapy: 63% relapse;
– placebo without psychotherapy: 73% relapse.

These results clearly confirm the efficacy of neuroleptic therapy in preventing new schizophrenic episodes, whereas the protective benefit of psychotherapeutic efforts was demonstrable, but quantitatively less impressive. A second evaluation after a further 12 months, i.e., after a total follow-up of two years, confirmed the first year's findings: at this point in time considerably fewer of the patients being treated with neuroleptics had suffered a relapse in comparison to those treated with placebo and there was further, albeit numerically less important, confirmation of the efficacy of psychotherapy. In a subsequent publication (Hogarty et al., 1976) the authors considered whether the effect of the psychotherapeutic measures in the group receiving combined therapy was at best due to the fact that the respective patients took their medication more regularly than did the remaining patients, with the result that the presumed effect of the psychotherapy was in reality a consequence of the more reliable intake of the neuroleptics. It emerged that there was no difference between the average daily doses prescribed for the groups and that the compliance reported by patients and relatives was also more or less the same for both groups. The protective effect of the psychotherapy was consequently deemed a real one and not merely the result of a more regular intake of the medication.

May et al. (1976) published catamnestic results of a study which was both quantitatively and qualitatively impressive: follow-up examinations over several years were carried out in a sample of initially 228 patients participating in a comparative study conducted in the 1960s. During their stay in hospital the patients (schizophrenics of both sexes hospitalized for the first time) had received one of the following therapies according to a randomized experimental design:

– analytically orientated individual psychotherapy;
– a neuroleptic (trifluoperazine);
– psychotherapy plus neuroleptic;
– electroshocks;
– environmental therapy, i.e. none of the four therapies named.

After three, four and five years the long-term effects of these treatments were examined. The criterion of success was taken to be the number of days spent by the patients in psychiatric hospitals (a) since the first hospitalization; (b) since their discharge from first hospitalization.

– *After three years*, 203 patients could be followed up: the total number of days spent in hospital in the case of the groups treated with psychotherapy and with environmental therapy alone was very significantly greater than in the other three groups. The results were similar when the number of

hospital days since discharge were considered: patients who had received analytical psychotherapy had on average to be rehospitalized more frequently and/or for longer periods than did the other patients.
– *After four years*, when it was still possible to examine 113 patients, the result was equivalent to that after three years, and a similar tendency was observed in 61 patients five years after commencement of the study: in all cases the catamnestic findings were least favourable for those patients treated with psychotherapy or environmental therapy.

In this study, psychotherapy was clearly inferior to both drug therapy and to electroshock therapy; the patients treated with psychotherapy and environmental therapy were on average hospitalized for 50% longer than the other groups and, as noted by the authors, this clearly contradicts a popular prejudice against neuroleptics: 'it was simply *not* true that patients who had been initially treated with drugs relapsed more rapidly and spent more time in hospital in the end than non-drug-treated patients. On the contrary, the initial advantages of drug treatment seemed to persist for at least three years and, to a lesser extent, up to five years' (May *et al.*, 1976, p. 486).

A critical remark that should be made in this context is that the authors merely took as independent variables the treatments applied at the time of first hospitalization, neglecting other factors which had arisen in subsequent years. If the patients really were schizophrenics, it is almost certain that the majority of them would have received further treatment which – contrary to the original experimental design – could no longer be introduced in the sense of a controlled trial. The results after four and five years at least must thus be regarded rather cautiously for this reason.

Studies published in the last fifteen years

In more recent studies, the therapeutic efforts have probably emphasized more than before the individual requirements of the patients and their social relationships. As an example of a project directed to individual requirements and thus 'uncontrolled' in various respects, the therapeutic study published by Alanen *et al.* (1986) in 100 schizophrenic patients in Turku, Finland, can be cited. Three-quarters of these cases were hospitalized initially and almost all received neuroleptics, at least at the start of treatment, mostly in rather low doses. They were subsequently incorporated into various psychotherapeutic and sociotherapeutic programmes that were greatly individualized and adapted to the resources available in the participating institutions: intensive individual psychotherapy, occasional psychotherapy of an essentially supportive nature, care in day clinics, family and husband/wife therapy, support in occupational rehabilitation. Five years after the start of this programme, more than half of all patients and about one-third of the typical schizophrenics were asymptomatic, and clear psychotic features could be detected only in a minority. In many cases the neuroleptics had been discontinued without a relapse occurring, a result that was particularly clear in those patients who had received occasional or intensive individual psychotherapy. In all, this study which, owing to its structure, can only partially be summarized in figures, provides a rather optimistic picture of the therapeutic outcome for schizophrenic patients.

Schooler and Hogarty (1987) summarized a large proportion of the works published since 1978 in which drug treatment and psychotherapy or sociotherapy were combined for the treatment of schizophrenic patients, and drew the following conclusions with regard to each therapeutic approach:

Individual psychotherapy: Apart from a barely valid study comparing two psychotherapeutic methods (insight-orientated versus adaptation-orientated), a controlled comparative study with four treatment groups (depot neuroleptic or orally administered neuroleptic, intensive or less intensive psychotherapy directed to interpersonal problems) has been published. Marked differences could not be detected between the four treatments during the course of two years, although the group with depot neuroleptics plus intensive psychotherapeutic care tended to do best: none of the patients in this group suffered further relapses after the first eight months of study.

Social and life skills training: The four cited studies were of short duration (five days, seven weeks, nine weeks, 12 weeks) and showed an improvement in the parameters of interest (eye contact, self-assertion). There is no detailed information on the neuroleptics administered and, according to the authors, it is also unclear how long the stated behavioural changes lasted.

Group psychotherapy: in this area there is a well-documented study by Malm (1982) in 80 recently hospitalized schizophrenics. All patients were receiving depot neuroleptics and underwent a three-month course to improve their social skills; half the patients also participated in communication-orientated group therapy for one year. In this group there was an additional improvement in features relating to ability for emotional contact, general well-being, leisure activities and social contacts.

Particularly interesting are treatment trials that are directed to the *relatives of schizophrenic patients* and have the objective of modifying family dynamics. Four of the six studies cited by Schooler and Hogarty were based on the concept of expressed emotions (EE); i.e., they started from the observation that schizophrenic patients who return from the hospital to families with markedly expressed feelings of criticism, hostility or even excessive care suffer relapses more frequently than others. In a study by Leff *et al.* (1982) it emerged that the relapse rate was reduced from 50% to 9% within nine months by breaking down this behaviour of the relatives and the simultaneous administration of neuroleptics to patients.

Müller and Schöneich (1992) also reported on favourable experience with intensive outpatient psychotherapy combined with neuroleptic treatment. On the basis of a before–after comparison over 2 × 5 years in a university outpatient clinic, they were able to show that the duration of rehospitalizations required by 89 patients could be reduced from a mean of 10 weeks to two weeks per year when a special schizophrenia outpatient service offering individualized psychotherapy and psychosocial treatment was available to the patients instead of the routine psychiatric outpatient service. A beneficial effect of psychotherapy was demonstrated both in those patients taking neuroleptics continuously for long-term prophylaxis and in those taking the drugs intermittently when prodromal symptoms appeared in order to prevent relapse.

The view of combined drug therapy and psychotherapy in schizophrenia has thus changed clearly since May's review (1968) classified psychotherapy as being of very little value. Whether given orally or in depot form, whether used for long-term prophylaxis or intermittently, neuroleptics form the backbone of schizophrenia therapy, but at the same time it is now considered that individualized psychotherapy and psychosocial therapy of hospitalized patients and especially of outpatients is essential since these measures decisively improve the quality of life of patients and their families, help to prevent rehospitalizations and thus improve the long-term prognosis of schizophrenic psychoses (see Katschnig et al., 1992, for additional references and a presentation of various psychosocial treatment models).

8.3   ANTIDEPRESSANTS AND THE TREATMENT OF DEPRESSION

8.3.1   Treatment of depressive episodes

The drug therapy of depression differs in a number of critical points from that given to schizophrenics. Depressions are phasically occurring deviations from the norm which, in the majority of cases, show spontaneous remission, although this may often only be after a period of some months. The majority of depressives can be treated as outpatients – a fact which explains why the illness generally does not make as severe an encroachment into the family and social surroundings of the patient as does schizophrenia. Outsiders are able to imagine what a depression must be like, or at least believe that they can: everyone is occasionally sad, disappointed, devoid of hope. In the eyes of his fellow men and women a depressive consequently tends to be a person to be pitied, but not one who is necessarily mad.

The efficacy of antidepressants has been demonstrated statistically (Table 1.5 in Chapter 1) and confirmed also in a recently published meta-analysis of about 300 published clinical studies (Davis et al., 1993): a positive therapeutic result is to be expected in almost two-thirds of cases with imipramine, amitriptyline, amoxapine and some newer drugs, whereas a good one-third of all patients show a clinically relevant improvement with placebo. According to Davis et al. (1993), these figures prove the therapeutic utility of antidepressants 'beyond the shadow of a doubt' and also show that there are hardly any quantitative differences between the various substances licensed as antidepressants. But what is to be done with the 35% or so of patients who do not obtain a beneficial effect within six weeks of medication and who are thus 'refractory to therapy'? Poor compliance must be assumed in some of these patients, perhaps as a result of side effects of antidepressants, and in others the prescribed dose may be inadequate; both these factors could be monitored by measuring drug levels in the plasma (p. 153 f.). In the other cases with 'true refractoriness to treatment', leading authors first advise a change of antidepressant, then combined drug therapy and finally a change to other forms of treatment. Suitable staged plans or strategies are reported by Möller (1991) and by Janicak et al. (1993; Chapter 7).

None of today's antidepressants are completely devoid of side effects which, for their own part, can intensify the feeling of illness and concern felt by the patient. Doctors consequently will not prescribe antidepressants unnecessarily, especially in older patients who react particularly sensitively to the central and peripheral effects of these substances.

Many doctors even seem to tend to insufficient prescriptions: according to a survey by Keller et al. (1982), in the USA more than half of patients suffering from a depressive illness for at least one month were either receiving no, or only insufficiently dosed, antidepressants. Two-thirds of these patients were receiving psychotherapy and more than half were taking tranquillizers, but only about one-third had been treated with antidepressants for at least four weeks. Whether this situation is the consequence of insufficient familiarity with the diagnosis and therapy of depression (as the authors of the study assume), or whether it reflects wise restraint (Uhlenhuth, 1982) cannot be determined from this study by Keller et al. In contrast, it is interesting to note that the nature and intensity of antidepressant treatment prescribed depended only slightly on the sociodemographic features of the patients but was determined by the tradition prevailing in the clinics and hospitals attended by the patients (Keller et al., 1986). A Swedish study (Isaacson et al., 1992) showed the potentially tragic consequences of inadequate antidepressant prescription. Of 80 representative suicide victims selected in the period 1970–1984, at least 40 had consulted a doctor in the three months before their death. Of these, 27 received a prescription for psychopharmaceuticals, mostly tranquillizers or sleeping pills (i.e. the patients must have complained of mental symptoms), but an antidepressant was prescribed in only eight cases. The authors of this study therefore saw a clear relationship between inadequate psychopharmaceutical prescription and successful suicide, and they demanded an improvement in the training of general practitioners with regard to psychiatric diagnosis and drug therapy.

8.3.2 Problems of maintenance therapy

According to modern treatment guidelines, episodes of endogenous depression are treated with antidepressants for 6–12 months, both in hospital and at home. In cases of doubt the medication is given for a longer period since the restored subjective feeling of well-being does not necessarily reflect the abatement of a depressive episode, but is often only the expression of transient neutralization of the illness. Short-term prospects are good for the acutely depressive, since remission occurs within one year in 85% of patients. In the medium and long term the prognosis is less favourable: up to 65% of all patients receiving no further treatment suffer a relapse of greater or lesser severity within one year. About half of all depressives experience more than one severe depressive episode in the course of their lives and are thus at risk for years (Klerman and Weissman, 1992), and about 15% of all depressed patients commit suicide. In view of the fact that depression is a recurring, or even a chronic illness in a proportion of patients, the question of maintenance therapy arises in many cases.

Prien (1987) differentiated three forms of long-term drug treatment of depressions: (1) continuation therapy with the aim of maintaining the symptomatic improvement obtained in an acute episode; (2) preventive treatment with the aim of avoiding or attenuating further episodes (secondary prevention); (3) chronic treatment of dysthymia, cyclothymia or other affective disorders. These three forms of treatment will be discussed briefly below.

Continuation therapy of depressive episodes

Controlled discontinuation trials show that about half of all depressive patients suffer a serious relapse within six months if their antidepressant medication is withdrawn shortly after the disappearance of acute symptoms; with continuation therapy, only about one-fifth of patients experience a relapse in the same period. The difficulty for the treating doctor is to estimate reliably how long he should continue to prescribe antidepressants for his patients who have overcome depression. The results of a study particularly devoted to this question (Prien and Kupfer, 1986) suggest that this period should be *at least four to five months*; even mild continuing symptoms may indicate that a depressive episode has not yet completely ceased and that the treatment should be continued further.

Since the continued symptoms of a treated episode cannot be clearly separated from the prodromal symptoms of a subsequent episode (Fava and Kellner, 1991), the continuation or rapid resumption of drug therapy is advisable in all such cases. A prerequisite is close cooperation between doctors, patients and relatives so that symptoms are recognized early and reported, and the necessary measures can then be taken (CINP Task Force, 1993).

Preventive therapy

Some 10–15% of all affective illnesses are manic-depressive or bipolar psychoses (ICD No. F31). In these patients, lithium prevents the appearance of manic phases although its efficacy is somewhat less pronounced in the case of depressive episodes. In controlled studies of between five and 28 months duration involving patients with bipolar psychoses, the relapse rate was an average of 79% with placebo and 35% with lithium (Prien and Caffey, 1977). Whereas lithium is at present the drug of choice in the treatment of manic-depressive psychoses it by no means represents the ideal solution since there is a failure rate of over 20% (see Kaschka, 1993) and has a late onset of action. Its use is recommended when manic and depressive phases are known to follow each other in rapid succession. A practical advantage of lithium therapy lies in the fact that plasma levels are easy to monitor, thus making it possible to prevent over- or underdosage. A disadvantage is the limited therapeutic range of the preparation (Greil and van Calker, 1983).

Unipolar depressions occur much more frequently than manic-depressive psychoses and are aetiologically heterogeneous. The question of maintenance therapy is consequently a more complex one in such cases and some aspects are as yet unsolved. Lithium provides a certain amount of protection against further episodes of unipolar endogenous depression (ICD No. F33), but it is still unclear whether depressive episodes can really be prevented or merely attenuated sufficiently to prevent the need for hospitalization. Many clinicians regard the protective effect of lithium in cases of unipolar depression to be too weak to merit its routine use. Instead, the long-term administration of antidepressants is frequently recommended today. Several studies have shown that these drugs not only suppress or curtail acute depressive phases, but can also prevent the reappearance of previously resolved episodes or, when administration is continued for years, the appearance of new episodes (Kupfer *et al.*, 1992). *Chronic treatment* with antidepressants is generally considered to be justified when episodes of depression have occurred at least twice in five years within the context of unipolar psychosis (CINP Task Force, 1993). Both the older, 'classical' antidepressants and the newer substances with more specific mechanisms of action (SSRIs, etc.) can be considered for this application.

The anticonvulsant *carbamazepine* is used with some success in patients with bipolar psychoses who do not respond to lithium (Post, 1987), but further clarification is needed to determine if it is also useful in unipolar illness (Prien and Gelenberg, 1989). A combination of lithium and carbamazepine or other anticonvulsants is recommended under certain conditions if an adequate preventive effect cannot be obtained with the substances individually (Kaschka, 1993; Emrich and Dose, 1993).

With the aid of lithium, antidepressants, carbamazepine and various combinations of these drugs, the great majority of patients can be protected from recurring episodes of affective illness. Unsatisfactory features of current therapy and prophylaxis include not only the limited tolerability and safety of some antidepressants and lithium, but also the fact that not all patients can be protected completely against recurrence of depression, and that apart from the frequency of depressive episodes, there are no reliable prognostic factors which can simplify the decisions regarding the introduction and duration of maintenance drug therapy (Calabrese *et al.*, 1995).

8.3.3 Drug therapy and psychotherapy of depressions

Numerous investigations have been published concerning the question of the contributions which psychotherapy and drug therapy can make to the treatment of depressions, which psychotherapeutic procedures are particularly suitable for depressions and whether combined drug therapy and psychotherapy is sensible for depressions. In view of the care and the effort expended in most of these studies, a rather more extensive discussion is indicated.

Studies from the early 1970s

The first such investigation, the so-called Boston–New Haven Study, has been described in several complementary individual reports (Klerman *et al.*, 1974; Weissman *et al.*, 1974; Paykel *et al.*, 1976). This started out with 150 ambulatory female depressed patients and involved a comparison between six forms of treatment.

- For at least 1 hour per week, 75 of the patients saw psychotherapeutically trained female social workers with whom they were able to discuss the problems preoccupying them at the time. These therapies were supportive and not primarily analytically orientated (high contact group). The remaining 75 patients saw a psychiatrist for about 15 minutes per month, told him how they felt and discussed any changes in the medication (low contact group).
- One-third of the patients in each of the two groups were then given an antidepressant (amitriptyline) in doses of 100–200 mg per day and a third were given placebo, the remaining third receiving no tablets at all.

Cells were formed on the basis of these 2 x 3 groups receiving different forms of treatment (the cells show the respective numbers of patients at the beginning and at the end of the trial):

	Amitriptyline	*Placebo*	*No medication*	*Total*
High contact	25→19	25→18	25→18	75→55
Low contact	25→20	25→15	25→16	75→51
Total	50→39	50→33	50→34	150→106

The patients were suffering from depression of moderate severity most of which were classified as neurotic, i.e., not endogenous. The majority had low or middle class backgrounds; their average age was 38 years. The women had been selected from an original sample of 278 depressive patients, the selection criterion being a pronounced symptomatic improvement under amitriptyline therapy within four to six weeks (Fig. 8.1). After four and eight months the trial was evaluated on the basis of the criteria 'relapse rate' and 'social adjustment and satisfaction'; relapse was defined as the renewed return of a depression rating score to the pretreatment level, social adjustment being assessed on the basis of an extensive interview. Results were as follows:

(1) At the end of the trial (six months after randomization) the relapse rate in both amitriptyline groups was more than 50% lower than in the four non-drug groups. In the high-contact groups the relapse rate was some 25% lower than in the low-contact groups (this difference was not statistically significant). Both forms of therapy – drug and psychotherapy – consequently had favourable effects on the relapse rate, amitriptyline being numerically superior.

(2) After four months' treatment (two months in the assigned group) there was no difference between the groups in respect of social adjustment and satisfaction. After eight months, significantly better results were observed in the high-contact groups than in the other patients, there being no difference between those patients receiving medication and those receiving no medication.

In the authors' views drug therapy was clearly superior to psychotherapy with regard to the prevention of relapses, although social adjustment – and hence also long-term prognosis – was improved in those patients receiving psychotherapy. It was striking to note the difference in the effect between the two forms of treatment over time: amitriptyline worked more rapidly and strongly on the actual depressive symptoms, psychotherapy acted more slowly and on different mental aspects. The two therapies were additive as seen in the amitriptyline–high-contact group. The authors concluded: 'Psychotherapy is not an alternative to antidepressant treatment and does not prevent relapse or the recurrence of symptoms. Alternatively, continued amitriptyline has no effect on social adjustment and is no better or worse than a placebo or no pill' (Weissman et al., 1974, p. 778).

Several points need to be noted in the interpretation of this study. Firstly, it should be pointed out that the 150 female patients included in the study constituted a selection in that they had responded favourably to amitriptyline given in a trial of several weeks' duration, thus implying that drug treatment was favoured from the outset. Secondly, as the experimental plan shows, it was not the immediate, antidepressive action of the two forms of treatment which was compared, but their maintenance effect once symptomatic improvement had already occurred. The higher incidence of relapses in the groups receiving placebo or no medication could consequently have been the result of the premature discontinuation of the medicament to which the patients had favourably responded. It is consequently all the more interesting to note the effect, found as a trend but not statistically significant, of psychotherapy on the relapse rate. On the other hand, the improved social adjustment in the groups treated with psychotherapy is not surprising (Spitzer, 1976): these patients had been treated for six months

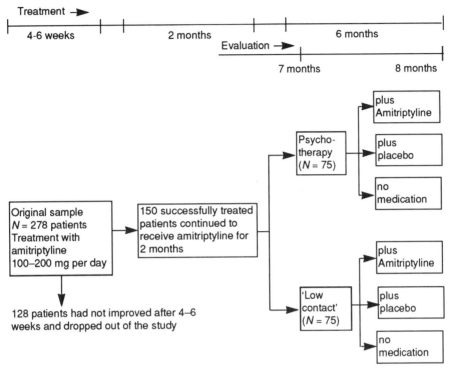

Figure 8.1.   Design of the study by Klerman *et al.* (1974)

with a view to their social adjustment and the resolution of interpersonal conflicts, and they evaluated themselves at the end of the study; their hopes and expectations therefore must have spilled over into the assessments.

Despite these limitations, the following conclusions can be drawn from the Boston–New Haven study and two other, similarly extensive studies published at the same time (with analytically orientated group therapy: Covi *et al.*, 1974; with family therapy: Friedman, 1975):

(1) The treatment of depressives using either drugs or psychotherapy appears to influence different symptoms or personality areas. The antidepressants used acted in particular on symptoms in the somatic, drive and mood sectors, psychotherapy affecting more the relationship between the patients and their families and their wider surroundings.

(2) Combined treatments had mainly additive effects. Patients being treated pharmacologically and psychotherapeutically benefited in two ways. There was certainly no negative interaction between drug treatment and psychotherapy.

Both conclusions apply to outpatients with neurotic, i.e., rather lighter and generally non-endogenous forms of depression. Two of the three investigations dealt with maintenance therapy of patients who had already shown pronounced symptomatic improvement with antidepressant treatment.

In the following studies, psychotherapeutic techniques were applied that had been specifically developed for the treatment of depressions, namely cognitive therapy, interpersonal therapy and a behaviourally orientated technique, social skills training.

Studies with cognitive therapy

Cognitive therapy (CT) is based on a theory developed by A. Beck according to which some typical symptoms of depression (despair, sadness, suicidal tendencies) reflect pathological changes in the cognitive organization of an individual (Beck, 1991). These patients regard themselves, their world and the future in a negative light (= depressive triad). Their distorted thinking is a result of logical and conceptual errors including arbitrary conclusions, over-extensive and thus false generalizations and simplifications. The purpose of CT is to make the patients aware of their cognitive errors on the basis of specific examples and, by means of specific training and guidance, to enable them to correct their false attitude.

A first comparative study between CT and imipramine in 41 patients (Rush *et al.*, 1977) revealed a clear superiority of CT over drug therapy in the short term; however, a follow-up examination of the patients 1 year later no longer found any significant difference between the treatment groups (Kovacs *et al.*, 1981). Since the study exhibits various methodological defects (see Spiegel and Aebi, 1983, p. 209), the following three works with CT in depressions are of greater significance.

Blackburn *et al.* (1981) studied 49 patients with mild to moderately severe depressions in a psychiatric outpatient department and 39 patients from a general practice in Edinburgh, i.e., a total of 88 patients, of whom 64 (14 men, 50 women) completed the study. The patients were selected on the basis of the Research Diagnostic Criteria (Spitzer *et al.*, 1978) as well as various rating and self-rating scales; one-third of the patients each received one of the following, randomly allocated treatments for a maximum of 20 weeks:

– CT: 2 hours per week for three weeks, then 1 hour per week;
– drug therapy: generally amitriptyline or chlorimipramine at 150 mg per day;
– CT plus drug therapy: a combination of both procedures.

Patients who showed a decrease in their symptoms by less than 50% after 12 weeks were considered to be therapeutic failures. The major results of the rather complex statistical evaluation were as follows:

(1) Patients from both the psychiatric outpatient unit and from general practice showed the best results with combined CT and drug therapy.

(2) The poorest results in both subgroups were obtained with drug therapy alone.
(3) In the general practice patients, CT was significantly better than drug therapy.
(4) Endogenous and non-endogenous depressives showed similar rates of success or failure with the three types of treatment.

In all, this study clearly suggests the *suitability of CT in mild to moderately severe depressions* and tends to speak against drug treatment of patients whose mental illness is conditioned primarily by their life situation. It also confirmed that drug therapy and non-drug treatments can be combined in depressions.

In a study carried out by Beck *et al.* (1985) in Philadelphia, the efficacy of CT alone was compared with that of CT plus drug treatment. Eighteen of the 33 outpatients (nine men, 24 women) with mild to moderately severe depressions received a maximum of 2 hours CT in 12 weeks; 15 patients also received CT with additional amitriptyline individually dosed within a range of 50–200 mg per day. At the end of treatment there were no significant differences between the two groups with regard to the various rating scales, i.e., the antidepressant administered in addition to CT had in total neither a beneficial nor an adverse effect. A follow-up examination 12 months later showed a slight tendency in favour of combined CT plus antidepressant treatment.

Murphy *et al.* (1984) could only partially confirm these results in a study involving 87 depressive outpatients. Their mostly middle class, predominantly female and rather young patients with moderately severe to severe depression were randomly allocated to one of the following treatment groups:

– CT: two sessions of 50 minutes per week for eight weeks, then one session per week for four weeks;
– drug therapy: an individually adjusted dose of the antidepressant nortriptyline up to a previously established therapeutic window;
– CT plus drug therapy;
– CT plus 'active placebo' (atropine and phenobarbitone in very small doses to imitate the concomitant effects of the antidepressant).

Seventy of 87 patients ended the study as intended, and most of the premature terminations concerned patients given the antidepressant or CT plus antidepressant. Comparisons within the four groups undertaken at the end of treatment and then again four weeks later showed a highly significant decrease in symptoms relative to baseline in all four groups, but no difference between the groups. This means that all four treatments were approximately equally effective and that the combination of an antidepressant with CT provided no additional benefit, unlike the observations of Blackburn *et al.* (1981). Also of interest are the results published by Simons *et al.* (1986) concerning a follow-up of these patients 12 months after the completion of treatment: most relapses occurred in the group of patients treated with drugs alone, whereas the patients treated with CT (with or without additional anti-depressant) showed relevant deterioration less frequently.

In all, despite the considerable differences between the cited studies, these results suggest that *CT is effective as a therapeutic procedure for ambulatory patients with mild to moderately severe depressions*: CT and drug therapy seem to have roughly the same efficacy in these cases. It remains to be determined whether a combination of CT with an antidepressant provides a significant additional benefit, and it is also unclear what the precise indications are for both forms of therapy (see Hollon *et al.*, 1991). Two more recent studies have also not provided definitive answers to these questions:

- In a multicentre study with exemplary methodology involving 250 patients, Elkin *et al.* (1989) found that drug therapy with imipramine together with the usual clinical care tended to be more effective than 16 weeks of treat-ment with CT (one session per week) in patients with 'major depressive disorder', and that CT in turn had greater efficacy than placebo therapy plus the usual clinical care. The superiority of drug therapy was particularly seen in severely ill patients, as is also confirmed by a recalculation of the results by Klein and Ross (1993). CT was equivalent to drug therapy in milder cases.
- On the other hand, the results of a study by Hollon *et al.* (1992) suggest that 12 weeks of CT is as effective as the same duration of treatment with imipramine. In this comparison between CT, imipramine and a combina-tion of CT plus imipramine in 107 ambulatory depressives, the combination treatment tended to be superior to the two single therapies, but without achieving the threshold of statistical significance. The superiority of drug therapy reported by Elkin *et al.* (1989) was not confirmed in this study. However, the high dropout rate (about 40% of all patients) was a notable feature and affected all three treatment groups to roughly the same degree.

In another study which is of interest in this connection, Mercier *et al.* (1992) noted that the majority of patients with so-called atypical depression not responding to CT did respond favourably to treatment with a MAO inhibitor or imipramine following CT. From these results they concluded that both CT and drug therapy can be considered effective treatments for different groups of depressed patients and possibly have differential indications. However, the small number of cases in this study does not allow a conclusion to be reached regarding possible prognostic factors for successful therapy with CT or antidepressants.

Studies with 'interpersonal therapy'

The method of interpersonal therapy (IPT) developed by Klerman, Weissman and other authors is based on the concept that depressions have their origin in the area of interpersonal relationships and that they also run their course in that area (see Klerman *et al.*, 1984). The purpose of IPT is to restore the patients within a short time to a position in which they can better understand their interpersonal problems and can change their unsatisfactory behaviour towards others that leads to conflicts and frustrations.

A first study with separate and combined use of IPT and antidepressants was published by Weissman *et al.* (1979). The participants were 81 outpatients (12 men, 69 women) aged 18–65 years (mean approximately 30 years) suffering from moderately severe unipolar depressions classified as neurotic depressions according to the nomenclature at the time. Half the patients received at least one session of 50 minutes IPT per week for 16 weeks, and the other patients could make 'free appointments': they were given the name and telephone number of a psychiatrist at the clinic and could call him whenever they wanted to make an appointment. They were granted a maximum of one therapy session per month. Half of each of the two psychotherapy groups received amitriptyline in individually adjusted daily doses of between 100 and 200 mg, or placebo.

Clinical assessments were made by psychiatrists or psychologists not involved in the treatment after one, four, eight, 12 and 16 weeks had elapsed. The study was intended to cover 96 patients, 15 of whom withdrew at the very beginning when they heard what treatment they were to be given. Most of those withdrawing were in the psychotherapy group. In addition, patients who failed to show any pronounced improvement in their symptoms within eight weeks or whose condition even deteriorated were withdrawn from the study. In the case of those patients withdrawing from the study, scores recorded at the time of withdrawal were used for purposes of evaluation (last observation carried forward = LOCF analysis). Withdrawals from the study occurred rather frequently and showed the following distribution:

	Withdrew	*Withdrew during the first week*	*% completed*
Psychotherapy	13/25	8	48
Drug therapy	16/24	4	33
Psychotherapy plus drug therapy	8/24	1	67
Free appointments	16/23	2	30
Total	53/96	15	45

According to this criterion, the combined therapy was superior to the other three treatments, and drug therapy alone was little different from the control conditions with free appointments. An additional assessment directed at target symptoms (DiMascio *et al.*, 1979) showed that the drug therapy had a particularly rapid and thorough effect on sleep disorders, whereas anxiety and other affective symptoms only showed a significant improvement at a later stage. The effect of psychotherapy on anxious and depressive mood was of rapid onset, whilst vegetative and somatic symptoms showed little change. No negative interactions were observed between the two forms of therapy, the treatment effects thus being differential and additive. These results indicate that drug therapy was particularly suitable for those patients whose symptoms were mainly vegetative–somatic in nature. Furthermore, the authors concluded from their findings that a patient rejecting one of the two forms of therapy (drug or psychotherapy) can be offered the other form of therapy with good prospects of success.

Prusoff *et al.* (1980) and Klerman *et al.* (1982) analysed the outcome of this investigation in still another way by classifying the patients according to their type of depression. On the basis of Research Diagnostic Criteria (Spitzer *et al.*, 1978) they formed several subgroups, the most important of which was a group of endogenous depressive patients ($N = 20$) and a group of depressives whose illness was labelled situative ($N = 31$). Situative depressions were diagnosed when the illness developed after an event or in a situation which probably contributed to the appearance of the depressive episode at that particular time. This led to the following insights:

– Endogenous depressives responded best to a combination of drug and psychotherapy. Drug therapy alone was only marginally better than free appointments. Psychotherapy alone was less effective than free appointments.
– In the case of situative depressives, psychotherapy and combined drug and psychotherapy achieved approximately the same result and both were markedly better than drug therapy alone which latter was, in turn, better than free appointments.

Viewed as a whole, this investigation supports the view that tricyclic antidepressants are particularly effective in cases of endogenous depression, whilst psychotherapy, possibly in conjunction with drug therapy, constitutes the best solution in cases of situative depression (which would probably be termed reactive depression in the terminology used hitherto). It is interesting to note that the combination of drug therapy with psychotherapy provided additional benefit in patients with endogenous depression. It must, however, be stated that this final conclusion is only based on a fairly small subsample.

In the comparative study published by Elkin *et al.* (1989) (see the section on CT), IPT was used as the fourth form of treatment in addition to CT, imipramine treatment and placebo treatment. According to Elkin *et al.*, IPT was about as effective as imipramine treatment and rather more effective than CT, especially in more severe cases. According to a subsequent calculation by Klein and Ross (1993), however, the drug therapy was significantly superior to both CT and IPT in the more severe cases. The trend in favour of IPT compared to CT was also confirmed in this additional analysis.

Social skills therapy

This behaviour-orientated form of therapy is based on the assumption that depressions are attributable to the inability of the patients to provide themselves with positive 'reinforcement' through suitable modes of behaviour (Kovacs, 1980). As Bellack *et al.* (1981) have stated, depressive persons often have disturbed relationships within their marriage or families, cannot affirm themselves and create widespread unease in their surroundings and thereby induce hostile feelings and rejection in others. Social skills therapy or training (SST) attempts to overcome the behavioural deficit and thereby to increase affectively satisfactory social contacts with family members, friends, colleagues and others.

Bellack *et al.* (1981) reported on a comparative study involving 72 women with non-psychotic unipolar depressions, of whom 60% came from a psychiatric outpatient clinic and 40% answered advertisements in the press and radio for treatment. They were aged 20–60 years with a mean age of 36 years. The patients were divided into the following treatment groups at random:

- Amitriptyline: the antidepressant dose was increased from an initial 50 mg per day to 200 mg per day within two weeks. The patients saw their psychiatrist for 15–20 minutes each week, mainly to discuss the medication.
- SST plus placebo: the patients received 1 hour of SST with an experienced and dedicated SST therapist each week for 12 weeks. They also received placebo tablets.
- SST plus amitriptyline: in addition to SST, the patients received amitriptyline in individually adjusted doses.
- Psychotherapy plus placebo tablets: the patients in this group received 1 hour of individual, generally psychodynamically orientated psychotherapy by experienced and dedicated psychotherapists each week for 12 weeks.

The most striking result of this study was the high dropout rate in the two groups treated with amitriptyline: more than 50% of the amitriptyline patients and almost 30% of those receiving SST plus amitriptyline interrupted the treatment prematurely, whereas only 15% of the SST plus placebo group and only 24% of the psychotherapy plus placebo group dropped out. The patients remaining in the study showed similar degrees of improvement in their symptoms after 12 weeks. In their discussion of the results, the authors considered the possibility that the numerous dropouts in the amitriptyline groups resulted from the recruitment procedure and the disappointed expectations of the patients: presumably many of them had wanted a helper or ally and were disappointed when only medication and an occasional short interview were offered to them.

Concluding comments on drug therapy and psychotherapy of depressions

As Weissman *et al.* (1987) emphasized in a review, the utility of several psychotherapeutic procedures in the treatment of unipolar non-psychotic depressions has been shown convincingly in controlled studies. Clearly structured procedures with time limits, such as CT, IPT and SST, represent a valuable alternative or a supplement to drug therapy with antidepressants, especially in outpatients. As found in a meta-analysis by Conte *et al.* (1986), combined drug therapy and psychotherapy can be even more effective than each of these therapies alone, but the difference is not very impressive in quantitative terms when seen as a whole.

Meterissian and Bradwein (1989) came to a rather different conclusion after they had critically analysed a large number of studies comparing drug therapy and psychotherapy. Although they did not generally question the value of non-drug procedures, they highlighted the fact that in most comparisons the drug treatment was not applied with the same care and the necessary specialist knowledge as used in the case of psychotherapy. Depending on the study, either inadequate antidepressant doses were used, plasma levels of the drug were not monitored, or hardly any of the known methods for improving the therapeutic success of drugs (change of drug, combination with lithium, etc.) were used. Since it is a matter of finding the precise place, the specific indication for various treatments, these authors consider it essential to apply all the compared procedures optimally. Obviously, psychotherapy and drug therapy cannot be compared blind, and it is thus all the more important to create the best possible conditions for all procedures that are compared. According to Meterissian and Bradwein, this was not the case in most of the available studies.

Another aspect worth mentioning is that there have been only sporadic comparative studies between the various psychotherapeutic procedures (see Grawe, 1992), so that their precise indication and relative utilities are not very well known. In view of the difficulties discussed in Chapter 6 in identifying reliable predictors of therapeutic success, even large-scale comparative studies between different psychotherapeutic procedures are not likely to provide clear answers.

Drug therapy with antidepressants cannot be avoided even in the future in the case of hospitalized patients with severe depressions. There have been only sporadic controlled studies performed so far to determine whether psychotherapeutic measures provide a significant effect in these cases. Tölle (1985, p. 252 ff.) emphasized the need for psychotherapeutic effort specifically in melancholic patients, who often consider themselves not to require treatment or not to be worthy of treatment. Although these patients often feel themselves to be lost, rejected and valueless, this therapeutic attention can get through to them and give them the feeling that they are not entirely alone, given up by everybody and fully misunderstood.

A study by Miller *et al.* (1989) in 45 hospitalized patients with mainly severe depressions seems to support this view; patients who had received CT or social skills therapy in addition to drug therapy responded better to the antidepressant treatment and after one year also showed fewer relapses than patients who had received only antidepressants in addition to the usual hospital care.

8.4 THE TREATMENT OF ANXIETY SYNDROMES AND NEUROTIC DISORDERS

Introductory comments on nomenclature

In Chapter 1 we learned of benzodiazepine tranquillizers as drugs with a very broad, not always clearly delimited range of indications in almost all branches of medicine. In the present connection we are concentrating on the most common uses of these drugs in psychiatry. According to the ICD-10 nomenclature (WHO, 1992), these are:

- phobic anxiety disorders (F 40);
- other anxiety disorders (F 41), especially panic disorders (F 41.0) and generalized anxiety disorder (GAD: F 41.1);
- reactions to severe stress and adjustment disorders (F 43).

Neurotic and stress-related disorders are included in the ICD-10 category obsessive-compulsive disorder OCD (F 42), and are increasingly being treated with antidepressants today. The ICD-10 was published in 1992, but most of the studies mentioned below come from an earlier time, so that for this reason alone almost all the studies are either based on other classification schemes or the patients were allocated to different treatment groups on the basis of specific target symptoms.

8.4.1 Typical indications for tranquillizers

About one-third of all adults suffer at some time in their lives from states of anxiety and tension which can considerably impair their quality of life (Lader, 1981b). The majority of these seek medical help sooner or later, about half of them within a year after the outbreak of the symptoms. English statistics show that some 10% are referred to a psychiatrist. Psychiatrists consequently only see a small proportion of patients suffering from states of anxiety, generally the rather severe, chronic, neurotic, socially decompensated cases. The remaining 90% of patients mostly turn to their general practitioner; they are predominantly persons who react to burdensome circumstances with acute anxiety or stress symptoms. States of this nature are generally known to wane after some six weeks, although this remission can be accelerated by taking a tranquillizer.

Most of these patients belong to ICD-10 categories F 43 (reactions to severe stress and adjustment disorders) or F 41.1 (generalized anxiety disorder, GAD). Clinically, intensive or apparently exaggerated anxiety and worries about the existing circumstances of life are most prominent, and they often also have physically experienced tension and stress, vegetative disturbances of all types, hypervigilance and irritability. These patients almost always respond rapidly to benzodiazepine tranquillizers with marked improvement of symptoms (Shader and Greenblatt, 1993).

Panic disorders (F 41.0) are sudden attacks of severe anxiety accompanied or even dominated by physical symptoms such as heart palpitations, difficulty in breathing and a constrictive feeling in the chest, which can intensify the anxiety attack and put the subject in fear of his life. Panic attacks often arise spontaneously without detectable cause (F 41.0) or are associated with particular situations such as being in a crowd, in a small, enclosed space or on an exposed street (F 40.01: agoraphobia, associated with panic disorder). Both syndromes can be treated successfully with benzodiazepines. Alternatives to tranquillizers include certain antidepressants and non-drug therapeutic procedures (see below).

Independently of these specific indications, the symptomatic efficacy of tranquillizers on mental and physical anxiety and tension symptoms has been demonstrated in hundreds of individual investigations. According to a survey by Freedman (1980), 80–90% of all controlled studies with tranquillizers show a clear superiority as compared to placebo. The success rate appears to be independent of the nature of the functional symptoms.

8.4.2 Alternatives to tranquillizers

Beta-receptor blockers

An alternative to the use of tranquillizers is the administration of beta-receptor blockers, generally called beta-blockers for short, to control the vegetative concomitant symptoms of anxiety and tension states (Kelly, 1980; Suzman, 1981). Affective arousal is accompanied by an increased release of adrenaline and noradrenaline into the blood, which, in turn, produce physical signs such as palpitations, trembling, sweating and irregular breathing. These individually variable vegetative changes are perceived by the subject and may potentiate the excitement; they can thus become detached from their original cause and become a problem as such. With beta-blockers, i.e., substances which occupy a subgroup of adrenergic receptors and protect them against the action of released catecholamines, the vegetative arousal is reduced, so that a state of excitement can lose much of its severity.

In experiments with ski jumpers it has been shown that beta-blockers dampen the emotional tachycardia that arises before a jump. Public speakers and singers can overcome their stage fright during public appearances by means of these substances. While the vegetative symptoms of stress can be eliminated with beta-blockers, mental clarity or artistic performance are not adversely affected (Neftel *et al.*, 1982). In controlled trials, students with exam nerves achieved better results with beta-blockers than with diazepam and placebo since, although they still felt the tension of the examination, they were not additionally disturbed by palpitations, tremor and other symptoms. Beta-blockers are generally well tolerated, but contraindications include asthma, bronchospasm and certain cardiac arrhythmias.

Alprazolam and antidepressants

Alprazolam is a benzodiazepine derivative with a rather short half-life which is used as an anxiolytic and, in larger doses, for the treatment of *panic attacks*. As the first substance of its class, it was licensed by the American health authority, the FDA, in this indication. However, a comprehensive literature survey by Jonas and Cohon (1993) indicates that other benzodiazepines are just as effective as alprazolam for panic attacks and also do not differ from the latter with regard to onset of action and tolerability.

As alternatives to tranquillizers and especially benzodiazepines, antidepressants have recently been recommended for the treatment of panic attacks (with or without agoraphobia) and obsessive-compulsive disorders (OCD). Studies by Gentil *et al.* (1993) with chlorimipramine, by Hoehn-Saric *et al.* (1993) with fluvoxamine and by other authors suggest that SSRIs are particularly suitable for the treatment of *panic disorders* and, according to observations by Hoehn-Saric *et al.*, mainly reduce the number of panic attacks but have little effect on the severity of the remaining anxiety attacks. Severe *OCD* which is not amenable to psychotherapy and may be accompanied by depressive symptoms is today treated with serotoninergic antidepressants in many centres. According to McDougle *et al.* (1993), SSRIs are to be considered the drugs of first choice in this indication, and a meta-analysis by Cox *et al.* (1993) of 25 controlled therapeutic trials shows that equally good effects on compulsive symptoms of OCD patients can be obtained with chlorimipramine and fluoxetine as with behavioural therapy, but that the two serotoninergic antidepressants are clearly superior with regard to their action on depressive symptoms.

Psychotherapy and/or drug therapy?

According to older surveys by Luborsky *et al.* (1975) and Freedman (1980), drug treatments with tranquillizers are more effective overall than psychotherapy in anxiety and tension states. However, the comparative studies considered here were mostly of short duration and thereby favoured the drug therapy. It is also interesting that combined drug therapy and psychotherapy in these older studies usually produced higher success rates than treatment with tranquillizers alone, and that there were no reports of adverse interactions, e.g. no adverse effect of drug therapy on the psychotherapeutic process. A more recent analysis by Wardle (1990), which was directed particularly to the question of whether benzodiazepines could have an adverse effect on the results of behavioural therapy (e.g. as a result of state-dependent learning within the context of flooding or exposure techniques), came to a very similar conclusion as the older authors. In four of six studies considered, the results with combined behavioural and tranquillizer therapy were better than with behavioural therapy alone, in one study there was no difference and in only one study (in which barbiturate infusions had been used, not a tranquillizer) was there evidence of a superior action of behavioural therapy without concomitant drug therapy.

In the meantime, both the psychotherapeutic approaches and the possible drug therapies for the treatment of anxiety and obsessional syndromes have progressed further and several models have been developed for the interplay of the two approaches which initially appear so different (see Hersen, 1986; Coryell and Winokur, 1991). A recently published review of several meta-analyses of non-drug treatment studies shows that in many indications, including the anxiety syndromes of interest to us here, psychotherapeutic procedures of various types can be expected to produce therapeutic effects of the same magnitude as with psychopharmaceuticals in the corresponding disorders (Lipsey and Wilson, 1993). Behavioural therapy, cognitively orientated therapies and many combinations and variants of these procedures clearly produce results which open up an alternative to drug therapy for patients and their doctors or psychotherapists (see also Gelernter et al., 1991; Cox et al., 1993).

A study by Welkowitz et al. (1991) shows that positive therapeutic results with non-drug procedures can also be obtained in institutions and by therapists who initially were less familiar with psychotherapeutic techniques. In a psychiatric centre traditionally orientated toward drug therapy in New York, several psychiatrists, nurses and psychologists were introduced to a cognitively orientated behavioural therapy technique on the basis of instruction books and video tapes and then treated a group of 24 patients with panic disorders. These were patients, mainly women, who had previously responded insufficiently to drugs or who desired non-drug therapy. After concluding the programme of 12 sessions that were highly structured in time and content, 14 of the 24 patients were assessed as asymptomatic, and another three had far fewer panic attacks than before or even none at all. As the authors admit, the favourable therapeutic result may partly be attributable to the positive motivation of the 'experimental therapists' and the special selection of patients, but also clearly shows that non-drug methods of treatment can be quickly learned and be used successfully in indications for which tranquillizers conventionally tend to be used.

8.4.3 Recommended treatments

It is generally recommended that tranquillizers be prescribed for not more than 6–12 weeks for states of anxiety, unrest and tension not arising within the context of psychosis (Rickels and Schweizer, 1987). One advantage of these drugs is their rapid onset of action. On the other hand, a non-drug treatment should be introduced whenever possible in the case of more prolonged disturbances. Practically all leading authors stress the need to adapt drug therapy, psychotherapy and combined therapies to match the individual symptoms and requirements of each patient and not to approach each individual case with a predetermined regimen (review by Roy-Byrne et al., 1993).

Table 8.1. Scheme of preferred forms of therapy for anxiety syndromes. The procedures preferred today are shown *in italics*, but the individual therapy must be guided by the symptoms and responses of the patient as well as the means available in practice

	Severity of physical symptoms	
	Severe symptoms	Mild symptoms
Syndromes with strong 'cognitive' component	**Panic disorder**	**Generalized anxiety disorder**
	Tranquillizers Psychotherapy (various methods) Antidepressants, especially in more severe cases	*Psychotherapy* Tranquillizers (at start of treatment)
Syndromes with weak 'cognitive' component	**Vegetative symptoms, e.g. stage fright**	**Transient states of unrest**
	Beta-blockers Psycho- therapy (behavioural therapy)	*Advice, calming* Possibly tranquillizers

Despite these limitations, some general recommendations shown in Table 8.1, based on a scheme by Freedman (1980), can be given.

8.4.4   Hypnotics and the treatment of sleep disturbances

The efficacy of preparations such as nitrazepam, flurazepam, triazolam and temazepam in combating sleep onset disorders and difficulties in sleeping through the night has been comprehensively documented in a large number of controlled trials against placebo, some of which also incorporated objective sleep polygraphic methods (Borbély, 1992). Contrary to older views, these preparations do not lose their efficacy even after weeks and months of regular use, except in the case of insomnia related to severe mental disorders. This is, however, not the case in the majority of patients suffering from impaired sleep. In young people sleeplessness occurs mostly at times of increased emotional strain or professional worries. It also occurs temporarily after transcontinental flights in an easterly or westerly direction (jet lag syndrome). The short-term use of hypnotics in such situations can be in the interest of the sleep-disturbed individual and is also widely accepted. The chronic use of hypnotics in the under-60s should, on the other hand, only be resorted to after alternative possibilities have been exhausted (relaxation exercises, autogenic training, short-term psychotherapy).

In all cases the patients must be informed that withdrawal symptoms can arise after several days of using hypnotics and be expressed in the form of transiently intensified insomnia.

Sleep disturbances are more frequent in the elderly: since human sleep alters greatly during the course of life (depth of sleep decreases with advancing age, sleep interruptions become more frequent and longer) there are more grounds for functional sleep disturbances than there are in the young. There has been hardly any investigation at to whether relaxation exercises, and possibly also psychotherapeutic measures, can be of benefit here (Spiegel *et al.*, 1991). Sleep disturbances in advanced age are almost exclusively treated today by means of drugs, preference being given to compounds having a shorter biological half-life, such as temazepam and triazolam. The continuous administration of long-acting medicaments such as nitrazepam and flurazepam can result in drug accumulation in elderly patients and thus lead clinically to impairment of attentiveness, memory and motor functions (Shader and Greenblatt, 1993).

Non-drug therapy of patients with functional sleep disorders is still the exception today, although some behavioural therapy techniques can be used with good prospects of success, especially in patients with difficulty in falling asleep. The study by McClusky *et al.* (1991) may be cited as an example of a controlled comparison in which the actions of standardized stimulus control and relaxation training were compared with those of a short-acting hypnotic (0.5 mg triazolam 30 minutes before going to bed for seven nights, then reducing to 0.25 mg for three nights and 0.125 mg for four nights). The 30 (2 × 15) patients, mostly young persons with severe difficulty in falling asleep, responded positively but differently to the two treatments. Triazolam had a clear effect with immediate onset on the time taken to fall asleep and the duration of sleep, and this action persisted during the two weeks of treatment but had disappeared at follow-up five weeks later. Behavioural training had a slower action with a latency of one to two weeks, but its effects persisted to the time of the follow-up examination. Among other things, the authors concluded from these results that the two forms of therapy could also be combined in urgent cases in order to combine the advantages of a fast onset of action and prolonged efficacy. It remains to be seen whether behavioural therapy is also suitable for the often stubborn insomnias of older and elderly patients. According to today's knowledge, individual advice associated with moderate use of hypnotics still plays the major role in these cases.

8.5 PSYCHOSTIMULANTS AND THE TREATMENT OF THE HYPERKINETIC SYNDROME IN CHILDREN

One of the few acknowledged indications for amphetamine-like stimulants is the hyperkinetic syndrome in children (ADHD; p. 22). Methylphenidate, the drug most used today in this indication, leads to a significant improvement of symptoms in up to 75% of cases, whereas 25–35% of children show no significant change or even show a deterioration in their state. The view expressed in older works that patients with an organic brain disorder respond particularly well to psychostimulants has not been confirmed. Caffeine, a psychostimulant with a mechanism of action different from that of amphetamines, has no effect on the hyperkinetic syndrome.

8.5.1   Questions of long-term medication

Since the hyperkinetic syndrome represents a severe disorder lasting for years, which makes prolonged treatment necessary, questions arise about the long-term action and safety of psychostimulants used in this indication. The therapeutic action of amphetamines and methylphenidate seems to be maintained for years in the majority of patients, and there is no need to increase the dose to a relevant degree (Safer and Allen, 1989). Controlled discontinuation studies have shown that a proportion of children can do without psychostimulants temporarily or entirely. Because of this, it is advisable to withdraw the medication from time to time so that the patient does not continue to take a product which is no longer effective or no longer necessary.

Amphetamines and methylphenidate inhibit appetite and modify various endocrine processes, so that the question arises as to whether the physical development and growth of patients treated long term with these drugs runs a normal course. Children undergoing long-term treatment with methylphenidate grow somewhat slower but make up the deficit during adolescence and achieve normal stature in adulthood. As Gittelman Klein (1987) commented, this observation applies to children whose treatment was discontinued during adolescence. There have been only a few studies dealing with the question of the positive long-term actions of psychostimulants on the hyperkinetic syndrome. After weighing up the available clinical evidence, Gittelman Klein came to the conclusion that treatment with psychostimulants is certainly effective during prolonged periods of time, but it cannot be said with certainty whether the ultimate outcome is modified to a significant degree. This rather cautious evaluation contrasts with the positive results of long-term observations of drug-treated hyperkinetic children as published by Weiss and Hechtman (1986).

8.5.2   Drug therapy and psychotherapy of the hyperkinetic syndrome

In her review, Gittelman Klein (1987) considered nine studies published between 1977 and 1985 and dealing with combined drug therapy and psychotherapy of hyperkinetic children. The non-drug treatments included cognitive training (five studies), various forms of behavioural therapy (five studies) and parent training (one study); more than one method was used in some studies.

The results are unanimous and surprising in that not one of the therapeutic studies showed a clearly detectable advantage of combined treatment over drug therapy with stimulants alone in everyday or school behaviour.

In contrast to Kauffmann and Hallahan's conclusion (1979) that behavioural therapy techniques have an important role to play, it may be assumed on the basis of this more recent analysis that none of the non-drug procedures have a clinically detectable action on ADHD. Nevertheless, experienced therapists have no doubt that drug therapy by itself, without supportive sociotherapy or psychotherapy, is virtually pointless in the treatment of the hyperkinetic syndrome. Although it is still not known which children are more likely to respond and to what degree to different treatment regimens, family counselling, medical–pedagogical or behavioural therapy are considered advisable. In addition, changes in attitude on the part of the family and teachers are essential if therapy is to succeed in correcting these disturbances, which are so extremely unpleasant for all concerned.

8.6 CONCLUDING COMMENTS TO CHAPTER 8

In the preceding pages an attempt has been made to discuss the position of drug therapy of various types of mental disorders within a wider perspective, and especially to clarify the relationship between drug therapy and non-drug treatments. It was necessary to deal separately with the various classes of psychopharmaceuticals and the disorders treated with them, and for our purposes it was also sensible to refer as far as possible to controlled, i.e., comparative studies. The drawback of this approach is obvious: comparative studies of therapeutic procedures almost necessarily favour one of the compared treatments since they can never be carried out with completely identical preconditions for all treatments (Elkin *et al.*, 1988). The value of a summary such as presented here is that results obtained in different places by different authors with different preconditions can be compared and related one to the other.

As Karasu (1982) has stated some time ago, the relative positions of drug therapy and psychotherapy have changed several times over recent decades. In the 1950s most psychiatrists and psychotherapists were chiefly interested in psychoanalytically orientated psychotherapy of predominantly neurotic disorders. 'Drug treatment was considered as inhibitory or, at best, superfluous.' Some of the critical arguments represented in the upper right quadrant of Fig. 8.2 therefore derive from this period. Over the following decade neuroleptics became established as the therapy of choice for schizophrenic psychoses, whereas psychotherapy, mainly in the form of group therapy or social measures, initially proved to be a not very effective adjuvant in these patients. A certain arrogance on the part of drug therapists, expressed by statements such as those in the lower right quadrant of Fig. 8.2, also derived from that period. During the 1970s the advantages of a combined approach to therapy were recognized, initially in the treatment of affective disorders, and thoughts of synergistic effects arose, at least in certain indications. This positive aspect is summarized on the left-hand side of Fig. 8.2, even though it is accepted that additive or even supra-additive actions of drug therapy and psychotherapy have not been demonstrated in all indications.

In the course of the treatment of schizophrenia, depressive and various neurotic syndromes, it has repeatedly been found that psychopharmaceuticals and psychotherapies are likely to influence different types of symptoms and stages of illness which in fact could – to simplify matters very considerably and possibly over-optimistically – pave the way to the more efficient use of

Effects of drug therapy on psychotherapy

Positive

1. The symptomatic improvement (calming, reduction of anxiety) makes patients more accessible to therapy

2. Autonomous ego functions such as attention, speech, memory are strengthened, especially in psychotics

3. Drugs have a symbolic significance: 'The doctor has given me something, he is helping me'

4. Drugs are part of the usual interaction between doctor and patient; a mental illness is no different in this respect

Negative

1. The rapid symptomatic improvement inhibits confrontation with problems and conflicts

2. The patient believes that nothing can be done any more without drugs, and he becomes dependent on them

3. The undesirable dependency on the doctor is strengthened; an authoritarian attitude is encouraged

4. The patient's feeling of being ill is intensified

Effects of psychotherapy on drug therapy

1. Psychotherapeutic efforts (which are anyway useless) signify for the patient an undesirable intrusion into his privacy

2. Psychotherapy induces anxiety and conflict, and hazards a painfully restored balance

1. The patient receives the impression of being perceived as a person and not just as a patient

2. Thanks to the improved relationship between doctor and patient, the latter takes his medicine reliably

Figure 8.2. Arguments for and against combined drug therapy and psychotherapy (Pfefferbaum, 1977; Weissman, 1978; Karasu, 1982)

therapy. Of practical significance is the statement by DiMascio *et al.* (1979) that, in the course of the treatment of depression, patients having different expectations and practical possibilities of therapy *can today be offered various forms of treatment with good prospects of success*, without the therapist having to work within the framework of a specific psychotherapeutic or pharmaco-therapeutic school of thought.

Have all the fears and critical questions raised at the beginning of this chapter been reassuringly and satisfactorily answered? Within the scope of empirical and quantitatively orientated studies the answer is presumably yes – but it is not possible to go any further. Some of the negative interactions formulated in Fig. 8.2 are derived not simply from the envy of jealous psycho-therapists or from the arrogance of pharmacotherapists spoiled by success, but from practical experience made by many doctors and psychotherapists. They can, however, only be exemplified by means of a qualitative analysis of individual cases (therapeutic failures) and are lost in the global success figures typical for comparative investigations. In other words, even if the left-hand side of Fig. 8.2 appears to be largely supported by the statistical data put forward, this does not definitively refute the right-hand side thereof.

Psychopharmaceuticals can – if used incorrectly or at the wrong moment (or if not used at all!) – impede or wreck the psychotherapeutic process, and the same applies to psychotherapeutic intervention introduced at the wrong moment or in a substantially incorrect manner in the context of psychophar-macotherapies. Whilst the possible synergy between the two forms of therapy, which has been demonstrated in several indications, does increase the pros-pects of success from a statistical point of view, it is by no means a guarantee of success in the individual case.

CHAPTER 9

Epilogue

9.1 ECONOMIC ASPECTS OF PSYCHOPHARMACOLOGY

In Europe, North America and Japan, which together represent between 80% and 85% of the world pharmaceutical market, the turnover in 1993 for psycho-pharmaceuticals was about 14 billion Swiss francs (SFr.). Relative to the total drugs market, which comes to over 200 billion SFr., this amounted to about 7%. The turnover per psychopharmaceutical class in the stated regions was as follows:

Neuroleptics:	2.2 billion SFr.
Antidepressants:	4.7 billion SFr.
Anxiolytics:	3.9 billion SFr.
Anti-dementia drugs, nootropics:	2.1 billion SFr.

The turnover for psychostimulants, lithium and other small groups was slightly more than one billion SFr. It is now interesting to relate these turnover figures to the estimated prevalence of the mental illnesses treated with these drugs:

	Prevalence	*Of which, treated with drugs*	
Schizophrenia	4.7 million	80%	3.8 million persons
Depression	65 million	23%	15 million persons
Anxiety disorders	72.6 million	17%	12.3 million persons
Dementias	7–9 million	23%	1.8 million persons

Several conclusions can be drawn from these figures, which are based on WHO information and the estimates of a market research company:

(1) Schizophrenia is less common than the other disorders listed here, but the great majority of sufferers are treated with drugs.
(2) Depressions, especially non-endogenous and of mild to moderate severity, are very common but in the majority of cases are not treated with drugs, at least not with antidepressants. Nevertheless, antidepressants have the highest turnover of all psychopharmaceuticals at the present time.
(3) Anxiety disorders are about as common as depressions and are still less frequently treated with drugs. Despite this, anxiolytics achieve a very high turnover.

(4) In the countries considered here, with their high life expectancy, dementias are about twice as common as schizophrenia but are treated with drugs in only about 20% of cases.

If the 1993 yearly turnover figures for neuroleptics, antidepressants, etc. are related to the numbers of patients treated, a roughly estimated sequence is obtained for the mean cost of drug treatment per patient per year. This runs: dementia (about 1150 SFr.) > schizophrenia (about 600 SFr.) > depressions and anxiety disorders (both about 300 SFr.). However, the introduction of new and generally more expensive drugs into further markets will presumably produce rapid changes.

Psychopharmaceuticals in the modern sense have been available for about 40 years and have greatly altered psychiatric practice. Disorders and illnesses which were considered incurable for centuries can be symptomatically improved, prevented and at times cured with drugs, and many patients with a previously gloomy prognosis can today lead a largely normal life in society. Can the undoubted benefits of psychopharmaceuticals be quantitatively represented even better than by descriptions of a clinical type? As a consequence of efforts to limit the costs of health care in most countries, many authors have been concerned with the quantifiable benefits of drug treatments and other forms of therapy (review by Warner and Luce, 1982). Whereas the costs of therapeutic interventions can usually be calculated very accurately, quantification of the benefits of these measures takes us quickly into a field which is only partly accessible to economic considerations. The respective analyses are known by the following names (Drummond et al., 1987):

– *Cost-effectiveness analysis*: The effectiveness of therapeutic procedures is expressed here in units as close as possible to clinical practice, e.g. 'number of days less in hospital' or 'symptomatic improvement by X points on the BPRS score'. The therapeutic result is not converted into a money value, but the quantified clinical efficacy is left at the centre.
– *Cost–utility analysis*: In this instance an attempt is made to relate the results achieved as a result of a therapeutic procedure with the criterion that is perceived by patients and their environment as 'quality of life', e.g. prolongation of life by cancer chemotherapy with the simultaneous loss of quality of life as a result of the side effects of cytostatic drugs. One application of this procedure in psychiatry would be an attempt to equate the years lived without depressive episodes during lithium medication with the perceived quality of life during that time. With cost–utility analysis also there is no conversion of the therapeutic result into a money value since the difficulties in quantifying and weighting the subjective factors which all go to make up the construct 'quality of life' are obvious even without this additional step.
– The so-called *cost–benefit analysis* attempts to convert the therapeutic results into money values. It is clear even to the adherents of this analysis that

only some specific aspects of a therapeutic result can be converted into parameters such as Swiss francs, German marks, US dollars and English pounds. Examples are the number of days in hospital spared, the time for which a patient remains available for work or is unable to work, and the time demanded from relatives to care for a family member. On the other hand, conversion into financial parameters takes no account of emotional factors such a suffering, agitation, worry and also care, support and love.

A cost–benefit analysis was performed for antidepressants over 20 years ago (Brand *et al.*, 1975). This exemplary study showed that the savings in nursing costs and the earlier return of patients to work were many times greater than the cost of treatment, including drugs. Similar studies have meanwhile been performed for neuroleptics (e.g. clozapine; see Meltzer *et al.*, 1993) and other psychopharmaceuticals. Nevertheless, authors such as Klerman and Weissman (1992) and Montgomery *et al.* (CINP Task Force, 1993) have expressed the view that the economic consequences of mental illnesses and especially depression are still largely overlooked and the economic benefits of suitable prophylaxis and therapy of mental illnesses are still poorly known. This situation could presumably be turned around if one were to compile the available but largely ignored results of cost–benefit analyses and put them into a suitable form for public presentation. In this way, cost–benefit analysis could not only justify drug prices but could become a significant factor in improving public health. Aspects of economic outcome are increasingly being incorporated into clinical trial protocols for new drugs once they are approaching registration and market introduction (Zarkin *et al.*, 1995).

9.2 EFFECTS OF PSYCHOPHARMACOLOGY ON PSYCHIATRY

How has the introduction of psychopharmaceuticals affected psychiatry and what are the consequences of psychopharmacology in relation to psychology? The following two sections deal with some aspects of these questions.

Apart from the repeatedly mentioned practical consequences for the work of the psychiatrist (more frequent and better therapeutic successes, even with schizophrenia and depression, shorter stay of patients in hospitals, more outpatient treatment, increase in interventive activity, combinations of drug therapy and psychotherapy), the possible consequences for certain theoretical aspects of psychiatry and especially the understanding of mental illnesses are of interest.

Seen in a very general way, the success of treatment with psychopharmaceuticals has promoted the view that at least some mental illnesses are curable and that healing can be obtained or promoted with medicines, i.e., by material and scientifically comprehensible means. Previously, and chiefly under the influence of psychoanalytical theories, views on the genesis of mental illnesses had become increasingly psychodynamic and thus immaterial: life history and social factors were considered decisive for schizophrenias and depressions (and certainly for neuroses), whereas the biological side of the process was viewed as inaccessible and correspondingly attracted little attention. A change started after the discovery of neuroleptics and antidepressants: the biological substrate of mental disorders returned to centre-stage and *biological psychiatry* increased in significance. Klerman (1987) speaks of a paradigm shift in psychiatry and by this means the return from psychodynamically accentuated thinking to biologically orientated views and back to the nosological categories introduced by Kraepelin and Bleuler at the turn of the twentieth century: since neuroleptics are effective in schizophrenia and antidepressants act on depressions, and since they have different pharmacological profiles, different biological mechanisms must also underlie schizophrenias and affective psychoses. This insight signified a rejection of the tendency, detectable until about 1955, to consider neuroses, depressions and schizophrenias as poorly delimited parts of a psychopathological continuum and not as separate nosological categories.

The new orientation of psychiatry also had consequences for its *methodology*: study design and the statistical evaluation of trials, the use of objective methods for the clinical evaluation of patients also, the use of electrophysiological, biochemical, neuroendocrinological and, recently, imaging procedures are among the everyday matters of biological psychiatry. Research activity is multidisciplinary and psychiatrists have to talk with chemists, endocrinologists, psychologists, statisticians and even physicists and engineers. However, criticism of this technological form of psychiatry and research is not lacking even among biologically orientated authors: Goodwin and Roy Byrne (1987) spoke of a 'decline in scholarship' and by this mean the tendency of many researchers to carry out expansive studies with the widest possible range of modern apparatus and techniques in the hope that something useful will emerge in any case. They correctly urge the execution of studies that either derive from and are planned on the basis of reasoned and formulated hypotheses or are characterized as exploratory and, in the service of finding hypotheses, are interpreted as such.

The opinion is sometimes heard or read that the advent of psychopharmaceuticals has brought back psychiatric thinking to the *medical model*. Mental disorders are again considered to be due to one, perhaps a few, biological causes that can be corrected by suitable means. A multifactorial way of thinking (the view that genetic, historical, social, familial and individual life history factors interact in a complex way until a mental disorder arises) is said to be hindered if not made impossible by the medical model. A typical example of this monocausal and, in the final analysis, materialistic way of thinking (according to this view) is the dopamine hypothesis of schizophrenia, which places the emphasis on a single neurotransmitter and neglects all other important elements, so that in its turn it is discordant even with biological reality, especially the interaction between different neurotransmitter systems. Here is not the place to discuss further or even refute this fundamental criticism of biologically orientated psychiatry, but a statement made earlier will merely be repeated, namely that the stressing and scientific study of one or a few hypothetical pathogenetic factors does not necessarily mean that other factors should be ignored or denied (see p. 115). Feer (1985) discusses this fundamental conflict further. Apart from its scientific rigour, the rejection of ever-recurring scientific obscurantism in the field also speaks in favour of biological psychiatry.

9.3 EFFECTS OF PSYCHOPHARMACOLOGY ON PSYCHOLOGY

Psychotherapists who are not medical doctors may not prescribe any medicines, so that their therapeutic means have not been immediately improved by the introduction of modern psychopharmaceuticals. On the contrary, thanks to the possibility of choosing between or even combining psychopharmaceuticals and non-drug therapies, medically qualified psychiatrists gained an advantage that led many psychologists to a violent and not always justified rejection of drug therapies and combined treatments (see Pfefferbaum, 1977). Soon, however, the number of patients accessible to psychotherapy and who requested it increased as a result of the de-institutionalization of psychiatry and other social changes, so that the demand for the services of non-medical psychotherapists increased. The rise of psychopharmaceuticals has therefore also indirectly promoted the chances of psychologists active in therapy.

In a Presidential Address to the 1993 Congress of the APA (American Psychological Association), Wiggins (1994) examined some aspects of these developments. In 1952 (the year in which chlorpromazine was discovered) the APA had 10 000 members and affiliates; in 1993 the figure was 124 000. In the USA, the number of practising psychologists exceeds that of psychiatrists and is predicted to rise by another 64% by the year 2005. According to Wiggins, psychologists make a decisive contribution to public health in the USA and, in the opinion of the APA President, this should also be taken into due account in laws and regulations. He thus proposed that, after suitable further training, psychologists be empowered to prescribe psychopharmaceuticals – an idea which should attract attention in other countries also.

With the rise of psychopharmacology, new opportunities have arisen for psychologists to work in hospitals, universities and industry. In the experimental and clinical study of psychotropic substances in subjects and patients, psychologists can fruitfully use their knowledge of methodology and play a suitable part in the mostly multidisciplinary working groups. Examples of activities of this type include the study of new psychopharmaceuticals in healthy subjects and patients, the testing of anxiolytics in experimental models of anxiety (Kohnen and Krüger, 1986) and the investigation of the effects of drugs on driving behaviour (e.g. Hobi, 1983).

A new practical question arising from the advent of psychopharmaceuticals, and one which often confronts psychologists involved in diagnostic work, relates to the assessment of patients receiving psychopharmaceuticals. How reliable are psychological test results or other diagnostic findings acquired under such circumstances? Knowing the nature and dosage of the medication, as well as the duration of therapy, notable disturbances of alertness and unusual fatigue can be understood and weighted better in psychodiagnostic examinations. The results of pharmacopsychological experiments set out in Chapter 3 should be of assistance here. Assessment is more difficult when patients do not know which drug they are taking, or when they conceal the fact that they are taking CNS-active medication. It is in any case advisable for the psychologist to discuss unusual test results with the doctor in charge, including a discussion of the prescribed medication. It may sometimes be necessary to take a blood sample in order to determine the plasma levels of medicines being taken so that unexpected and perplexing test results can be interpreted.

Apart from these political and practical aspects, another question of interest in this context is also how far psychology as a science has been influenced by psychopharmacology, for example whether psychological theory has profited in some areas from modern psychopharmacology. Ornstein (1972) has expressed the view that preoccupation with hallucinogenic drugs such as LSD and marihuana, the so-called drug culture of the 1960s, has contributed to the reawakening of interest in questions of the psychology of consciousness. However, he provides no direct evidence for the coupling of experimental or even anecdotally acquired knowledge with new psychological insights into consciousness. From the history of psychology it is known that 'big names' in psychology, such as Freud, Kraepelin and James, experimented to various degrees with psychotropic drugs, but it is difficult here to prove direct relationships between these experiments and these authors' theories.

Especially in the early years of the modern psychopharmaceutical era, authors such as Eysenck (1962), Lienert (1964) and Janke (1964) performed pharmacopsychological experiments with primarily theoretical objectives. Drugs were used since they made it possible to create reproducible, qualitatively different and quantitatively graded modifications of the mental state in healthy test subjects under controlled conditions. Manipulations of this type can hardly be produced in ethical ways by other means (sleep deprivation, frustration and other challenging situations). Eysenck (1962) checked specific predictions of his personality theory by modifying the drive level of healthy subjects with the aid of stimulant and sedative substances. Lienert (1964) hoped to clarify some ontogenetic aspects of the development of intelligence by using LSD. From today's viewpoint, however, the theoretical yield of these experiments was modest and they were subsequently virtually abandoned (see Chapter 3, Section 3.5.3). Particular interest at present attaches to the pharmacopsychology of memory processes even though, as discussed in Chapter 7, methodological difficulties are especially pronounced in this field.

On the other hand, pharmacopsychology has brought some practical benefit to applied psychology. From pharmacopsychological experiments we now know the sensitivities of various methods for measuring modifications of drive and mood, and the methodological experience gained can be transferred to other fields such as occupational and traffic psychology as well as therapeutic research. A surprising finding in this context, and one that merits further study, is the fact that so-called higher intellectual functions are affected by drugs to a lesser extent than are simple and, in particular, repetitive processes.

However, in the opinion of this author the main relevance of psychopharmacology to psychology lies in the recognition that psychological theories and psychological practice are incomplete and not appropriate to their subject unless they consider the biological substrate underlying all mental processes (mood, affect, drive, cognition, actions and reflection). It is biological processes, controlled and influenced partly internally and partly externally, that underlie our mental life. A small fraction of these processes and their carriers are accessible today by technical means: we study cells, cell constituents, synapses; we measure concentrations of neurotransmitters, enzymes and intracellular messengers in the living organism. EEG and EP recordings give an insight into the electrical correlates of mental processes. Tomorrow there will be other, better measurement methods, other things to measure and other concepts. An essential and particularly exciting element of these activities is the oscillation between various levels of study and measurement, all covering a part of reality, and in some way the interdisciplinary approach to working and thinking also answers the old question of the primacy of material and spirit: there is no primacy, we need both.

References

Ackerknecht, E.H.: *Kurze Geschichte der Psychiatrie*. Enke, Stuttgart, 1967.

Adam, K., Allen, S., Carruthers-Jones, J., Oswald, I., Spence, M.: Mesoridazine and human sleep. *Br. J. Clin. Pharmacol.* **3**, 157–163, 1976.

Adam, K., Oswald I.: Effects of repeated ritanserin on middle-aged poor sleepers. *Psychopharmacology* **99**, 219–221, 1989.

Aitken, R.C.B.: Measurement of feelings using visual analogue scales. *Proc. Roy. Soc. Med.* **62**, 989–996, 1969.

Alanen, Y.O., Räkköläinen, V., Laakso, J., Rasimus, R., Kaljonen, A.: *Towards Need-Specific Treatment of Schizophrenic Psychoses*. Springer, New York, 1986.

Aldrich, M.S.: Narcolepsy. *New Engl. J. Med.* **323**, 389–394, 1990.

Allen, D., Lader, M.: The interactions of ethanol with single and repeated doses of suriclone and diazepam on physiological and psychomotor functions in normal subjects. *Eur. J. Clin. Pharmacol.* **42**, 499–505, 1992.

Allgulander, C.: History and current status of sedative–hypnotic drug use and abuse. *Acta Psychiatr. Scand.* **73**, 465–478, 1986.

Alpern, H.P., Jackson, S.J.: Stimulants and depressants: Drug effects on memory. In: Lipton, M.A., DiMascio, A., Killam, K.F. (eds): *Psychopharmacology: A Generation of Progress*. Raven, New York, 1978, pp. 663–675.

Aman, M.G., Sprague, R.L.: The state-dependent effects of methylphenidate and dextroamphetamine. *J. Nerv. Ment. Dis.* **158**, 268–279, 1974.

Angrist, B., Peselow, E., Rubinstein, M., Corwin, J., Rotrosen, J.: Partial improvement in negative schizophrenic symptoms after amphetamine. *Psychopharmacology* **78**, 128–130, 1982.

Angst, J. (and 15 co-authors): Das Dokumentationssystem der Arbeitsgemeinschaft für Methodik und Dokumentation in der Psychiatrie (AMP). *Arzneimittelforschung* **19**, 399–405, 1969.

APA: American Psychiatric Association: *Diagnostic and Statistical Manual of Mental Disorders* (DSM-III-R). Washington, DC, 1987, 3rd edn, revised.

APA: American Psychiatric Association: *Diagnostic and Statistical Manual of Mental Disorders* (DSM-IV). Washington, DC, 1994, 4th edn.

APA Task Force: The dexamethasone suppression test: An overview of its current status in psychiatry. *Am. J. Psychiatry.* **144**, 1253-1262, 1987.

Asberg, M, Cronholm, B., Sjöqvist, F., Tuck, D.: Relationship between plasma level and therapeutic effect of nortriptyline. *Br. Med. J.* **iii**, 333–334, 1971.

Asberg, M., Thoren, P., Trasknan, L.: 'Serotonin depression': a biochemical subgroup within the affective disorders? *Science* **191**, 478–480, 1976.

Awad, A.G.: Methodological and design issues in clinical trials of new neuroleptics: an overview. *Br. J. Psychiatry.* **163** (Suppl.) 21–57, 1993.

Bachmann, P.: *Das hyperkinetische Syndrom im Kindesalter*. Huber, Bern/Stuttgart/Wien, 1976.

Baddeley, A.: *The Psychology of Memory*. Basic Books, New York, 1976.

Balant-Gorgia, A.E., Balant, L.P., Andreoli, A.: Pharmacokinetic optimisation of the treatment of psychosis. *Clin. Pharmacokinet.* **25**, 217–236, 1993.

Baldessarini, R.J.: *Chemotherapy in Psychiatry: Principles and Practice*. Harvard University Press, Cambridge, MA, 1985.

Baldessarini, R.J., Davis, J.M.: What is the best maintenance dose of neuroleptics in schizophrenia? *Psychiatry Res.* **3**, 115–122, 1980.

Baldessarini, R.J., Frankenberg, F.R.: Clozapine: A novel antipsychotic agent. *N. Engl. J. Med.* **324**, 746–754, 1991.

Ban, T.A.: *Psychopharmacology*. Williams & Wilkins, Baltimore, 1969.

Barkley, R.A.: *Attention Deficit Hyperactivity Disorder: A Handbook for Diagnosis and Treatment*. Guilford Press, New York, 1990.

Barrett, K., McCallum, W.C., Pocock, P.V.: Brain indicators of altered attention and information processing in schizophrenic patients. *Br. J. Psychiatry.* **148**, 414–420, 1986.

Bartel, P., Blom, M., Robinson, E. *et al.*: Effects of chlorpromazine on pattern and flash ERGs and VEPs compared to oxazepam and to placebo in normal subjects. *Electroencephalogr. Clin. Neurophysiol.* **77**, 330–339, 1990.

Bartus, R.T., Dean, R.L., Beer, B., Lippa, A.S.: The cholinergic hypothesis of geriatric memory dysfunction. *Science* **217**, 408–417, 1982.

Baumann, P.: Therapeutisches Drug Monitoring. In: Riederer, P., Laux, G., Pöldinger, W. (eds): *Neuro-Psychopharmaka Bd.I*. Springer, Vienna, 1992a, pp. 291–310.

Baumann, P.: Clinical pharmacokinetics of citalopram and other selective serotoninergic reuptake inhibitors (SSRI). *Int. Clin. Psychopharm.* **6** (Suppl. 5): 13–20, 1992b.

Baumann, P.: Pharmakogenetik. In: Riederer, P., Laux, G., Pöldinger, W. (eds): *Neuro-Psychopharmaka, Bd.I*. Springer, Vienna, 1992c, pp. 311–321.

Beck, A.T.: Cognitive therapy, a 30-year restrospective. *Am. Psychologist* **46**, 368–375, 1991.

Beck, A.T., Hollon, S.D., Young, J.E., Bedrosian, R.C., Budenz, D.: Treatment of depression with cognitive therapy and amitriptyline. *Arch. Gen. Psychiatry* **42**, 142–148, 1985.

Becker, R.E., Giacobini, E.: Mechanisms of cholinesterase inhibition in senile dementia of the Alzheimer type: Clinical, pharmacological and therapeutic aspects. *Drug Dev. Res.* **12**, 163–195, 1988.

Beckmann, H., Holzmüller, B., Fleckenstein, P.: Clinical investigation into antidepressive mechanisms. II. Dexamethasone suppression test predicts response to nomifensine or amitriptyline. *Acta Psychiatr. Scand.* **70**, 342–353, 1984.

Bellack, A.S., Hersen, M., Himmelhoch, J.: Social skills training compared with pharmacotherapy and psychotherapy in the treatment of unipolar depression. *Am. J. Psychiatry* **138**, 1562–1567, 1981.

Benkert, O., Hippius, H.: *Psychiatrische Pharmakotherapie*. Springer, Berlin/Heidelberg/New York, 1980.

Benowitz, N.L.: Clinical pharmacology of caffeine. *Annu. Rev. Med.* **41**, 277–288, 1990.

Bensimon, G., Benoit, D., Lacomblez, L. *et al.*: Antagonism by modafinil of the psychomotor and cognitive impairment induced by sleep-deprivation in 12 healthy volunteers. *Eur. Psychiatry* **6**, 93–97, 1991.

Bente, D.: Elektroencephalographische Gesichtspunkte zur Klassifikation neuro- und thymoleptischer Pharmaka, 1. Teil. *Med. Exp.* **5**, 337–346, 1961.

Bente, D.: Vigilance and evaluation of psychotropic drug effects on EEG. *Pharmakopsychiat.* **12**, 137–147, 1979.

Bergen, J., Kitchin, R., Berry, G.: Predictors of the course of tardive dyskinesia in patients receiving neuroleptics. *Biol. Psychiatry* **32**, 580–594, 1992.

Berger, F.M.: Anxiety and the discovery of the tranquillizers. In: Ayd, F.J., Blackwell, B. (eds): *Discoveries in Biological Psychiatry*. Lippincott, Philadelphia, 1970, pp. 115–129.

Berger, F.M., Potterfield, J.: The effect of antianxiety tranquillizers on the behavior of normal persons. In: Evans, W.O., Kline, N.S. (eds): *The Psychopharmacology of the Normal Human*. Thomas, Springfield IL, 1969, pp. 38–113.

Berger, H.: Über das Elektrenkephalogramm des Menschen. 2. Mitteilung. *J. Psychol. Neurol.* **40**, 160–179, 1930.

Berger, H.: Über das Elektrenkephalogramm des Menschen. 3 Mitteilung. *Arch. Psychiatr. Nervenkr.* **94**, 16–60, 1931.

Berger, M. (ed.): *Handbuch des normalen und gestörten Schlafs*. Springer, Berlin, Heidelberg, New York, 1992.

Berger M., Doerr, P., Lund, R. *et al.*: Neuroendocrinological and neurophysiological studies in major depressive disorders: Are these biological markers for the endogeneous subtype? *Biol. Psychiatry* **17**, 1217–1242, 1982.

Berkhout, J., Walter, D.O., Ross Adey, W.: Alterations of the human electroencephalogram induced by stressful verbal activity. *Electroencephalogr. Clin. Neurophysiol.* **27**, 457–469, 1969.

Berrios, G.E.: Neuroleptic-refractory patients and their drug plasma levels. *Encéphale* **8**, 465–485, 1982.

Bianchine, J.R.: Drugs for Parkinson's disease: Centrally acting muscle relaxants. In: Goodman Gilman, A., Goodman, L.S., Gilman, A. (eds): *The Pharmacological Basis of Therapeutics*, Macmillan, New York/Toronto/London, 1980, pp. 475–493.

Biederman, J.: Attention Deficit Hyperactivity Disorder (ADHD). *Ann. Clin. Psychiatry* **3**, 9–22, 1991.

Bielski, R.J., Friedel, R.O.: Prediction of tricyclic antidepressant response. A critical review. *Arch. Gen. Psychiatry* **33**, 1479–1489, 1976.

Birbaumer, N., Schmidt, R.F.: *Biologische Psychologie*. Springer, Berlin, Heidelberg, New York, 1991.

Bixler, E.O., Kales, A., Manfredi, R.L. *et al.*: Next-day memory impairment with triazolam use. *Lancet* **337**, 827–831, 1991.

Blackburn, I.M., Bishop, S., Glen, A.I.M., Whalley, L.J., Christie, J.E.: The efficacy of cognitive therapy in depression: A treatment trial using cognitive therapy and pharmacotherapy, each alone and in combination. *Br. J. Psychiatry* **139**, 181–189, 1981.

Blackwell, B., Sternberg, M.S.: Trial management in psychopharmacology: The roles and tasks of an industry physician. *J. Clin. Pharmacol.* **11**, 83–90, 1971.

Blaschke, T.F., Melmon, K.L.: Antihypertensive agents and the drug therapy of hypertension. In: Goodman Gilman, A., Goodman, L.S., Gilman, A. (eds): *The Pharmacological Basis of Therapeutics*. Macmillan, New York/Toronto/London, 1980, pp. 793–818.

Bleuler, E.: *Dementia praecox oder Gruppe der Schizophrenien*. Deuticke, Leipzig/Wien, 1911.

Bleuler, E.: *Lehrbuch der Psychiatrie*. Springer, Berlin 1916 ff.

Bleuler, M.: Psychiatrische Irrtümer in der Serotonin-Forschung. *Dtsch. Med. Wschr.* **81**, 1078–1081, 1956.

Blois, R., Gaillard, J.M.: Effects of moclobemide on sleep in healthy human subjects. *Acta Psychiatr. Scand. Suppl.* **360**, 73–75, 1990.

Bloom, F.E.: Neurohumoral transmission and the central nervous system. In: Goodman Gilman, A., Goodman, L.S., Gilman, A. (eds): *The Pharmacological Basis of Therapeutics*. Macmillan, New York, 1980, pp. 235–257.

Bloom, F.E., Kupfer, D.J. (eds): *Psychopharmacology: The Fourth Generation of Progress*. Raven Press, New York, 1995.

Bond, A.J., Lader, M.H.: Comparative effects of diazepam and buspirone on subjective feelings, psychological tests and the EEG. *Int. Pharmacopsychiatry* **16**, 212–220, 1981.

Bonnet, M.H., Kramer, M., Roth, T.: A dose response study of the hypnotic effectiveness of alprazolam and diazepam in normal subjects. *Psychopharmacology* **75**, 258–261, 1981.

Borbély, A.: *Das Geheimnis des Schlafs.* Ullstein Sachbuch. Frankfurt, Berlin, 1991.
Borbély, A.A.: Die Beeinflussung des Schlafs durch Hypnotika. In: Berger, M. (ed.): *Handbuch des normalen und gestörten Schlafs.* Springer, Berlin, Heidelberg, New York, 1992, pp. 120–139.
Borbély, A.A., Schläpfer, B., Trachsel, L.: Effect of midazolam on memory. *Arzneim. Forsch.* **38**, 824–827, 1988.
Bowen, D.M., Davison, A.N.: Biochemical studies of nerve cells and energy metabolism in Alzheimer's disease. *Br. Med. Bull.* **42**, 75–80, 1986.
Bowen, D.M., Smith, C.B., White, P., Davison, A.N.: Neurotransmitter-related enzymes and indices of hypoxia in senile dementia and other abiotrophies. *Brain* **99**, 459–496, 1976.
Braddock, L.: The dexamethasone suppression test. Fact and artefact. *Br. J. Psychiatry* **148**, 363–374, 1986.
Branconnier, R.J.: The efficacy of the cerebral metabolic enhancers in the treatment of senile dementia. *Psychopharmacol. Bull.* **19**, 212–219, 1983.
Branconnier, R.J., Harto, N.E., Dessain, E.C. *et al.*: Speech blockage, memory impairment, and age: A prospective comparison of amitriptyline and maprotiline. *Psychopharmacol. Bull.* **23**, 230–234, 1987.
Brand, M., Menzl, A., Escher, M., Harisberger, B.: *Kosten-Nutzen-Analyse Antidepressiva.* Springer, Berlin/Heidelberg/New York, 1975.
Brewin, T.B.: Consent to randomized treatment. *Lancet* **ii**, 919–921, 1982.
Brown, A.S., Gershon, S.: Dopamine and depression. *J. Neural Transm.* **91**, 75–109, 1993.
Brownell, K.D., Stunkard, A.J.: The double-blind in danger: untoward consequences of informed consent. *Am. J. Psychiatry.* **139**, 1487–1489, 1982.
Bruce, M., Scott, N., Lader, M., Marks, V.: The psychopharmacological and electrophysiological effects of single doses of caffeine in healthy human subjects. *Br. J. Clin. Pharmacol.* **22**, 81–87, 1986.
Bunney, W.E., Garland-Bunney, B., Patel, S.B.: Biological markers in depression. *Psychopathology* **19**, Suppl. 2: 72–78, 1986.
Burley, D.M., Binns, T.B. (eds): *Pharmaceutical Medicine.* Arnold, London, 1985.
Buros, O.K. (ed.): *The Eighth Mental Measurement Yearbook.* Gryphon Press, Highland Park, NJ, 1978.
Buschke, H.: Selective reminding for analysis of memory and learning. *J. Verb. Learn. Verb. Behav.* **12**, 543–550, 1973.
Buschke, H., Fuld, P.A.: Evaluating storage, retention and retrieval in disordered memory and learning. *Neurology* **11**, 1019–1025, 1974.
Busto, U., Sellers, E.M., Naranjo, C.A. *et al.*: Withdrawal reaction after long-term therapeutic use of benzodiazepines. *N. Engl. J. Med.* **315**, 854–859, 1986.
Bye, C., Munro-Faure, A.D., Peck, A.W., Young, P.A.: A comparison of the effects of *1*-Benzylpiperazine and dexamphetamine on human performance tests. *Eur. J. Clin. Pharmacol.* **6**, 163–169, 1973.
Bye, C., Clubley, M., Peck, A.W.: Drowsiness, impaired performance and tricyclic antidepressant drugs. *Br. J. Clin. Pharmacol.* **6**, 155–161, 1978.
Cade, J.F.J.: The story of lithium. In: Ayd, F.J., Blackwell, B. (eds): *Discoveries in Biological Psychiatry.* Lippincott, Philadelphia, 1970, pp. 218–229.
Calabrese, J.R., Bowden, Ch., Woyschville, M.J.: Lithium and the anticonvulsants in the treatment of bipolar disorder. In: Bloom, F.E., Kufper, D.J. (eds): *Psychopharmacology: The Fourth Generation of Progress.* Raven Press, New York, 1995, pp. 1099–1111.
Caldwell, A.E.: *Origins of Psychopharmacology: From CPZ to LSD.* Thomas, Springfield, IL, 1970.
Caldwell, A.E.: History of psychopharmacology. In: Clark, W.G., del Giudice, J. (eds): *Principles of Psychopharmacology.* Academic Press, New York, 1978, pp. 9–40.

Carlsson, A.: Perspectives on the discovery of central monoaminergic neurotransmission. *Ann. Rev. Neurosci.* **10**, 19–40, 1987.

Carlsson, A., Lindquist, M.: Effect of chlorpromazine or haloperidol on formation of 3-methoxytyramine and normetanephrine in mouse brain. *Acta Pharmacol. (Kobenhavn)* **20**, 140–144, 1963.

Carroll, B.J., Feinberg, M., Greden, J.F. *et al.*: A specific laboratory test for the diagnosis of melancholia: Standardization, validation, and clinical utility. *Arch. Gen. Psychiatry* **38**, 15–22, 1981.

Carroll, K.M., Rounsaville, B.J., Nich, C.: Blind man's bluff: Effectiveness and significance of psychotherapy and pharmacotherapy blinding procedures in a clinical trial. *J. Consult. Clin. Psychol.* **62**, 276–280, 1994.

Cassens, G., Inglis A.K., Appelbaum, P.S., Gutheil, T.G.: Neuroleptics: Effects on neuropsychological function in chronic schizophrenic patients. *Schizophr. Bull.* **16**, 477–499, 1990.

Chassan, J.B.: Statistical inference and the single case in clinical design. *Psychiatry* **23**, 173–184, 1960.

Chen, C-N.: Sleep, depression and antidepressants. *Br. J. Psychiatry.* **135**, 385–402, 1979.

Chen, Y., Lader, M.: Long-term benzodiazepine treatment: is it ever justified? *Hum. Psychopharmacol.* **5**, 301–312, 1990.

Chiappa, K.H.: *Evoked Potentials in Clinical Medicine.* Raven Press, New York, 1983.

Chiarello, R.J., Cole, J.O.: The use of psychostimulants in general psychiatry–a reconsideration. *Arch. Gen. Psychiatry* **44**, 286–295, 1987.

Cigánek, L.: The EEG response (evoked potential) to light stimulus in man. *Electroencephalogr. Clin. Neurophysiol.* **13**, 165–172, 1961.

CINP Task Force: Impact of neuropharmacology in the 1990s: Strategies for the therapy of depressive illness. *Eur. Neuropsychopharmacol.* **3**, 153–156, 1993.

CIPS Internationale Skalen für Psychiatrie. Collegium internationale scalarum, dritte Auflage. Beltz, Weinheim, 1986.

Claridge, G.S.: *Personality and Arousal: A Psychophysiological Study of Psychiatric Disorder.* Pergamon Press, Oxford/London, 1967.

Cleghorn, J.M., Kaplan, R.D., Szechtman, B., Szechtman, H., Brown, G.M.: Neuroleptic drug effects on cognitive function in schizophrenia. *Schizophr. Res.* **3**, 211–219, 1990.

Clubley, M., Bye, C., Henson, T.A., Peck, A.W., Riddington, C.J.: Effects of caffeine and cyclizine alone and in combination on human performance, subjective effects and EEG activity. *Br. J. Clin. Pharmacol.* **7**, 157–163, 1979.

Clyde, D.J.: *Manual for the Clyde Mood Scale.* Biometric Lab., University of Miami, Coral Gables, FL, 1963.

Cohen, I.M.: The benzodiazepines. In: Ayd, F.J., Blackwell, B. (eds): *Discoveries in Biological Psychiatry.* Lippincott, Philadelphia, 1970, pp. 130–141.

Conte, H.R., Plutchik, R., Wild, K.V., Karasu, T.B.: Combined psychotherapy and pharmacotherapy for depression. *Arch. Gen. Psychiatry* **43**, 471–479, 1986.

Coper, H., Kanowski, S.: Nootropika-Grundlagen und Therapie. In: Langer, G., Heimann, H. (eds): *Psychopharmaka. Grundlagen und Therapie.* Springer, Wien/New York, 1983, pp. 409–433.

Coper, H., Heimann, H., Kanowski, S., Künkel, H. (eds): *Hirnorganische Psychosyndrome im Alter III: Methoden zum klinischen Wirksamkeitsnachweis von Nootropika.* Springer, Berlin/Heidelberg/New York, 1987a.

Coper, H., Herrmann, W.M., Woite, A.: Psychostimulanten, Analeptika, Nootropika. *Deutsches Ärzteblatt,* **84**, 337–342, 1987b.

Coppen, A.: Biochemistry of affective disorders. *Br. J. Psychiatry* **113**, 1237–1264, 1967.

Coryell, W., Winokur, G. (eds): *The Clinical Management of Anxiety Disorders.* Oxford University Press, New York, 1991.

Costall, B., Naylor, R.J., Tyers, M.B.: The psychopharmacology of 5-HT$_3$ receptors. *Pharmacol. Ther.* **47**, 181–202, 1990.

Covi, L., Lipman, R.S., Derogatis, L.R., Smith, J.E., Pattison, J.: Drugs and group psychotherapy in neurotic depression. *Am. J. Psychiatry* **131**, 191–198, 1974.

Cowdry, R.W., Goodwin, F.K.: Biological and physiological predictors of drug response. In: van Praag, H.M., Lader, M., Rafaelson, O.J., Sachar, E.J. (eds): *Handbook of Biological Psychiatry*. Marcel Dekker, New York, 1981, pp. 263–308.

Cox, B.J., Swinson, R.P., Morrison, B., Lee, P.S.: Clomipramine, fluoxetine, and behavior therapy in the treatment of obsessive-compulsive disorder: A meta-analysis. *J. Behav. Ther. Exp. Psychiatry* **24**, 149–153, 1993.

Craik, F.I.M.: Age differences in human memory. In: Birren, J.E., Schaie, W.K. (eds): *Handbook of the Psychology of Aging*. Van Nostrand Reinhold, New York, 1977, pp. 384–414.

Craik, F.I.M., Lockhart, R.S.: Levels of processing: A framework for memory research. *J. Verb. Learn. Behav.* **11**, 671–684, 1972.

Craik, F.I.M., Salthouse, T.A. (eds): *The Handbook of Aging and Cognition*, L. Erlbaum, Hillsdale, NJ, 1992.

Creese, I., Burt, D.R., Snyder, S.H.: Dopamine receptor binding predicts clinical and pharmacological potencies of antischizophrenic drugs. *Science* **192**, 481–483, 1976.

Creutzfeldt, O.D.: *Cortex Cerebri*. Springer, Berlin/Heidelberg/New York, 1983.

Crook, Th., Ferris, S., Bartus, R. (eds): *Assessment in Geriatric Psychopharmacology*. Mark Powley Assoc., New Canaan, CT, 1983.

Crow, T.J.: Positive and negative schizophrenic symptoms and the role of dopamine. *Br. J. Psychiatry* **137**, 383–386, 1980.

Crow, T.J.: The biology of schizophrenia. *Experientia* **38**, 1275–1282, 1982.

Crow, T.J.: The dopamine hypothesis survives, but there must be a way ahead. *Br. J. Psychiatry* **151**, 460–465, 1987.

Crow, T.J., Macmillan, J.F., Johnson, A.L., Johnstone, E.C.: A randomised controlled trial of prophylactic neuroleptic treatment. *Br. J. Psychiatry* **148**, 120–127, 1986.

Curran, H.V.: Benzodiazepines, memory and mood: A review. *Psychopharmacology* **105**, 1–8, 1991.

Curran, H.V.: Antidepressant drugs, cognitive function and human performance. In: Smith, A., Jones, D. (eds): *Handbook of Human Performance*. Academic Press, New York, Vol. 2, pp. 319–336, 1992a.

Curran, H.V.: Memory functions, alertness and mood of long-term benzodiazepine users: A preliminary investigation of the effects of a normal daily dose. *J. Psychopharmacol.* **6**, 69–75, 1992b.

Curran, H.V., Lader, M.: The psychopharmacological effects of repeated doses of fluvoxamine, mianserin and placebo in healthy subjects. *Europ. J. Clin. Pharmacol.* **29**, 601–607, 1986.

Curran, H.V., Sakulsripong, M., Lader, M.: Antidepressants and human memory: An investigation of four drugs with different sedative and anticholinergic profiles. *Psychopharmacology* **95**, 520–527, 1988.

Curran, H.V., Schifano, F., Lader, M.: Models of memory dysfunction? A comparison of the effects of scopolamine and lorazepam on memory, psychomotor performance and mood. *Psychopharmacology* **103**, 83–90, 1991.

Dahl, S.G.: Plasma level monitoring of antipsychotic drugs: Clinical utility. *Clin. Pharmacokinetics* **11**, 36–61, 1986.

Danion, J.M., Peretti, S., Grangé, D. et al.: Effects of chlorpromazine and lorazepam on explicit memory, repetition priming and cognitive skill learning in healthy volunteers. *Psychopharmacology* **108**, 345–351, 1992.

Davies, A.P. Maloney, A.J.F.: Selective loss of cholinergic neurons in Alzheimer's disease. *Lancet* **ii**, 1403–1404, 1976.

Davis, J.M.: A two factor theory of schizophrenia. *J. Psychiatr. Res.* **11**, 25–29, 1974.

Davis, J.M., Casper, R.C.: General principles of the clinical use of neuroleptics. In: Clark, W.G., Del Giudice, J. (eds): *Principles of Psychopharmacology*. Academic Press, New York/San Francisco, 1978, pp. 511–536.

Davis, J.M., Wang, Z., Janicak, Ph.G.: A quantitative analysis of clinical drug trials for the treatment of affective disorders. *Psychopharmacol. Bull.* **29**, 175–181, 1993.

Davis, K.L., Kahn, R.S., Ko, G., Davidson, M.: Dopamine in schizophrenia: A review and reconceptualization. *Am. J. Psychiatry* **148**, 1474–1486, 1991.

Davis, K.L., Thal, L.J., Gamzu, E.R. *et al.*: A double-blind, placebo-controlled, multi-center study of tacrine for Alzheimer's disease. *N. Engl. J. Med.* **327**, 1253–1259, 1992.

Debus, G., Janke, W.: Psychologische Aspekte der Psychopharmakotherapie. In: Pongratz, L.J. (ed.): *Handbuch der Psychologie*, Bd. 8: Klinische Psychologie, 2. Halbband. Hogrefe, Göttingen, 1978, pp. 2161–2227.

Debus, G., Janke, W.: Allgemeine und differentielle Wirkungen von Tranquillantien bei gesunden Personen in Hinblick auf Angstreduktion. In: Janke, W., Netter, P. (eds): *Angst und Psychopharmaka*. Kohlhammer, Stuttgart, 1986, pp. 135–149.

Degkwitz, R.: *Leitfaden der Psychopharmakologie*. Wissenschaftliche Verlagsgesellschaft, Stuttgart, 1967.

Deijen, J.B., Loriaux, S.M. Orlebeke, J.F., De Vries, J.: Effects of paroxetine and maprotiline on mood, perceptual-motor skills and eye movements in healthy volunteers. *J. Psychopharmacol.* **3**, 149–155, 1989.

Delay, J., Deniker, P.: Les neuroplégiques en thérapeutique psychiatrique. *Thérapie* **8**, 347–364, 1953.

Delay, J., Deniker, P., Harl, J.-M.: Utilisation en thérapeutique psychiatrique d'une phénothiazine d'action centrale élective (4560 RP). *Ann. Méd.-Psychol.* **110**, 112–117, 1952.

Delay, J., Pichot, P., Nicolas-Charles, P., Perse, J.: Etude psychométrique des effets de l'amobarbital (amytal) et de la chlorpromazine sur des sujets normaux. *Psychopharmacologia* **1**, 48–58, 1959.

Delgado, P.L., Charney, D.S., Price, L.H. *et al.*: Serotonin function and the mechanism of antidepressant action. *Arch. Gen. Psychiatry* **47**, 411–418, 1990.

De Oliveira, I.R., Do Prado-Lima, P.A.S., Samuel-Lajeunesse, B.: Monitoring of tricyclic antidepressants plasma levels and clinical response: A review of the literature. Part I. *Psychiatr. Psychobiol.* **4**, 43–60, 1989a.

De Oliveira, I.R., Do Prado-Lima, P.A.S., Samuel-Lajeunesse, B.: Monitoring of tricyclic antidepressants plasma levels and clinical response: A review of the literature. Part II. *Psychiatr. Psychobiol.* **4**, 81–90, 1989b.

Deptula, D., Pomara, N.: Effects of antidepressants on human performance: A review. *J. Clin. Psychopharmacol.* **10**, 105–111, 1990.

Deutch, A.Y., Moghaddam, B., Innis, R.B. *et al.*: Mechanisms of action of atypical antipsychotic drugs. *Schizophr. Res.* **4**, 121–156, 1991.

Dietmaier, O., Laux G.: Übersichtabellen [Neuroleptika]. In: Riederer, P., Laux, G., Pöldinger, W. (eds): *Neuro-Psychopharmaka, Bd.4, Neuroleptika*. Springer, Wien, pp. 197–215, 1992.

Dietmaier, O., Laux, G.: Übersichtabellen [Antidepressiva]. In: Riederer, P., Laux, G., Pöldinger, W. (eds): *Neuro-Psychopharmaka, Bd.3: Antidepressiva und Phasenprophylaktika*. Springer, Wien, pp. 579–600, 1993.

DiMascio, A., Haven, L.L., Klerman, G.L.: The psychopharmacology of phenothiazine compounds: A comparative study of the effects of chlorpromazine in normal males. *J. Nerv. Ment. Dis.* **136**, 15–28 and 168–186, 1963.

DiMascio, A., Heninger, G., Klerman, G.L.: Psychopharmacology of imipramine and desipramine: A comparative study of their effects in normal males. *Psychopharmacologia* **5**, 361–371, 1964.

DiMascio, A., Brown, J., Kline, J.: Psychological testing in psychopharmacology: A review. (Unpublished manuscript, 1965.)

DiMascio, A., Weissman, M.M., Prusoff, B.A. *et al.*: Differential symptom reduction by drugs and psychotherapy in acute depression. *Arch. Gen. Psychiatry* **36**, 1450–1456, 1979.

Dixon, A.K.: Ethological aspects of psychiatry. *Schweiz. Arch. Neurol. Psychiat.* **137**, 151–163, 1986.

Dörner, K.: *Bürger und Irre. Zur Sozialgeschichte und Wissenschaftssoziologie der Psychiatrie.* Fischer, Frankfurt/Main, 1975.

Dorow, R., Horowski, R., Paschelke, G., Amin, M., Braestrup, C.: Severe anxiety induced by FG 7142, a beta-carboline ligand for benzodiazepine receptors. *Lancet* **i**, 98–99, 1983.

Douglas, W.W.: Histamine and 5-hydroxytryptamine (serotonin) and their antagonists. In: Goodman Gilman, A., Goodman, L.S., Gilman, A. (eds): *The Pharmacological Basis of Therapeutics, sixth edition.* Macmillan, New York/Toronto/London, 1980, pp. 609–646.

Drummond, M.F., Stoddart, G.L., Torrance, G.W.: *Methods for the Economic Evaluation of Health Care Programmes.* Oxford University Press, Oxford, 1987.

Duerr, H.P.: *Traumzeit: über die Grenze zwischen Wildnis und Zivilisation.* Syndikat, Frankfurt, 1979.

Dunleavy, D.L.F., Brezinova, V., Oswald, I., Maclean, A.W., Tinker, M.: Changes during weeks in effects of tricyclic drugs on the human sleeping brain. *Br. J. Psychiatry* **120**, 663–672, 1972.

ECDEU Assessment Manual. Guy, W., Bonato, R.B. (eds): US Department of Health, Education, and Welfare: National Institute of Mental Health. US Government Printing Office, 1976.

Eiff, A.W., von Jesdinsky, H.J.: Etude clinico-pharmacologique du halopéridol chez des personnes normales. *Acta Neurol. Belg.* **60**, 63–69, 1960.

Eitan, N., Levin, Y., Ben-Artzi, E., Levy, A., Neumann, M.: Effects of antipsychotic drugs on memory functions of schizophrenic patients. *Acta Psychiatr. Scand.* **85**, 74–76, 1992.

Elkin, I., Pilkonis, P.A., Docherty, J.P., Sotsky, S.M.: Conceptual and methodological issues in comparative studies of psychotherapy and pharmacotherapy, I: Active ingredients and mechanisms of change. *Am. J. Psychiatry* **145**, 909–917, 1988.

Elkin, I., Shea, T., Watkins, J.T. *et al.*: National Institute of Mental Health Treatment of Depression Collaborative Research Program. *Arch. Gen. Psychiatry.* **46**, 971–982, 1989.

Elomaa, A.: Long-term 'treatment' of schizophrenics with typical neuroleptics: A crime against humanity? *Med. Hypotheses* **41**, 434, 1993.

Emrich, H.M., Dose, M.: Carbamazepin und andere Antikonvulsiva. In: Riederer, P., Laux, G., Pöldinger, W. (eds): *Neuro-Psychopharmaka, Bd.3*: Antidepressiva und Phasenprophylaktika. Springer, Wien, 1993, pp. 529–555.

Emrich, H.M., Berger, M., Riemann, D., von Zerssen, D.: Serotonin reuptake inhibition vs. norepinephrine reuptake inhibition: A double-blind differential-therapeutic study with fluvoxamine and oxaprotiline in endogeneous and neurotic depressives. *Pharmacopsychiatry* **20**, 60–63, 1987.

Engelsmann, F., Katz, J. Ghadirian M., Schachter, D.: Lithium and memory: a long-term follow-up study. *J. Clin. Psychopharmacol.* **8**, 207–212, 1988.

Enna, S.J., Möhler, H.: Gamma-aminobutyric acid (GABA) receptors and their association with benzodiazepine recognition sites. In: Meltzer, H.Y. (ed.): *Psychopharmacology: The Third Generation of Progress.* Raven, New York, 1987, pp. 265–272.

Eysenck, H.J. (ed.): *Experiments with Drugs.* Pergamon, Oxford/New York, 1962.

Fagan, D., Scott, D.B., Mitchell, M., Tiplady, B.: Effects of remoxipride on measures of psychological performance in healthy volunteers. *Psychopharmacology* **105**, 225–229, 1991.

Farlow, M., Gracon, S.I., Hershey, L.A. *et al.*: A controlled trial of tacrine in Alzheimer's disease. *JAMA* **268**, 2523–2528, 1992.

Farmer, A.E., Blewett, A.: Drug treatment of resistant schizophrenia. *Drugs* **45**, 374–383, 1993.

Fava, G.A., Kellner, R.: Prodromal symptoms in affective disorders. *Am. J. Psychiatry* **148**, 823–830, 1991.

FDA Guidelines: General Considerations for the Clinical Evaluation of Drugs. US Department of Health, Education, and Welfare. Public Health Service, Food and Drug Administration. US Government Printing Office, Washington, DC, 1977a.

FDA Guidelines: Guidelines for the Clinical Evaluation of Antianxiety Drugs. US Department of Health, Education, and Welfare. Public Health Service, Food and Drug Administration. US Government Printing Office, Washington, DC, 1977b.

Feer, H.: *Biologische Psychiatrie. Eine Standortbestimmung.* Enke, Stuttgart, 1985.

Feinberg, I., Fein, G., Walker, J.M. *et al.*: Flurazepam effects on sleep EEG. *Arch. Gen. Psychiatry* **36**, 95–102, 1979.

Fink, M.: EEG classification of psychoactive compounds in man: A review and theory of behavioral associations. In: Efron, D.H., Cole, J.O., Levine, J., Wittenborn, J.R. (eds): *Psychopharmacology: A Review of Progress 1957–1967.* US Public Health Service Publication No. 1836. US Government Printing Office, Washington, DC, 1968, pp. 497–507.

Fink, M.: Psychoactive drugs and the waking EEG, 1966–1976. In: Lipton, M.A., DiMascio, A., Killam, K.F. (eds): *Psychopharmacology: A Generation of Progress.* Raven, New York, 1978, pp. 691–698.

Fink, M.: Classification of psychoactive drugs: Quantitative EEG analysis in man. In: Van Praag, H.M. *et al.* (eds): *Handbook of Biological Psychiatry*, Part VI. Marcel Dekker, New York/Basel, 1981, pp. 309–326.

Fitzgerald, J.D.: The influence of the medication on compliance with therapeutic regimens. In: Sackett, D.L., Haynes, R.B. (eds): *Compliance with Therapeutic Regimens.* Johns Hopkins University Press, Baltimore, MD, 1976, pp. 119–128.

Fleischmann, U.M.: *Gedächtnis und Alter.* Huber, Bern, Stuttgart, 1989.

Fleischmann, U.M.: Wirkeffekte nootroper Substanzen bei Alterspatienten: Eine Sekundäranalyse am Beispiel von Piracetam. *Zeitschr. Gerontopsychol. -psychiatr.* **4**, 285–304, 1990.

Fleishman, E.A.: Psychomotor tests in drug research. In: Uhr, L., Miller, J.G. (eds): *Drugs and Behavior.* Wiley, New York, 1964, pp. 273–296.

Fleishman, E.A.: Structure and measurement of psychomotor abilities. In: Singer, R.N. (ed.): *The Psychomotor Domain: Movement Behavior.* Lea & Febiger, New York, 1972.

Folstein, M.F., Folstein, S.E., McHugh, P.R.: Mini-Mental State: A practical method for grading the cognitive state of patients for the clinician. *J. Psychiatr. Res.* **12**, 189–201, 1975.

Foreman, N., Barraclough, S., Moore, C. *et al.*: High doses of caffeine impair performance of a numerical version of the Stroop test in man. *Pharmacol. Biochem. Behav.* **32**, 399–403, 1989.

Foucault, M.: *Wahnsinn und Gesellschaft (Histoire de la folie), third edition.* Suhrkamp, Frankfurt/Main, 1978.

Frankenburg, F.R.: History of the development of antipsychotic medication. *Psychiatr. Clin. North Am.* **17**, 531–546, 1994.

Freedman, A.M.: Psychopharmacology and psychotherapy in the treatment of anxiety. *Pharmakopsychiat.* **13**, 277–289, 1980.

Friedman, D., Squires-Wheeler, E.: Event-related potentials (ERPs) as indicators of risk for schizophrenia. *Schizophr. Bull.* **20**, 63–74, 1994.

Friedman, A.S.: Interaction of drug therapy with marital therapy in depressive patients. *Arch. Gen. Psychiatry* **32**, 619–637, 1975.

Fritze, J.: Neurobiochemie, Wirkungsmechanismen. In: Riederer, P., Laux, G., Pöldinger, W. (eds): Neuro-Psychopharmaka, Bd.3, Neuroleptika. Springer, Wien, 1992, pp. 59–80.

Fritze, J., Deckert, J., Lanczik, M. *et al.*: Zum Stand der Aminhypothesen depressiver Erkrankungen. *Nervenarzt* **63**, 3–13, 1992.

Gardos, G., Cole, J.O.: Maintenance antipsychotic therapy. For whom and how long? In: Lipton, M.A., Di Mascio, A., Killam, K.F. (eds): *Psychopharmacology: A Generation of Progress*. Raven, New York, 1978, pp. 1169–1178.

Garfield, E.: Patient compliance: A multifaceted problem with no easy solution. *Curr. Contents* **37**, 5–14, 1982.

Gastpar, M., Rimpel, J.: Klinik [der Beta-Rezeptoren-Blocker]. In: Riederer, P., Laux, G., Pöldinger, W. (eds): *Neuro-Psychopharmaka, Bd.6: Notfalltherapie, Antiepileptika, Beta-Rezeptoren-Blocker und sonstige Psychopharmaka*. Springer, Wien, 1993, pp. 111–124.

Gelernter, Ch.Sh., Uhde, T.W., Cimbolic, P. *et al.*: Cognitive-behavioral and pharmacological treatments of social phobia. *Arch. Gen. Psychiatry* **48**, 938–945, 1991.

Gentil, V., Lotufo-Neto, F., Andrade, L. *et al.*: Clomipramine, a better reference drug for panic/agoraphobia. I. Effectiveness comparison with imipramine. *J. Psychopharmacol.* **7**, 316–324, 1993.

George, K.A., Dundee, J.W.: Relative amnesic actions of diazepam, flunitrazepam and lorazepam in man. *Br. J. Clin. Pharmacol.* **4**, 45–50, 1977.

Geyer, M.A., Markou, A.: Animal models of psychiatric disorders. In: Bloom, F.E., Kupfer, D.J. (eds): *Psychopharmacology: The Fourth Generation of Progress*. Raven Press, New York, 1995, pp. 787–798.

Ghoneim, M.M.: The reversal of benzodiazepine-induced amnesia by flumazenil: A review. *Curr. Ther. Res.* **52**, 757–767, 1992.

Ghoneim, M.M., Mewaldt, S.P.: Benzodiazepines and human memory: A review. *Anesthesiology* **72**, 926–938, 1990.

Ghoneim, M.M., Hinrichs, J.V., Mewaldt, S.P.: Dose–response analysis of the behavioral effects of diazepam: I. Learning and memory. *Psychopharmacology* **82**, 291–295, 1984a.

Ghoneim, M.M., Mewaldt, S.P., Hinrichs, J.V.: Dose–response analysis of the behavioral effects of diazepam: II. Psychomotor performance, cognition and mood. *Psychopharmacology* **82**, 296–300, 1984b.

Gillin, J.Ch., Mendelson, W.B., Sitaram, N., Wyatt, R.J.: Neuropharmacology of sleep and wakefulness. *Annu. Rev. Pharmacol. Toxicol.* **18**, 563–579, 1978.

Gillin, J.Ch., Sitaram, N.: Rapid eye movement (REM) sleep: Cholinergic mechanisms. *Psychol. Med.* **14**, 501–506, 1984.

Gittelman Klein, R.: Pharmacotherapy of childhood hyperactivity: An update. In: Meltzer, H.Y. (ed.): *Psychopharmacology: The Third Generation of Progress*. Raven, New York, 1987, pp. 1215–1224.

Glass, R.M., Uhlenhuth, E.H., Hartel, F.W., Matuzas, W., Fischman, M.W.: Cognitive dysfunction and imipramine in outpatient depressives. *Arch. Gen. Psychiatry* **38**, 1048–1051, 1981.

Glenny, H., Nelmes, Ph. (eds): *Handbook of Clinical Drug Research*. Blackwell, Oxford/London/Edinburgh, 1986.

Gloor, P.: Hans Berger and the electroencephalogram of man. *Electroencephalogr. Clin. Neurophysiol.* 1969, Suppl. 28.

Goedert, M., Spillantino, M.G., Cairns, N.J., Gowther, A.A.: Tau proteins of Alzheimer paired helical filaments; abnormal phosphorylation of all six brain isoforms. *Neuron* **8**, 159–168, 1992.

Goldberg, S.C.: Persistent flaws in the design and analysis of psychopharmacology research. In: Meltzer, H.Y. (ed.): *Psychopharmacology: The Third Generation of Progress*. Raven, New York, 1987, pp. 1005–1012.

Goldberg, T.E., Greenberg, R.D., Griffin, S.J. *et al.*: The effect of clozapine on cognition and psychiatric symptoms in patients with schizophrenia. *Br. J. Psychiatry* **162**, 43–48, 1993.

Golombok, S., Moodley, P. Lader, M.: Cognitive impairment in long-term benzodiazepine users. *Psychol. Med.* **18,** 365–374, 1988.

Goodnick, M.D., Gershon, S.: Chemotherapy of cognitive disorders in geriatric subjects. *J. Clin. Psychiatry* **45,** 196–209, 1984.

Goodwin, D.W., Powell, B., Bremer, D., Hoine, H., Stern, J.: Alcohol and recall: State-dependent effects in man. *Science* **163,** 1358–1360, 1969.

Goodwin, F.K., Roy-Byrne, P.P.: Future directions in biological psychiatry. In: Meltzer, H.Y. (ed.): *Psychopharmacology: The Third Generation of Progress.* Raven, New York, 1987, pp. 1691–1698.

Grawe, K.: Psychotherapieforschung zu Beginn der neunziger Jahre. *Psychol. Rundschau.* **43,** 132–163, 1992.

Gray, J.A., Enz, A., Spiegel, R.: Muscarinic agonists for senile dementia: Past experience and future trends. *Pharmacol. Sci.* **10** (Suppl.), 85–88, 1989.

Greenberg, G.: Logistics and management of clinical trials. *Br. J. Clin. Pharmacol.* **14,** 25–30, 1982.

Greenblatt, D.J., Friedman, H.L., Shader, R.I.: Correlating pharmacokinetics and pharmacodynamics of benzodiazepines: Problems and assumptions. In: Dhal, S.G., Gram, L.F., Paul, S.M., Potter, W.Z. (eds): *Clinical Pharmacology in Psychiatry.* Springer, Berlin/Heidelberg/New York, pp. 62–71.

Greil, W., Van Calker, D.: Lithium: Grundlagen und Therapie. In: Langer, G., Heimann, H. (eds): *Psychopharmaka. Grundlagen und Therapie.* Springer, Wien/New York, 1983, pp. 161–202.

Griesinger, W.: *Die Pathologie and Therapie der psychischen Krankheiten, zweite Auflage.* Stuttgart, 1861.

Griffiths, R.R., Sannerud, Ch.A.: Abuse of and dependence on benzodiazepines and other anxiolytic sedative drugs. In: Meltzer, H.Y. (ed.): *Psychopharmacology: The Third Generation of Progress.* Raven, New York, 1987, pp. 1535–1541.

Guldner, J. Rothe, B., Lauer, C. *et al.*: Effects of a 5-HT-3-receptor antagonist on sleep EEG and sleep-associated secretion of cortisol and growth hormone. *Biol. Psychiatr.* **29,** 326–327S, 1991.

Gupta, U.: Differential effects of caffeine on free recall after semantic and rhyming tasks in high and low impulsives. *Psychopharmacology* **105,** 137–140, 1991.

Guttmann, G.: *Einführung in die Neuropsychologie.* Huber, Bern/Stuttgart/Wien, 1972.

Haefely, W.: Psychopharmacology of anxiety. *Eur. Neuropsychopharmacol.* **1,** 89–95, 1991.

Haider, M., Groll-Knapp, E., Ganglberger, J.A.: Event-related slow (DC) potentials in the human brain. *Rev. Physiol. Biochem. Pharmacol.* **88,** 125–197, 1981.

Hamilton, M.: A rating scale for depression. *J. Neurol. Neurosurg. Psychiatry* **23,** 56–62, 1960.

Hamilton, M.J., Smith, P.R., Peck, A.W.: Effects of bupropion, nomifensine and dexamphetamine on performance, subjective feelings, autonomic variables and electroencephalogram in healthy volunteers. *Br. J. Clin. Pharmacol.* **15,** 367–374, 1983.

Hamon, J., Paraire, J., Velluz, J.: Remarques sur l'action du 4560 RP sur l'agitation maniaque. *Ann. Med-Psychol.* **110,** 331–335, 1952.

Harrison, P.J.: Pathogenesis of Alzheimer's disease: Beyond the cholinergic hypothesis: Discussion paper. *J. R. Soc. Med.* **79,** 347–352, 1986.

Hartmann, E.: Effects of psychotropic drugs in sleep: The catecholamines and sleep. In: Lipton, M.A., DiMascio, A., Killam, K.F. (eds): *Psychopharmacology: A Generation of Progress.* Raven, New York, 1978, pp. 711–728.

Hechtman, L., Weiss, G.: Das hyperkinetische Kind. In: Nissen, G. (ed.): *Die Bedeutung der medikamentösen Therapie bei Verhaltensstörungen im Kindesalter.* Huber, Bern/Stuttgart/Wien, 1977, pp. 17–30.

Heiberg, J.L.: *Geisteskrankheiten im klassischen Altertum.* De Gruyter, Berlin/Leipzig, 1927.

Heimann, H.: Essai d'objectivation expérimentale et clinique de l'émotionalité. *Schweiz. Arch. Neurol. Neurochir. Psychiatr.* **100**, 475–486, 1967.

Heimann, H.: Effects of psychotropic drugs on normal man. *Confinia Psychiatr.* **12**, 205–221, 1969.

Heimann, H.: Prüfung psychotroper Substanzen am Menschen. *Arzneimittel Forsch.* **24**, 1341–1346, 1974.

Heinrich, K.: *Psychopharmaka in Klinik und Praxis.* Thieme, Stuttgart, 1976.

Heinze, H.J., Münte, T.F., Künkel, H., Dickmann, K.: Methodische Aspekte bei der Analyse von Pharmakaeffekten (Diazepam and Koffein) auf die Contingent Negative Variation. *Z. EEG–EMG.* **16**, 69–74, 1985.

Hellman, S., Hellman, D.S.: Problems of the randomized clinical trial. *N. Engl. J. Med.* **324**, 1585–1589, 1991.

Helsinki Declaration. Declaration of Helsinki recommendations guiding doctors in clinical research. *Fed. Register*, **40**, No. 69, 16056, 1975.

Henderson, A.S.: Epidemiology of mental illness. In: Häfner, L., Moschel, G., Sartorius, N. (eds): *Mental Health in the Elderly.* Springer, Berlin, Heidelberg, 1986, pp. 29–34.

Herrmann, W.M.: Development and critical evaluation of an objective procedure for the electroencephalographic classification of psychotropic drugs. In: Herrmann, W.M. (ed.): *Electroencephalography in Drug Research.* Fischer, Stuttgart 1982, pp. 249–351.

Herrmann, W.M., Hofmann, W., Kubitzki, St.: Psychotropic drug induced changes in auditory averaged evoked potentials: Results of a double-blind trial using an objective fully automated AEP analysis method. *Int. J. Clin. Pharmacol. Therapy Toxicol.* **19**, 55–62, 1981.

Herrmann, W.M., Kropf, D., Fichte, K., Müller-Oerlinghausen, B.: Elektroenzephalographische und psychoexperimentelle Untersuchungen mit Lithium an gesunden Probanden. *Pharmakopsychiat.* **13**, 200–212, 1980.

Herrmann, W.M., Schärer, E.: *Pharmako-EEG: Grundlagen, Methodik, Anwendungen.* Ecomed, Langsberg/Lech, 1987.

Herrmann, W.M., Schärer, E., Delini-Stula, A.: Predictive value of pharmacoelectroencephalography in early human-pharmacological evaluations of psychoactive drugs. First example: savoxepine. *Pharmacopsychiatry* **24**, 196–205, 1991a.

Herrmann, W.M., Schärer, E., Wendt, G., Delini-Stula, A.: Pharmaco-EEG profile of levoprotiline: Second example to discuss the predictive value of pharmacoelectroencephalography in early human pharmacological evaluations of psychoactive drugs. *Pharmacopsychiatry* **24**, 206–213, 1991b.

Herrmann, W.M., Schärer, E., Wendt, G., Delini-Stula, A.: Pharmaco-EEG profile of maroxepine: Third example to discuss the predictive value of pharmacoelectroencephalography in early human pharmacological evaluations of psychoactive drugs. *Pharmacopsychiatry* **24**, 214–224, 1991c.

Hersen, M. (ed.): *Pharmacological and Behavioral Treatment: An Integrative Approach.* Wiley, New York, 1986.

Hervé, F., Urien, S., Albengres, E., Duché, J.-C., Tillement, J.-P.: Drug binding in plasma: A summary of recent trials in the study of drug and hormone binding. *Clin. Pharmacokinet.* **26**, 44–58, 1994.

Herz, M.I., Melville, Ch.: Relapse in schizophrenia. *Am. J. Psychiatry* **137**, 801–805, 1980.

Hillyard, S.A., Kutas, M.: Electrophysiology of cognitive processing. *Ann. Rev. Psychol.* **34**, 33–61, 1983.

Hindmarch, I.: Psychomotor function and psychoactive drugs. *Br. J. Clin. Pharmacol.* **10**, 189–209, 1980.

Hindmarch, I.: The effects of paroxetine, with and without alcohol, on a battery of tests of psychomotor activity related to car driving. *Psychopharmacology* **96**, Suppl. 210, 1988.

Hindmarch, I., Bhatti, J.Z.: Psychopharmacological effects of sertraline in normal, healthy volunteers. *Eur. J. Clin. Pharmacol.* **35**, 221–223, 1988.

Hindmarch, I., Coleston, D.M., Kerr, J.S.: Psychopharmacological effects of pyritinol in normal volunteers. *Neuropsychobiology* **24**, 159–164, 1990.

Hinrichs, J.V., Ghoneim, M.M., Mewaldt, S.P.: Diazepam and memory: retrograde facilitation produced by interference reduction. *Psychopharmacology* **84**, 158–162, 1984.

Hinterhuber, H., Haring, Ch.: Unerwünschte Wirkungen, Kontraindikationen, Überdosierungen, Intoxikationen [von Neuroleptika]. In: Riederer, P., Laux, G., Pöldinger, W. (eds): *Neuro-Psychopharmaka*, Bd. 4: Neuroleptika. Springer, Wien, 1992, pp. 102–121.

Hobi, V., Psychopharmaka und Fahrverhalten. In: Langer, G., Heimann, H. (eds): *Psychopharmaka. Grundlagen und Therapie.* Springer, Wien/New York, 1983, pp. 649–661.

Hobi, V.: Psychopharmaka und Fahrtauglichkeit. In: Riederer, P., Laux, G., Pöldinger, W. (eds): *Neuro-Psychopharmaka*, Bd.I. Springer, Wien, 1992, pp. 335–352.

Hoehn-Saric, R., McLeod, D.R., Hipsley, P.A.: Effect of fluvoxamine on panic disorder. *J. Clin. Psychopharmacol.* **13**, 321–326, 1993.

Hogarty, G., Goldberg, S.: Drug and sociotherapy in the aftercare of schizophrenic patients: one year relapse rates. *Arch. Gen. Psychiatry* **28**, 54–64, 1973.

Hogarty, G.E., Ulrich, R., Goldberg, S., Schooler, N.: Sociotherapy and the prevention of relapse among schizophrenic patients: An artifact of drug? In: Spitzer, R.I., Klein, D.F. (eds): *Evaluation of Psychological Therapies.* Johns Hopkins University Press, Baltimore/London, 1976, pp. 285–293.

Hollister, L.E.: Tricyclic antidepressants (second of two parts). *N. Engl. J. Med.* **299**, 1168–1172, 1978.

Hollon, St.D., Shelton, R.C., Loosen, P.T.: Cognitive therapy and pharmacotherapy for depression. *J. Consult. Clin. Psychol.* **59**, 88–99, 1991.

Hollon, St.D., DeRubeis, R.J., Evans, M.D. *et al.*: Cognitive therapy and pharmacotherapy for depression. *Arch. Gen. Psychiatry* **49**, 774–781, 1992.

Holsboer-Trachsler, E., Hatzinger, M., Stohler, R. *et al.*: Effects of the novel acetylcholinesterase inhibitor SDZ ENA 713 on sleep in man. *Neuropsychopharmacology* **8**, 87–92, 1993.

Holttum, J.R., Gershon, S.: The cholinergic model of dementia, Alzheimer type: Progression from the unitary transmitter concept. *Dementia* **3**, 174–185, 1992.

Honigfeld, G.: NOSIE-30: History and current status of its use in pharmacopsychiatric research. In: Pichot, P. (ed.): Mod. Probl. Pharmacopsychiatry, Vol. 7. *Psychological Measurements in Psychopharmacology.* Karger, Basel, 1974, pp. 238–263.

Honigfeld, G., Patin, J.: Predictors of response to clozapine therapy. *Psychopharmacology* **99**, 64–S67, 1989.

Hordern, A.: Psychopharmacology: Some historical considerations. In: Joyce, C.R.B. (ed.): *Psychopharmacology: Dimensions and Perspectives.* Tavistock, London, 1968, pp. 95–148.

Hoyer, D., Clarke, D.E., Fozard, J.R. *et al.*: The IUPHAR classification of receptors for 5-hydroxytryptamine (serotonin). *Pharmacol. Rev.* **46**, 157–204, 1994.

Hsu, L.M.: Random sampling, randomization, and equivalence of contrasted groups in psychotherapy outcome research. In: Kazdin, A.E. (ed.): *Methodological Issues and Strategies in Clinical Research.* American Psychological Association, Washington, DC, 1992, pp. 91–105.

Huber, H.P.: Kontrollierte Fallstudie. In: Pongratz, L.J. (ed.): *Handbuch der Psychologie.* Band 8/2. Halbband. Hogrefe, Göttingen, 1978, pp. 1153–1199.

Hunter, B., Zornetzer, S.F., Jarvik, M.E., McGaugh, J.L.: Modulation of learning and memory: Effects of drugs influencing neurotransmitters. In: Iversen, L.L., Iversen, S.D., Snyder, S.H. (eds): *Handbook of Psychopharmacology*, Vol. 8. Plenum, New York, 1977, pp. 531–577.

Hurst, P.M., Radlow, R., Chubb, N.C., Bagley, S.K.: Effects of d-amphetamine on acquisition, persistence, and recall. *Am. J. Psychol.* **82**, 307–319, 1969.

Immich, H., Eckmann, F., Neumann, H. *et al.*: Grundlegende Probleme bei der Antidepressiva-Prüfung. *Arzneimittel-Forschung (Drug Res.)* **21**, 525–528, 1971.

Isacsson, G., Boëthius, G., Bergman, U.: Low level of antidepressant prescription for people who later commit suicide: 15 years of experience from a population-based drug database in Sweden. *Acta Psychiatr. Scand.* **85**, 444–448, 1992.

Itil, T.M.: Quantitative pharmaco-electroencephalography. In: Itil, T.M. (ed.): *Psychotropic Drugs and the Human EEG. Mod. Probl. Pharmacopsychiatr.*, Vol. 8. Karger, Basel, 1974, pp. 43–75.

Itil, T.M.: The discovery of psychotropic drugs by computer-analyzed cerebral bioelectrical potentials (CEEG). *Drug Dev. Res.* **1**, 373–407, 1981.

Jablensky, A.: Prediction of the course and outcome of depression. *Psychol. Med.*, **17**, 1–9, 1987.

Janicak, Ph.G., Davis, J.M., Preskorn, S.H., Ayd, F.J. (eds): *Principles and Practice of Psychopharmacotherapy*. Williams & Wilkins, Baltimore, 1993.

Janke, W.: *Experimentelle Untersuchungen zur Abhängigkeit der Wirkungen psychotroper Substanzen von Persönlichkeitsmerkmalen*. Akad. Verlagsgesellschaft, Frankfurt, 1964.

Janke, W.: *Psychodiagnostische Methoden in der Human-Psychopharmakologie*. Broschüre. Sandoz A.G., Nürnberg, 1977.

Janke, W.: Psychometric and psychophysiological actions of antipsychotics in men. In: Hoffmeister, F., Stille, G. (eds): *Handbook of Experimental Pharmacology*, Vol. 55/1. Springer, Berlin/Heidelberg, 1980, pp. 305–336.

Janke, W., Debus, G.: Experimental studies on antianxiety agents with normal subjects: Methodological considerations and review of the main effects. In: Efron, D.H., Cole, J.O., Levine, J.R., Wittenborn, J.R. (eds): *Psychopharmacology: A Review of Progress 1957–1967*. U.S. Public Health Service Publication No. 1836. US Government Printing Office, Washington, DC, 1968, pp. 205–230.

Janke, W., Debus, G.: EWL-K (Eigenschaftswörterliste). In: *Internationale Skalen für Psychiatrie*. CIPS – Collegium internationale psychiatriae scalarum, zweite Auflage, Berlin, 1981.

Janke, W., Erdmann, G.: Pharmakopsychologie. In: Riederer, P., Laux, G., Pöldinger, W. (eds): *Neuro-Psychopharmaka*, Bd. I, Springer, Wien, 1992, pp. 109–130.

Janowsky, D.S., Davis, J.M., El-Yousef, M.K., Sekerke, H.J.: A cholinergic–adrenergic hypothesis of mania and depression. *Lancet* **ii**, 632–635, 1972.

Jeste, D.V., Gillin, Ch., Wyatt, R.J.: Serendipity in biological psychiatry: a myth? *Arch. Gen. Psychiatry* **36**, 1173–1178, 1979.

Jeste, D.V., Wyatt, R.J.: Therapeutic strategies against tardive dyskinesia. *Arch. Gen. Psychiatry* **39**, 803–816, 1982.

Joffe, R.T., MacDonald, C., Kutcher, S.P.: Lack of differential cognitive effects of lithium and carbamazepine in bipolar affective disorder. *J. Clin. Psychopharmacol.* **8**, 425–428, 1988.

John, E.R., Prichep, L.S., Alper, K.L. *et al.*: Quantitative electrophysiological characteristics and subtyping of schizophrenia. *Biol. Psychiatr.* **36**, 801–826, 1994.

John, E.R., Prichep, L.S., Friedman, J., Eastan, P.: Neurometrics: Computer-assisted differential diagnosis of brain dysfunctions. *Science* **293**, 162–169, 1988.

Johnson, L.C., Chernik, D.A.: Sedative-hypnotics and human performance. *Psychopharmacology* **76**, 101–113, 1982.

Jolley, A.G., Hirsch, S.R., McRink, A., Manchanda, R.: Brief Trial of brief intermittent neuroleptic prophylaxis for selected schizophrenic outpatients: Clinical outcome at one year. *Br. Med. J.* **298**, 985–990, 1989.

Jonas, J.M., Cohen, M.S.: A comparison of the safety and efficacy of alprazolam versus other agents in the treatment of anxiety, panic and depression: a review of the literature. *J. Clin. Psychiat.* **54, Suppl. 10**, 25–45, 1993.

Jones, D.M., Allen, E.M., Griffiths, A.N., Marshall, R.W., Richens, A.: Human cognitive function following binedaline (50 mg and 100 mg) and imipramine (75 mg): Results with a new battery of tests. *Psychopharmacology* **89**, 198–202, 1986.

Jorm, A.F. Korten, A.E., Henderson, A.S.: The prevalence of dementia: A quantitative integration of the literature. *Acta Psychiatr. Scand.* **76**, 465–479, 1987.

Joseph, K.C., Sitaram, N.: The effect of clonidine on auditory P300. *Psychiatr. Res.* **28**, 255–262, 1989.

Joyce, P.R., Paykel, E.S.: Predictors of drug response in depression. *Arch. Gen. Psychiatry* **46**, 89–99, 1989.

Judd, L.L., Squire, L.R., Butters, N., Salmon, D.P., Paller, K.A.: Effects of psychotropic drugs on cognition and memory in normal humans and animals. In: Meltzer, H. (ed.): Psychopharmacology: The Third Generation of Progress. Raven, New York, 1987, 1467–1475.

Kalow, W. (ed.): Pharmacogenetics of Drug Metabolism. *International Encyclopedia of Pharmacology and Therapeutics*. Pergamon Press, New York, 1992.

Kammen, D.P. Van, Bunney, W.E., Docherty, J.P. *et al.*: *d*-Amphetamine-induced heterogeneous changes in psychotic behavior in schizophrenia. *Am. J. Psychiatry* **139**, 991–997, 1982.

Kane, J.M., Lieberman, J.A.: Maintenance therapy in schizophrenia. In: Meltzer, H.Y. (ed.): *Psychopharmacology: The Third Generation of Progress*. Raven, New York, 1987, pp. 1103–1109.

Kane, J., Honigfeld, G., Singer, J., Meltzer, H.: Clozapine for the treatment-resistant schizophrenic: A double-blind comparison with chlorpromazine. *Arch. Gen. Psychiatry* **45**, 789–796, 1988.

Kane, J.M., Smith, J.M.: Tardive dyskinesia. *Arch. Gen. Psychiatry* **39**, 473–481, 1982.

Karasu, T.B.: Psychotherapy and pharmacotherapy: toward an integrative model. *Am. J. Psychiatry* **139**, 1102–1113, 1982.

Karczmar, A.G.: Overview: Cholinergic drugs and behavior – what effects may be expected from a 'cholinergic diet?' In: Barbeau, A., Growdon, J.H., Wurtman, R.J. (eds): *Nutrition and the Brain*, Vol. 5. Raven, New York, 1979, pp. 141–175.

Karniol, I.G., Dalton, J., Lader, M.: Comparative psychotropic effects of trazodone, imipramine and diazepam in normal subjects. *Curr. Ther. Res.* **20**, 337–348, 1976.

Karoum, F., Karson, C.N., Bigelov, L.B., Lawson, W.B., Wyatt, R.J.: Preliminary evidence of reduced combined output of dopamine and its metabolites in chronic schizophrenia. *Arch. Gen. Psychiatry* **44**, 604–607, 1987.

Kaschka, W.P.: Lithium-Klinik. In: Riederer, P., Laux, G., Pöldinger, W. (eds): *Neuro-Psychopharmaka*, Bd. 3: Antidepressiva und Phasenprophylaktika. Springer, Wien, 1993, pp. 493–523.

Katschnig, H., Konieczna, I., Etzersdorfer, E.: Psychosoziale Massnahmen und Neuroleptika-Langzeitmedikation. In: Riederer, P., Laux, G., Pöldinger, W. (eds): *Neuro-Psychopharmaka*, Bd.4: Neuroleptika. Springer, Wien, 1992, pp. 169–183.

Katzman, R.: Alzheimer's disease. *N. Engl. J. Med.* **314**, 964–973, 1986.

Kauffmann, J.M., Hallahan, D.P.: Learning disability and hyperactivity (with comments on minimal brain dysfunction). In: Lahey, B.B., Kazoin, A.E. (eds): *Advances in Clinical Child Psychology*, Vol. 2. Plenum, New York, 1979, pp. 71–105.

Kay, D.C., Blackburn, A.C., Buckingham, J.A. Karacan, I.: Human pharmacology and sleep. In: Williams, R.L., Karacan, I. (eds): *Pharmacology of Sleep*. Wiley, New York, 1976, pp. 149–196.

Keck, P.E., Cohen, B.M., Baldessarini, R.J., McElroy, S.L.: Time course of antipsychotic effects of neuroleptic drugs. *Am. J. Psychiatry* **146**, 1289–1292, 1989.

Kellam, A.M.P.: The (frequently) neuroleptic (potentially) malignant syndrome. *Br. J. Psychiatry* **157**, 169–173, 1990.

Keller, M.B., Klerman, G.L., Lavori, P.W. *et al.*: Treatment received by depressed patients. *JAMA* **248**, 1848–1855, 1982.

Keller, M.B., Lavori, P.W., Klerman, G.L. et al.: Low levels and lack of predictors of somatotherapy and psychotherapy received by depressed patients. *Arch. Gen. Psychiatry* **43**, 458–466, 1986.

Kelly, D.: Clinical review of beta-blockers in anxiety. *Pharmakopsychiat.* **13**, 259–266, 1980.

Kielholz, P.: The classification of depressions, and the activity profile of the antidepressants. *Prog. Neuro-Psychopharmacol.* **3**, 59–63, 1979.

Kiloh, L.G.: The secondary dementias of middle and later life. *Br. Med. Bull.* **42**, 106–110, 1986.

King, D.J.: The effects of neuroleptics on cognitive and psychomotor function. *Br. J. Psychiatry* **157**, 799–811, 1990.

King, D.J.: Benzodiazepines, amnesia and sedation: Theoretical and clinical issues and controversies. *Hum. Psychopharmacol.* **7**, 79–87, 1992.

King, D.J., Henry, G.: The effect of neuroleptics on cognitive and psychomotor function: A preliminary study in healthy volunteers. *Br. J. Psychiatry* **160**, 647–653, 1992.

Kirchhoff, Th.: Geschichte der Psychiatrie. In: Aschaffenburg, G. (ed.): *Handbuch der Psychiatrie*, Bd. I., Deuticke, Wien, 1912.

Kirk, T., Roache, J.D., Griffiths, R.R.: Dose–response evaluation of the amnestic effects of triazolam and pentobarbital in normal subjects. *J. Clin. Psychopharmacol.* **10**, 160–167, 1990.

Kissling, W.: The current unsatisfactory state of relapse prevention in schizophrenic psychoses: Suggestions for improvement. *Clin. Neuropharmacol.* **14**, 33–44, 1991.

Klein, D.F., Ross, D.C.: Reanalysis of the National Institute of Mental Health treatment of depression collaborative research program general effectiveness report. *Neuropsychopharmacology* **8**, 241–251, 1993.

Klerman, G.L.: Future prospects for clinical psychopharmacology. In: Meltzer, H.Y. (ed.): *Psychopharmacology: The Third Generation of Progress*. Raven, New York, 1987, pp. 1699–1705.

Klerman, G.L., DiMascio, A., Weissman, M., Prusoff, B., Paykel, E.S.: Treatment of depression by drugs and psychotherapy. *Am. J. Psychiatry* **131**, 186–191, 1974.

Klerman, G.L., Weissman, M.M.: The course, morbidity, and costs of depression. *Arch. Gen. Psychiatry* **49**, 831–834, 1992.

Klerman, G.L., Weissman, M.M., Prusoff, B.A.: RDC endogenous depression as a predictor of response to antidepressant drugs and psychotherapy. In: Costa, E., Racagni, G. (eds): *Typical and Atypical Antidepressants: Clinical Practice*. Raven, New York, 1982, pp. 165–174.

Klerman, G.L., Weissman, M.M., Rounsaville, B.J. Chevron, E.S.: *Interpersonal Psychotherapy of Depression*. Basic Books, New York, 1984.

Klimt, C.R.: Principles of multi-center clinical studies. In: Boissel, J.P., Klimt, C.R. (eds): *Multicenter Controlled Trials. Principles and Problems*. INSERM, Paris, 1979.

Kline, N.S.: Monoamine oxydase inhibitors: An unfinished picaresque tale. In: Ayd, F.J., Blackwell, B. (eds): *Discoveries in Biological Psychiatry*. Lippincott, Philadelphia/Toronto, 1970, pp. 194–204.

Knapp, M.J., Knopman, D.S., Solomon, P.R. et al.: A 30 week randomized controlled trial of high-dose tacrine in patients with Alzheimer's disease. *JAMA*, **271**, 985–991, 1994.

Koelega, H.S.: Benzodiazepines and vigilance performance: a review. *Psychopharmacology* **98**, 145–156, 1989.

Koelega, H.S.: Stimulant drugs and vigilance performance: a review. *Psychopharmacology* **111**, 1–16, 1993.

Koella, W.: *Die Physiologie des Schlafes. Eine Einführung*. Fischer, Stuttgart, 1988.

Kohnen, R.: Über die Beeinflussung sozialer Verhaltensweisen durch Pharmaka. Bausteine einer Sozio-Pharmakopsychologie. In: Oldigs-Kerber, J., Leonard, J.P. (eds): *Pharmakopsychologie: experimentelle und klinische Aspekte*. G. Fischer, Jena, 1992, pp. 201–215.

Kohnen, R., Krüger, H.P.: Kurzfristige Wirkungen von Psychopharmaka–gezeigt am Vergleich eines Beta-Rezeptorenblockers. In: Janke, W., Netter, P. (eds): *Angst und Psychopharmaka*. Kohlhammer, Stuttgart, 1986, pp. 251–259.

Kooi, K.A.: *Fundamentals of Electroencephalography*. Harper & Row, New York, 1971.

Kovacs, M.: The efficacy of cognitive and behavior therapies for depression. *Am. J. Psychiatry* **137**, 1495–1501, 1980.

Kovacs, M., Rush, A.J., Beck, A.T., Hollon, S.D.: Depressed out-patients treated with cognitive therapy or pharmacotherapy. *Arch. Gen. Psychiatry* **38**, 33–39, 1981.

Kraepelin, E.: *Über die Beeinflussung einfacher psychischer Vorgänge durch einige Arzneimittel*. Jena, 1892.

Kraepelin, E.: *Psychiatrie. Bd.I: Allgemeine Psychiatrie, sechste Auflage*. Leipzig, 1899.

Kropf, D., Müller-Oerlinghausen, B.: Changes in learning, memory and mood during lithium treatment. *Acta Psychiatr. Scand.* **59**, 97–124, 1979.

Kuhn, R.: Über die Behandlung depressiver Zustände mit einem Iminodibenzylderivat (G22355). *Schweiz. Med. Wschr.* **87**, 1135–1140, 1957.

Kuhn R.: The imipramine story. In: Ayd, F.J., Blackwell, B. (eds): *Discoveries in Biological Psychiatry*. Lippincott, Philadelphia, 1970, pp. 205–217.

Kuitunnen, T., Mattila, M.J., Seppälä, T. *et al.*: Actions of zopiclone and carbamazepine, alone and in combination, on human skilled performance in laboratory and clinical tests. *Br. J. Clin. Pharmacol.* **30**, 453–461, 1990.

Kunsman, G.W., Manno, J.E., Manno, B.R., Kunsman, C.M., Przekop, M.A.: The use of microcomputer-based psychomotor tests for the evaluation of benzodiazepine effects on human performance: A review with emphasis on temazepam. *Br. J. Clin. Pharmacol.* **34**, 289–301, 1992.

Kupfer, D.J., Foster, F.G., Coble, P., McPortland, R.J., Ulrich, R.F.: The application of EEG sleep for the differential diagnosis of affective disorders. *Amer. J. Psychiat.* **135**, 69–74, 1978.

Kupfer, D.J., Frank, E., Perel., J.M. *et al.*: Five-year outcome for maintenance therapies in recurrent depression. *Arch. Gen. Psychiatry* **49**, 769–773, 1992.

Kupfer, D.J., Spiker, D.G., Coble, P.A. *et al.*: Sleep and treatment prediction in endogeneous depression. *Am. J. Psychiatry* **138**, 429–434, 1981.

Kupietz, S.S., Richardson, E., Gadow, K.D., Winsberg, B.G.: Effects of methylphenidate on learning a 'Beginning Reading Vocabulary' by normal adults. *Psychopharmacology* **69**, 69–72, 1980.

Labhardt, F.: Die Largactiltherapie bei Schizophrenien und anderen psychotischen Zuständen. *Schweiz. Arch. Neurol. Psychiatr.* **73**, 309–338, 1954.

Laborit, H., Huguenard, P., Alluaume, R.: Un nouveau stabilisateur végétatif (le 4560 R.P.). *Presse Med.* **60**, 206–208, 1952.

Lader, M.: The clinical assessment of depression. *Br. J. Clin. Pharmacol.* **11**, 5–14, 1981a.

Lader, M.: Clinical anxiety and the benzodiazepines. In: Palmer, G.C. (ed.): *Neuropharmacology of Nervous System and Behavioural Disorders*. Academic Press, New York, 1981b, pp. 225–241.

Lader, M., Petursson, H.: Rational use of anxiolytic/sedative drugs. *Drugs* **25**, 514–528, 1983.

Lamour, Y.: Alzheimer's disease: A review of recent findings. *Biomed. Pharmacother.* **48**, 312–318, 1994.

Lamping, D.L., Spring, B., Gelenberg, A.J.: Effects of two antidepressants on memory performance in depressed outpatients: a double-blind study. *Psychopharmacology* **84**, 254–261, 1984.

Lamy, P.P.: The role of cholinesterase inhibitors in Alzheimer's disease. *CNS Drugs* **1**, 146–165, 1994.

Langer, G., Schönbeck, G.: Klinische Pharmakokinetik der Antidepressiva. In: Langer, G., Heimann, H. (eds): *Psychopharmaka. Grundlagen und Therapie*. Springer, Wien/New York, 1983, pp. 111–118.

Langer, G., Koinig, G., Hatzinger, R. *et al.*: Response of thyrotropin to thyrotropin-releasing hormone as predictor of treatment outcome. *Arch. Gen. Psychiatry* **43**, 861–868, 1986.

Latz, A.: Cognitive test performance of normal human adults under the influence of psychopharmacological agents: A brief review. In: Efron, D.H., Cole, J.O., Levine, J., Wittenborn, J.R. (eds): *Psychopharmacology: Review of Progress, 1957–1967*. US Public Health Service Publication No. 1836. US Government Printing Office, Washington, DC, 1968, pp. 83–90.

Leff, J., Kuipers, L., Berkowitz, R., Eberlein-Vries, R., Sturgeon, D.: A controlled trial of social intervention in the families of schizophrenic patients. *Br. J. Psychiatry* **141**, 121–134, 1982.

Leonard, B.E.: The comparative pharmacology of new antidepressants. *J. Clin. Psychiatry* **54**, 3–15, 1993.

Leonard, B.E.: *Fundamentals of Psychopharmacology*. Wiley, Chichester, 1992.

Leonard, J.P., Ahlstich, S., Lohmann, H.: Kognitive Vigilanzkontrolle im Pharmako-EEG: Eine effektive, aufgabenbezogene Methode. In: Oldigs-Kerber, J., Leonard, J.P. (eds): *Pharmakopsychologie: experimentelle und klinische Aspeckte*. G. Fischer, Jena, 1992, pp. 265–284.

Lezak, M.D.: *Neuropsychological Assessment*. Oxford University Press, New York,1983.

Lieberman, H.R., Wurtman, R.J., Emde, G.G., Roberts, C., Coviella, I.L.G.: The effects of low doses of caffeine on human performance and mood. *Psychopharmacology* **92**, 308–312, 1987.

Lieberman, J.A., Kane, J.M., Sarantakos, S. *et al.*: Prediction of relapse in schizophrenia. *Arch. Gen. Psychiatry* **44**, 597–603, 1987b.

Lieberman, J., Jody, D., Geisler, St. *et al.*: Time course and biologic correlates of treatment response in first-episode schizophrenia. *Arch. Gen. Psychiatry* **50**, 369–376, 1993.

Lienert, G.A.: *Belastung und Regression–Versuch einer Theorie der systematischen Beeinträchtigung der intellektuellen Leistungsfähigkeit*. Anton Hain, Meisenheim, 1964.

Liljequist, R., Linnoila, A., Mattila, M.J., Saario, I., Seppala, T.: Effect of two weeks' treatment with thioridazine, chlorpromazine, sulpiride and bromazepam, alone or in combination with alcohol. *Psychopharmacologia (Berl.)* **44**, 205–208, 1975.

Liljequist, R., Linnoila, M., Mattila, M.J.: Effect of diazepam and chlorpromazine on memory functions in man. *Eur. J. Clin. Pharmacol.* **14**, 339–343, 1978.

Lingjaerde, O.: Benzodiazepines in the treatment of schizophrenia. An updated survey. *Acta Psychiatr. Scand.* **84**, 453–459, 1991.

Linnoila, M., Viukari, M.: Efficacy and side effects of nitrazepam and thioridazine as sleeping aids in psychogeriatric in-patients. *Br. J. Psychiatry* **128**, 566–569, 1976.

Lipsey, M.W., Wilson, D.B.: The efficacy of psychological, educational, and behavioral treatment. *Am. Psychologist*, **48**, 1181–1209, 1993.

Lister, R.G.: The amnesic action of benzodiazepines in man. *Neurosci. Biobehav. Rev.* **9**, 87–94, 1985.

Lucki, I., Rickels, K., Geller, A.M.: Chronic use of benzodiazepines and psychomotor and cognitive test performance. *Psychopharmacol.* **88**, 426–433, 1986.

R.,Luborsky, L., Singer, B., Luborsky, L.: Comparative studies of psychotherapies. *Arch. Gen. Psychiatry* **32**, 995–1008, 1975.

Lutzenberger, W., Elbert, B., Rockstroh, B., Birbaumer, N.: *Das EEG. Psychophysiologie und Methodik von Spontan-EEG und ereigniskorrelierten Potentialen*. Springer, Berlin/Heidelberg, 1985.

Maas, J.W.: Biogenic amines and depression: Biochemical and pharmacological separation of two types of depression. *Arch. Gen. Psychiatry* **32**, 1357–1361, 1975.

Maggini, C., Guazzelli, M., Ciapparelli, A. *et al.*: The effects of oxiracetam and D-amphetamine on all-night electronencephalogram sleep in young healthy subjects. *Curr. Ther. Res.* **43**, 979–990, 1988.

Mahendra, B.: *Dementia: A survey of the syndrome of dementia, second edition.* MTP Press, Lancaster, UK, 1987.

Maier, W., Benkert, O.: Methodenkritik des Wirkungsnachweises antidepressiver Pharmakotherapie. *Nervenarzt* **58**, 595–602, 1987.

Malla, A.K., Norman, R.M.G.: Prodromal symptoms in schizophrenia. *Br. J. Psychiatry* **164**, 487–493, 1994.

Malm, U.: The influence of group therapy on schizophrenia. *Acta Psychiatr. Scand.* **65**, (Suppl. 297), 1–65, 1982.

Marks, J.: Techniques of benzodiazepine withdrawal in clinical practice. *Med. Toxicol.* **3**, 324–333, 1988.

Markstein, R.: Bedeutung neuer Dopaminrezeptoren für die Wirkung von Clozapin. In: Naber, D., Müller-Spahn, F. (eds): *Clozapin. Pharmakologie und Klinik eines atypischen Neuroleptikums.* Springer, Berlin, Heidelberg, New York, 1994, pp. 5–15.

Matejcek, M.: Pharmaco-electroencephalography: The value of quantified EEG in psychopharmacology. *Pharmakopsychiat.* **12**, 126–136, 1979.

Matejcek, M., Irwin, P., Neff, G., Abt, K., Wehrli, W.: Determination of the central effects of the asthma prophylactic ketotifen, the bronchodilator theophylline, and both in combination. *Int. J. Clin. Pharmacol. Ther. Toxicol.* **23**, 258–266, 1985.

Matejcek, M., Neff, G., Tjeerdsma, H., Krebs, E.: Pharmaco-EEG studies with fluperlapine. *Arzneim.-Forschung* **34**, 114–120, 1984.

Mathieu, M.: *New Drug Development: A Regulatory Overview, third edition.* Parexel Int., Waltham, MA, 1994.

Mattila, M.J.: Interactions of benzodiazepines on psychomotor skills. *Br. J. Clin. Pharmacol.* **18** (Suppl. 1), 21S–26S, 1984.

Mattila, M.J., Mattila, M., Aranko, K.: Objective and subjective assessments of the effects of flupentixol and benzodiazepines on human psychomotor performance. *Psychopharmacology* **95**, 323–328, 1988.

Mattis, S.: Mental state examination for organic mental syndromes in the elderly patient. In: Bellak, L., Karasu, T.B. (eds): *Geriatric Psychiatry.* Grune & Stratton, New York 1976, pp. 77–121.

Maxwell, C.: Sensitivity and accuracy of the visual analogue scale: A psycho-physical classroom experiment. *Br. J. Clin. Pharmacol.* **6**, 15–24, 1978.

May, Ph.R.A.: Anti-psychotic drugs and other forms of therapy. In: Efron, D.H., Cole, J.O., Levine, J., Wittenborn, J.R. (eds): *Psychopharmacology: a Review of Progress.* US Government Printing Office, Washington, DC, PHS Publ. No. 1836, 1968, pp. 1155–1176.

May, Ph. R.A., Tuma, A.H., Yale, C., Potepan, P., Dixon, W.J.: Schizophrenia: A follow-up study of results of treatment. *Arch. Gen. Psychiatry* **33**, 481–486, 1976.

McClelland, G.R., Cooper, S.M., Pilgrim, A.J.: A comparison of the central nervous system effects of haloperidol, chlorpromazine and sulpiride in normal volunteers. *Br. J. Clin. Pharmacol.* **30**, 795–803, 1990.

McClusky, H.Y., Milby, J.B., Switzer, P.K., Williams, V., Wooten, V.: Efficacy of behavioral versus triazolam treatment in persistent sleep-onset insomnia. *Am. J. Psychiatry* **148**, 121–126, 1991.

McDougle, C.J., Goodman, W.K., Leckman, J.F., Price, L.H.: The psychopharmacology of obsessive compulsive disorder: Implications for treatment and pathogenesis. *Psychiatr. Clin. North Am.* **16**, 749–766, 1993.

McEvoy, J.P., Hogarty, G.E., Steingard, S.: Optimal dose of neuroleptic in acute schizophrenia. *Arch. Gen. Psychiatry* **48**, 739–745, 1991a.

McEvoy, J.P., Schooler, N.R., Wilson, W.H.: Predictors of therapeutic response to haloperidol in acute schizophrenia. *Psychopharmacol. Bull.* **27**, 97–101, 1991b.

McGuire, M.T., Raleigh, M.J., Brammer, G.L.: Sociopharmacology. *Annu. Rev. Pharmacol. Toxicol.* **22**, 643–661, 1982.

McKenna, P.J.: Pathology, phenomenology and the dopamine hypothesis of schizophrenia. *Br. J. Psychiatry* **151**, 288–301, 1987.

McKenna, P.J., Bailey, P.E.: The strange story of clozapine. *Br. J. Psychiatry* **162**, 32–37, 1993.

McKhann, G., Drachman, D., Folstein, M. *et al.*: Clinical diagnosis of Alzheimer's disease. Report of the NINCDS–ADRDA Work Group. *Neurology* **34**, 939–944, 1984.

McNair, D.M.: Antianxiety drugs and human performance. *Arch. Gen. Psychiatry* **29**, 611–617, 1973.

Mellinger, G.D., Balter, M.B., Uhlenhuth, E.H.: Prevalence and correlates of the long-term regular use of anxiolytics. *JAMA* **251**, 375–379, 1984.

Meltzer, H.Y. (ed.): *Psychopharmacology: The Third Generation of Progress*. Raven, New York, 1987.

Meltzer, H.Y.: Clinical studies on the mechanism of action of clozapine: The dopamine–serotonin hypothesis of schizophrenia. *Psychopharmacology* **99**, 518–527, 1989.

Meltzer, H.Y., Cola, P., Way, L. *et al.*: Cost effectiveness of clozapine in neuroleptic-resistant schizophrenia. *Am. J. Psychiatry* **150**, 1630–1638, 1993.

Mercier, M.A., Stewart, W., Quitkin, F.M.: A pilot sequential study of cognitive therapy and pharmacotherapy of atypical depression. *J. Clin. Psychiatry* **53**, 166–170, 1992.

Meterissian, G.B., Bradwejn, J.: Comparative studies on the efficacy of psychotherapy, pharmacotherapy, and their combination in depression: Was adequate pharmacotherapy provided? *J. Clin. Psychopharmacol.* **9**, 334–339, 1989.

Meyers, B.S., Mattis, S., Gabriele, M., Kakuma, T.: Effects of nortriptyline on memory self-assessment and performance in recovered elderly depressives. *Psychopharmacol. Bull.* **27**, 295–299, 1991.

Miller, I.W., Norman, W.H., Keitner, G.I.: Cognitive-behavioral treatment of depressed inpatients: Six- and twelve-month follow-up. *Am. J. Psychiatry* **146**, 1274–1279, 1989.

Modai, H., Rinsky, H., Cygielman, G.: The DST as a predictor of acute response to treatment with ECT, chlorimipramine, amitriptyline and phenelzine. *J. Clin. Psychiatry* **47**, 139–140, 1986.

Mohs, R.C., Davis, K.L., Levy, M.I.: Partial reversal of anticholinergic amnesia by choline chloride. *Life Sci.* **29**, 1317–1323, 1981.

Möller, H.J.: Therapieresistenz auf Antidepressiva: Risikofaktoren und Behandlungsmöglichkeiten. *Nervenarzt* **62**, 658–669, 1991.

Möller, H.J.: Klinische Prüfstudien. In: Riederer, P., Laux, G., Pöldinger, W. (eds): *Neuro-Psychopharmaka*, Bd.1. Springer, Wien, 1992, pp. 177–199.

Möller, H.J.: Niedrigdosierte Neuroleptika in Tranquilizer-Indikationen. *Sandorama* **1**, 22–25, 1993a.

Möller, H.J.: Neuroleptic treatment of negative symptoms in schizophrenic patients: Efficacy problems and methodological difficulties. *Eur. Neuropsychopharmacol.* **3**, 1–11, 1993b.

Montagu, J.D.: The effect of *d*-amphetamine on the EEG response to flicker in man. *Eur. J. Pharmacol.* **2**, 295–300, 1968.

Morris, J.B., Beck, A.T.: The efficacy of antidepressant drugs. *Arch. Gen. Psychiatry* **30**, 667–674, 1974.

Moskowitz, H., Burns, M.: The effects on performance of two antidepressants, alone and in combination with diazepam. *Prog. Neuro-Psychopharmacol. Biol. Psychiatry* **12**, 783–792, 1988.

Mueller, Ch. W., Lisman, S.A., Spear, N.E.: Alcohol enhancement of human memory: Tests of consolidation and interference hypotheses. *Psychopharmacology* **80**, 226–230, 1983.

Müller, Ch.: Psychotherapie und Soziotherapie der endogenen Psychosen. In: Kisker, K.P., Meyer, J.-E., Müller, M., Strömgren, E. (eds): *Psychiatrie der Gegenwart* Bd. II/1. Springer, Berlin/Heidelberg/New York, 1972, pp. 291–342.

Müller, P., Schöneich, D.: Einfluss kombinierter Pharmako- und Psychotherapie in einer Schizophrenie-Ambulanz auf Rehospitalisierungszeiten und Behandlungskosten. *Psychiatr. Prax.* **19**, 91–95, 1992.

Mungas, D., Magliozzi, R., Laubly, J.N., Blunden, D.: Effects of haloperidol on recall and information processing in verbal and spatial learning. *Prog. NeuroPsychopharmacol. Biol. Psychiatr.* **14**, 181–193, 1990.

Münte, T.F., Heinze, H.J., Künkel, H.: Use of endogenous event-related potentials (ERP) in the evaluation of psychotropic substances: Towards an ERP profile of drug effects. *Neuropsychobiology* **16**, 135–145, 1986.

Murphy, D.L., Aulakh, Ch.S., Garrick, N.A.: How antidepressants work: Cautionary conclusions based on clinical and laboratory studies of the longer-term consequences of antidepressant drug treatment. In: *Antidepressants and Receptor Function*. Ciba Foundation Symposium 123, Wiley, Chichester, 1986, pp. 106–125.

Murphy, G.E., Simons, A.D., Wetzel, R.D., Lustman, P.J.: Cognitive therapy and pharmacotherapy: Singly and together in the treatment of depression. *Arch. Gen. Psychiatry* **41**, 33–41, 1984.

Murphy, M.: The molecular pathogenesis of Alzheimer's disease: clinical prospects. *Lancet* **340**, 1512–1515, 1992.

Murray, J.B.: Psychophysiological effects of caffeine consumption. *Psychol. Rep.* **62**, 575–587, 1988.

Neftel, K.A., Adler, R.H., Kaeppeli, L. *et al.*: Stage fright in musicians: A model illustrating the effect of beta blockers. *Psychosom. Med.* **44**, 461–469, 1982.

Netter, P.: Effizienz: zur Methodik des Wirksamkeits-Nachweises, Placebo-Problematik. In: Riederer, P., Laux, G., Pöldinger, W. (eds): *Neuro-Psychopharmaka*, Bd.1. Springer, Wien, 1992, pp. 177–199.

Nicholson, A.N.: Visual analogue scales and drug effects in man. *Br. J. Clin. Pharmacol.* **6**, 3–4, 1978.

Nicholson, A.N., Pascoe, P.A.: Effects of fluoxetine on nocturnal sleep and daytime alertness in man. *Br. J. Pharmacol.* **89** (Suppl. 473P) 1986.

Nicholson, A.N., Pascoe, P.A.: Trimipramine, modulation of sleep in man. *Psychopharmacology* **96**, Suppl. 2, 1988.

Nigal, D., Calev, A., Kugelmass, S., Lerer, B.: Effect of four-week neuroleptic and anticholinergic drug withdrawal on memory function in chronic long-hospitalized schizophrenics. *Ann. Clin. Psychiat.* **3**, 141–145, 1991.

Norman, D.A.: *Memory and Attention*. Wiley, New York, 1969.

Nuechterlein, K.H., Dawson, M.E.: Neurophysiological and psychophysiological approaches to schizophrenia. In: Bloom, F.E., Kupfer, D.J. (eds.): *Psychopharmacology–The Fourth Generation of Progress*. Raven, New York (1995) pp. 1235–1244.

Odejide, D.A., Aderounmu, A.F.: Double-blind placebo substitution: withdrawal of fluphenazine decanoate in schizophrenic patients. *J. Clin. Psychiatry* **43**, 195–196, 1982.

O'Hanlon, J.F.: Review of buspirone's effects on human performance and related variables. *Eur. Neuropsychopharmacol.* **1**, 489–501, 1991.

O'Hanlon, J.F., Haak, T.W., Blaauw, G.J., Riemersma, J.B.J.: Diazepam impairs lateral position control in highway driving. *Science* **21**, 79–81, 1982.

O'Hara, M.W., Hinrichs, J.V., Kohut, F.J., Wallace, R.B., Lemke, J.H.: Memory complaint and memory performance in the depressed elderly. *Psychol. Aging* **1**, 208–214, 1986.

Olbrich, H.M.: Ereigniskorrelierte Hirnpotentiale und Psychopathologie. *Nervenartz* **58**, 471–480, 1987.

Oldigs-Kerber, J., Leonard, J.P. (eds): *Pharmakopsychologie: experimentelle und klinische Aspekte*. G. Fischer, Jena, 1992.

Orgogozo, J.M., Spiegel, R.: Critical review of clinical trials in senile dementia. *Postgrad. Med. J.* **63**, 237–240 and 337–343, 1987.

Ornstein, R.E.: *The Psychology of Consciousness*. Freeman, San Francisco, 1972.

Osmond, H., Smythies, J.: Schizophrenia: A new approach. *J. Ment. Sci.* **98**, 309–315, 1952.

Oswald, I.: Drugs and sleep. *Pharmacol. Rev.* **20**, 273–303, 1968.

Oswald, I., Adam, K.: Effects of paroxetine on human sleep. *Br. J. Clin. Pharmacol.* **22**, 97–99, 1986.

Oswald, I., Adam, K., Spiegel, R.: Human EEG slow-wave sleep increased by a serotonin antagonist. *Electroencephalogr. Clin. Neurophysiol.* **54**, 583–586, 1982.

Oswald, W.D., Roth, E.: Zusammenhänge zwischen EEG und Intelligenzvariablen. *Psychol. Beitr.* **16**, 1–47, 1974.

Overall, J.E., Gorham, D.R.: The brief psychiatric rating scale. *Psychol. Rep.* **10**, 799–812, 1962.

Overton, D.A.: Dissociated learning in drug states (state dependent learning). In: Efron, D.H., Cole, J.O., Levine, J., Wittenborn, J.R. (eds): *Psychopharmacology: A Review of Progress 1957–1967*. US Public Health Publication No. 1836. US Government Printing Office, Washington, DC, 1968, pp. 885–890.

Owen, R.T., Tyrer, P.: Benzodiazepine dependence: A review of the evidence. *Drugs* **25**, 385–398, 1983.

Padfield, J.M.: Making drugs into medicines. In: Burley, D.M., Binns, T.B. (eds): *Pharmaceutical Medicine*. Arnold, London, 1985, pp. 39–69.

Palfreyman, M., Kehne, J.H.: Does 5-HT have a role in anxiety and the action of anxiolytics? In: Sandler, M., Coppen, A., Harnett, S. (eds): *5-Hydroxytryptamine in Psychiatry: A Spectrum of Ideas*. Oxford University Press, Oxford, 1991, pp. 207–222.

Parker, E.S., Morihisa, J.M., Wyatt, R.J. *et al.*: The alcohol facilitation effect on memory: A dose–response study. *Psychopharmacology* **74**, 88–92, 1981.

Parkin, A.J.: *Memory and Amnesia: An Introduction*. Blackwell, Oxford, 1987.

Passouant, P., Cadilhac, J., Ribstein, M.: Les privations de sommeil avec mouvements oculaires par les antidepresseurs. *Rev. Neurol.* **127**, 173–192, 1972.

Paykel, E.S., Di Mascio, A., Klerman, G.L., Prusoff, B.A., Weissman, M.M.: Maintenance therapy of depression. *Pharmacopsychiatry* **9**, 127–136, 1976.

Peck, A.W., Bye, C.E., Clubley, M., Henson, T., Riddington, C.: Comparison of bupropion hydrochloride with dexamphetamine and amitriptyline in healthy subjects. *Br. J. Clin. Pharmacol.* **7**, 469–478, 1979.

Perlick, D., Stastny, P., Katz, I., Mayer, M., Mattis, S.: Memory deficits and anticholinergic levels in chronic schizophrenia. *Am. J. Psychiatry* **143**, 230–232, 1986.

Perry, E.: Cortical neurotransmitter chemistry in Alzheimer's disease. In: Meltzer, H.Y. (ed.): *Psychopharmacology: The Third Generation of Progress*. Raven, New York, 1987, pp. 887–895.

Perry, E.K., Tomlinson, B.E., Blessed, G. *et al.*: Correlation of cholinergic abnormalities with senile plaques and mental test scores in senile dementia. *Br. Med. J.* **ii**, 1457–1459, 1978.

Peters, R., McGee, R.: Cigarette smoking and state-dependent memory. *Psychopharmacology* **76**, 232–235, 1982.

Petersen, R.C.: Scopolamine induced learning failures in man. *Psychopharmacology* **52**, 283–289, 1977.

Pfefferbaum, A.: Psychotherapy and psychopharmacology. In: Barchas, J.D., Berger, Ph. A., Ciaranello, R.D., Elliott, G.R. (eds): *Psychopharmacology: From Theory to Practice*. Oxford University Press, New York, 1977, pp. 481–492.

Pflug, B., Hartung, M., Klemke, W.: Die Beeinflussung von Befindlichkeit und Leistungsfähigkeit gesunder Versuchspersonen durch Lithiumcarbonat. *Pharmakopsychiatrie* **13**, 175–181, 1980.

Pharmacopsychiatry (1982). Special Issue 1, Volume 15 of *Pharmacopsychiatry*, May 1982. Contains 13 contributions on critical flicker-fusion frequency and drug effects.

Philipp, M.: Psychometrie, Rating-Skalen, Evaluation. In: Riederer, P., Laux, G., Pöldinger, W. (eds): *Neuro-Psychopharmaka*, Bd.1. Springer, Wien, 1992, pp. 177–199.

Plutchik, R., Platman, S.R., Fieve, R.R.: Three alternatives to the double-blind. *Arch. Gen. Psychiatry* **20**, 428–432, 1969.

Poewe, W., Gerstenbrand, F.: Klinik der Dopamin-Agonisten. In: Riederer, P., Laux, G., Pöldinger, W. (eds): *Neuropsychopharmaka.*, Bd.5. Springer-Verlag, Wien, 1992, pp. 101–111.

Pöldinger, W.: Comparison between imipramine and desipramine in normal subjects and their action in depressive patients. *Psychopharmacologia* **4**, 302–307, 1963.

Pöldinger, W.: *Kompendium der Psychopharmakotherapie.* Editiones 'Roche', Basel, 1975.

Pollock, B.G., Perel, J.M., Shostak, M. *et al.*: Understanding the response lag to tricyclics. I. Application of pulse-loading regimens with intravenous clomipramine. *Psychopharmacol. Bull.* **22**, 214–219, 1986.

Pomara, N., Deptula, D., Medel, M. Block, R.I., Greenblatt, D.J.: Effects of diazepam on recall memory: Relationship to aging, dose and duration of treatment. *Psychopharmacol. Bull.* **25**, 144–148, 1989.

Pons, L., Trenque, T., Bielecki, M. *et al.*: Attentional effects of caffeine in man: comparison with drugs acting upon performance. *Psychiatr. Res.* **23**, 329–333, 1988.

Pope, H.G., Keck, P.E., McElroy, S.L.: Frequency and presentation of neuroleptic malignant syndrome in a large psychiatric hospital. *Am. J. Psychiatry* **143**, 1227–1233, 1986.

Post, R.M.: Mechanisms of action of carbamazepine and related anticonvulsants in affective illness. In: Meltzer, H.Y. (ed.): *Psychopharmacology: The Third Generation of Progress.* Raven, New York, 1987, pp. 567–576.

Preskorn, S.H.: Tricyclic antidepressants: the whys and hows of therapeutic drug monitoring. *J. Clin. Psychiatr.* **50** (Suppl.) 34–42, 1989.

Preskorn, S.H., Burke, M.J., Fast, G.A.: Therapeutic drug monitoring: principles and practice. *Psychiatr. Clin. North Am.* **16**, 611–641, 1993.

Preston, G.C., Brazell, C., Ward, C. *et al.*: The scopolamine model of dementia: determination of central cholinomimetic effects of physostigmine on cognition and biochemical markers in man. *J. Psychopharmacol.* **2**, 67–79, 1988.

Preston, G.C., Ward, C., Lines, C.R. *et al.*: Scopolamine and benzodiazepine models of dementia: Cross-reversal by Ro 15-1788 and physostigmine. *Psychopharmacology* **98**, 487–494, 1989.

Price, D.L., Whitehouse, P.J., Struble, R.G.: Cellular pathology in Alzheimer's and Parkinson's disease. *Trends Neurosci.* **9**, 29–33, 1986.

Prien, R.F.: Long-term treatment of affective disorders. In: Meltzer, H.Y. (ed.): *Psychopharmacology: The Third Generation of Progress.* Raven, New York, 1987, pp. 1051–1058.

Prien, R.F., Caffey, E.M.: Long-term maintenance drug therapy in recurrent affective illness: Current status and issues. *Dis. Nerv. Syst.* **38**, 981–992, 1977.

Prien, R.F. Gelenberg, A.J.: Alternatives to lithium for preventive treatment of bipolar disorder. *Am. J. Psychiatry* **146**, 840–848, 1989.

Prien, R.F., Kupfer, D.J.: Continuation drug therapy for major depressive episodes: How long should it be maintained? *Am. J. Psychiatry* **143**, 18–23, 1986.

Prusoff, B.A., Weissman, M.M., Klerman, G.L., Rounsaville, B.J.: Research diagnostic criteria subtypes of depression: Their role as predictors of differential response to psychotherapy and drug treatment. *Arch. Gen. Psychiatry* **37**, 796–801, 1980.

Putten Van, T., Marshall B.D., Liberman R. *et al.*: Systematic dosage reduction in treatment-resistant schizophrenic patients. *Psychopharmacol. Bull.* **29**, 315–320, 1993.

Putten Van, T., May, P.R.A., Marder, S.R.: Response to antipsychotic medication: The doctor's and the consumer's view. *Am. J. Psychiatry* **141**, 16–19, 1984.

Quitkin, F.M., Rabkin, J.G., Ross, D., McGrath, P.J.: Duration of antidepresant treatment. What is an adequate trial? *Arch. Gen. Psychiatry* **41**, 238–245, 1984.

Raskin, A.: The prediction of antidepressant drug effects: Review and critique. In: Efron, D.H., Cole, J.O., Levine, J., Wittenborn, J.R. (eds): *Psychopharmacology: A Review of Progress 1957–1967*. US Public Health Service Publication No. 1836. US Government Printing Office, Washington, DC, 1968, pp. 757–765.

Rechtschaffen, A., Kales, A. (eds): *A Manual of Standardized Terminology, Techniques and Scoring System for Sleep Stages of Human Subjects*. Public Health Service, US Government Printing Office, Washington, DC, 1968.

Regland, B., Gottfries, C.-G.: The role of amyloid ß-protein in Alzheimer's disease. *Lancet* **340**, 467–469, 1992.

Reisberg, B., Ferris, S.H., Gershon, S.: An overview of pharmacologic treatment of cognitive decline in the aged. *Am. J. Psychiatry* **138**, 593–600, 1981.

Reynolds, Ch.F. Kupfer, D.J.: Sleep research in affective illness: state of art circa 1987. *Sleep* **10**, 199–215, 1987.

Rickels, K., Schweizer, E.E.: Current pharmacotherapy of anxiety and panic. In: Meltzer, H.Y. (ed.): *Psychopharmacology: The Third Generation of Progress*. Raven, New York, 1987, pp. 1193–1203.

Rickels, K., Schweizer, E.E., Case, W.G., Greenblatt, D.J.: Long-term therapeutic use of benzodiazepines. I. Effects of abrupt discontinuation. *Arch. Gen. Psychiatry* **47**, 899–907, 1990.

Riederer, P., Laux, G., Pöldinger, W. (eds): *Neuro-Psychopharmaka: Ein Therapie-Handbuch*. 6 Bände. Springer-Verlag, Wien, 1992.

Riezen, H. van, Segal, M.: *Comparative Evaluation of Rating Scales for Clinical Psychopharmacology*. Elsevier, Amsterdam, 1988.

Rifkin, A., Doddi, S., Karajgi, B., Borenstein, M., Wachspress, M.: Dosage of haloperidol for schizophrenia. *Arch. Gen. Psychiat.* **48**, 166–170, 1991.

Rihmer, Z., Arato, M., Gyorgy, S., Reval, K., Demeter, E.: Dexamethasone suppression test as an aid for selection of specific antidepressant drugs in patients with endogeneous depression. *Pharmacopsychiatry* **18**, 306–308, 1985.

Robinson, D.S., Prien, R.F.: Clinical study design: Critical issues. In: Bloom, F.E., Kupfer, D.J. (eds): *Psychopharmacology: The Fourth Generation of Progress*. Raven Press, New York, 1995, pp. 829–838.

Robinson, S.: Relationship between EEG and behavior. In: Itil, T.M. (ed.): *Psychotropic Drugs and the Human EEG*. Karger, Basel, 1974, pp. 286–300.

Rogers, H.J., Spector, R.G.: Phase I studies. In: Glenny, H. Nelmes, Ph. (eds): *Handbook of Clinical Drug Research*. Blackwell, Oxford/London/Edinburgh, 1986, pp. 33–58.

Rohloff, A., Ott, H., Fichte, K.: ZNS-Profil von Bromergurid anhand von Pharmako-EEG, psychometrischen Tests und Fragebogen im Vergleich zu Haloperidol und Placebo nach einmaliger Gabe. In: Oldigs-Kerber, L.J., Leonard J.P. (eds): *Pharmakopsychologie: experimentelle und klinische Aspekte*. G. Fischer, Jena, 1992, pp. 285–304.

Rosen, G.: *Madness in Society*. Harper & Row, New York, 1969.

Rosen, W.G., Mohs, R.C., Davis, K.L.: A new rating scale for Alzheimer's Disease. *Am. J. Psychiatr.* **11**, 1356–1364, 1984.

Rosenberg, R.N.: A causal role for amyloid in Alzheimer's disease: The end of the beginning. *Neurology* **43**, 851–856, 1993.

Rösler, F.: Methoden der kognitiven Psychophysiologie: Spontan-EEG, ereigniskorrelierte Potentiale und Reaktionsgeschwindigkeiten im Rahmen der Pharmakopsychologie. In: Oldigs-Kerber, J., Leonard, J.P. (eds): *Pharmakopsychologie: experimentelle und klinische Aspekte*. G. Fischer, Jena, 1992, pp. 246–264.

Rossor, M.: Alzheimer's disease. *Br. Med. J.* **307**, 779–782, 1993.

Roth, M.: Senile dementia and its borderlands. In: Cole, J.O., Barrett, J.E. (eds): *Psychopathology in the Aged*. Raven, New York, 1980, pp. 205–232.

Roy-Byrne, P., Wingerson, D., Cowley, D., Dager, S: Psychopharmacologic treatment of panic, generalized anxiety disorder, and social phobia. *Psychiatr. Clin. North Am.* **16**, 719–735, 1993.

Rudorfer, M.V., Potter, W.Z.: Antidepressants: A comparative review of the clinical pharmacology and therapeutic use of the 'newer' versus the 'older' drugs. *Drugs* **37**, 713–738, 1989.

Rush, A.J., Beck, A.T., Kovacs, M., Hollon, S.: Comparative efficacy of cognitive therapy and pharmacotherapy in the treatment of depressed outpatients. *Cognitive Ther. Res.* **1**, 17–37, 1977.

Rush, A.J., Roffwarg, H.P., Giles, D.E. *et al.*: Psychobiological predictors of antidepressant drug response. *Pharmacopsychiatry* **16**, 192–194, 1983.

Sack, R.L., De Fraites, E.: Lithium and the treatment of mania. In: Barchas, J.D., Berger, Ph.A., Ciaranello, R.D., Elliott, G.R. (eds): *Psychopharmacology: From Theory to Practice.* Oxford University Press, New York, 1977, pp. 208–225.

Safer, D.J., Allen, R.P.: Absence of tolerance to the behavioral effects of methylphenidate in hyperactive and inattentive children. *J. Pediatr.* **115**, 1003–1008, 1989.

Sagales, T., Erril, S.: Effects of central dopaminergic blockade with pimozide upon the EEG stages of sleep in man. *Psychopharmacologia (Berl.)* **41**, 53–56, 1975.

Sakulsripong, M., Curran, H.V., Lader, M.: Does tolerance develop to the sedative and amnesic effects of antidepressants? *Eur. J. Clin. Pharmacol.* **40**, 43–48, 1991.

Saletu, B.: *Psychopharmaka, Gehirntätigkeit und Schlaf.* Bibl. Psychiat. Nr. 155. Karger, Basel, 1976.

Saletu, B.: Pharmaco-EEG profiles of typical and atypical antidepressants. In: Costa, E., Racagni, G. (eds): *Typical and Atypical Antidepressants: Clinical Practice.* Raven, New York, 1982, pp. 257–268.

Saletu, B., Frey, R., Krupka, M. *et al.*: Differential effects of a new central adrenergic agonist – Modafinil – and D-amphetamine on sleep and early morning behaviour in young healthy volunteers. *Int. J. Clin. Pharmacol. Res.* **9**, 183–195, 1989.

Sanger, D., Emmett-Oglesby, M., Willner, P. (eds.): Pharmacological approaches to learning and memory. *Behav. Pharmacol.* **3/4**, 283–421, 1992.

Sartorius, N., Ban, T.A. (eds): *Assessment of Depression.* Springer Verlag, Berlin, Heidelberg, New York, Tokyo, 1986.

Sartory, G., Maurer, J.: Benzodiazepine: Entzugsprobleme und unterstützende Behandlung des Entzugs. *Psychol. Rundschau* **42**, 187–194, 1991.

Satel, S.L., Nelson, J.C.: Stimulants in the treatment of depression: a critical overview. *J. Clin. Psychiatry* **50**, 241–249, 1989.

Schacter, D.: EEG theta waves and psychological phenomena: a review and analysis. *Biol. Psychol.* **5**, 47–82, 1977.

Schafer, A.: The ethics of the randomized clinical trial. *N. Engl. J. Med.* **307**, 719–724, 1982.

Schaie, K.W.: The Seattle longitudinal study: A 21-year exploration of psychometric intelligence in adulthood. In: Schaie, K.W. (ed.): *Longitudinal Studies of Adult Psychological Development.* Guilford, New York, 1983, pp. 64–135.

Schatzberg, A.F., Cole, J.O., Blumer, D.P.: Speech blockage: A tricyclic side effect. *Am. J. Psychiatry* **135**, 600–601, 1978.

Schatzberg, A.F., Orsulak, P.J., Rosenbaum, A.H. *et al.*: Toward a biochemical classification of depressive disorders, V: Heterogeneity of unipolar depressions. *Am. J. Psychiatry* **139**, 471–475, 1982.

Schied, H.W.: Psychiatrische Indikationen der Therapie mit Neuroleptika. In: Langer, G., Heimann, H. (eds): *Psychopharmaka: Grundlagen und Therapie.* Springer, Wien/New York, 1983, pp. 259–279.

Schildkraut, J.J.: The catecholamine hypothesis of affective disorders: A review of supporting evidence. *Am. J. Psychiatry* **122**, 509–522, 1965.

Schindel, L.: Placebo und Placeboeffekte in Klinik und Forschung. *Arzneimittel-Forschung* **17**, 892–917, 1967.

Schmidtke, A.: Statistische Auswertungen von Psychopharmaka-Prüfstudien. In: Riederer, P., Laux, G., Pöldinger, W. (eds): *Neuropsychopharmaka*, Bd.1. Springer, Wien, 1992, pp. 177–199.

Schneider, P.J.: *Entwurf zu einer Heilmittellehre gegen psychische Krankheiten–oder Heilmittel in Beziehung auf psychische Krankheitsformen*. Tübingen, 1824.

Schöny, W., Rittmannsberger, H.: Praktische Durchführung, allgemeine Behandlungsrichtlinien. In: Riederer, P., Laux, G., Pöldinger, W. (eds): *Neuro-Psychopharmaka*, Bd. 4: Neuroleptika. Springer, Wien, 1992, pp. 130–152.

Schooler, N.R.: Maintenance medication for schizophrenia: strategies for dose reduction. *Schizophr. Bull.* **17**, 311–324, 1991.

Schooler, N.R., Hogarty, G.E.: Medication and psychological strategies in the treatment of schizophrenia. In: Meltzer, H.Y. (ed.): *Psychopharmacology: The Third Generation of Progress*. Raven, New York, 1987, pp. 1111–1119.

Schöpf, J.: Psychische Abhängigkeit bei Benzodiazepin-Langzeitbehandlung. *Nervenarzt* **56**, 585–592, 1985.

Schou, M.: Lithium prophylaxis: Myths and realities. *Am. J. Psychiatry* **146**, 573–576, 1989.

Schrenk, M.: *Über den Umgang mit Geisteskrankheiten*. Springer, Berlin/Heidelberg/New York, 1973.

Schuurman, T., van der Stay, F.J., Traber, J.: Tierstudien. In: Riederer, P., Laux, G., Pöldinger, W. (eds): *Neuro-Psychopharmaka*, Bd.1. Springer, Wien, 1992, pp. 67–82.

Schweizer, E., Rickels, K., Case, W.G., Greenblatt, D.J.: Long-term therapeutic use of benzodiazepines. II. Effects of gradual taper. *Arch. Gen. Psychiatry* **47**, 908–915, 1990.

Scott, A.I.F., Whalley, L.J.: The onset and rate of the antidepressant effect of electroconvulsive therapy. *Br. J. Psychiatry* **162**, 725–732, 1993.

Seemann, P.: Brain dopamine receptors. *Pharmacol. Rev.* **32**, 229–313, 1980.

Shader, R.I., Greenblatt, D.J.: Use of benzodiazepines in anxiety disorders. *N. Engl. J. Med.* **328**, 1398–1405, 1993.

Shagass, Ch.: Electrical activity of the brain. In: Greenfield, N.S., Sternbach, R.A. (eds): *Handbook of Psychophysiology*. Holt, Rinehart & Winston, New York, 1972, pp. 263–328.

Shalev, A., Munitz, H.: The neuroleptic malignant syndrome: agent and host interaction. *Acta Psychiatr. Scand.* **73**, 337–347, 1986.

Shapiro, A.K.: The placebo effect. In: Clark, W.G., del Giudice, J. (eds): *Principles of Psychopharmacology*. Academic Press, New York, 1978, pp. 441–459.

Sharpley, A.L., Gregory, C.A., Solomon, R.A., Cowen, P.J.: Slow wave sleep and 5-HT2 receptor sensitivity during maintenance tricyclic antidepressant treatment. *J. Affect. Disord.* **19**, 273–277, 1990.

Sharpley, A.L., Walsh, E.S., Cowen, P.J.: Nefazodone – a novel antidepressant – may increase REM sleep. *Biol. Psychiatry* **31**, 1070–1073, 1992.

Sibley, D.R., Monsma, F.J.: Molecular biology of dopamine receptors. *Trends Pharmacol. Sci.* **13**, 61–69, 1992.

Siever, L.J., Davis, K.L.: Overview: Toward a dysregulation hypothesis of depression. *Am. J. Psychiatry* **142**, 1017–1031, 1985.

Simons, A.D., Murphy, G.E., Levine, J.L., Wetzel, R.D.: Cognitive therapy and pharmacotherapy for depression. *Arch. Gen. Psychiatry* **43**, 43–48, 1986.

Simpson, G.M., Yadalam, K.: Blood levels of neuroleptics: State of the art. *J. Clin. Psychiatry* **46**, 22–28, 1985.

Smiley, A.: Effects of minor tranquilizers and antidepressants on psychomotor performance. *J. Clin. Psychiatry* **48** (Suppl. 12), 22–28, 1987.

Smith, J.M., Misiak, H.: Critical flicker frequency (CFF) and psychotropic drugs in normal human subjects: A review. *Psychopharmacology* **47**, 175–182, 1976.

Smythies, J.R.: Biochemistry and the schizophrenias. *Southern Med. J.* **72**, 1272–1277, 1979.

Snyder, S.H.: Neurotransmitters and CNS disease. Schizophrenia. *Lancet* **ii**, 970–974, 1982.

Song, F., Freemantle, N., Sheldon, T.A. *et al.*: Selective serotonin reuptake inhibitors: meta-analysis of efficacy and acceptability. *Br. Med. J.* **306**, 683–687, 1993.

Sotsky, St. M., Glass, D.R., Shea, M.T. *et al.*: Patient predictors of response to psychotherapy and pharmacotherapy: Findings in the NIMH treatment of depression collaborative research program. *Am. J. Psychiatry* **148**, 997–1008, 1991.

Spiegel, R.: Effects of amphetamines on performance and on polygraphic sleep parameters in man. In: Passouant, P., Oswald, I. (eds): *Pharmacology of the States of Alertness.* Pergamon, Oxford, 1979, pp. 189–201.

Spiegel, R.: On predicting therapeutic usefulness of psychotropic drugs from experiments in healthy persons. *Rev. Pure Appl. Pharmacol. Sci* **1**, 215–291, 1980.

Spiegel, R.: Increased slow-wave sleep in man after several serotonin antagonists. Sleep 1980. *5th Eur. Congr. Sleep Res.*, Amsterdam, 1980. Karger, Basel, 1981a, pp. 275–278.

Spiegel, R.: *Sleep and Sleeplessness in Advanced Age.* Advances in Sleep Research, Vol. 5, Spectrum, New York, 1981b.

Spiegel, R.: Aspects of sleep, daytime vigilance, mental performance and psychotropic drug treatment in the elderly. *Gerontology* **28** (Suppl. 1), 68–82, 1982.

Spiegel, R.: Effects of RS 86, an orally active cholinergic agonist, on sleep in man. *Psychiatr. Res.* **11**, 1–13, 1984a.

Spiegel, R.: Zur Voraussage des Therapieerfolgs mit Antidepressiva: Sind kurze REM-Latenzen diagnostisch und prognostisch zuverlässige Merkmale? *Fortschr. Neurol. Psychiatr.* **52**, 302–11, 1984b.

Spiegel, R.: *Einführung in die Psychopharmakologie.* Huber, Bern, 1988.

Spiegel, R.: *Psychopharmacology – an Introduction, second edition*, Wiley, Chichester, 1989.

Spiegel, R.: Cholinergic drugs, affective disorders and dementia: problems of clinical research. In: Müller, W.E., Berger, M., Spiegel, R. (eds): *Cholinergic Drugs, Affective Disorders and Dementia. Acta Psychiatr. Scand.* **83**, Suppl. 366, pp. 66–69, 1991.

Spiegel, R.: Zur prädiktiven Validität von Phase-I-Studien mit Anti-Demenz-Substanzen (Nootropika). In: Oldigs-Kerber, J., Leonard, J.P. (eds): *Pharmakopsychologie-experimentelle und klinische Agente.* G. Fischer, Jena, 1992, pp. 445–458.

Spiegel, R., Aebi, H.-J.: *Psychopharmakologie.* Kohlhammer, Stuttgart, 1981.

Spiegel, R., Aebi, H.J.: *Psychopharmacology: An Introduction.* Wiley, Chichester, 1983.

Spiegel R., Azcona, A., Morgan, K.: Sleep and its disorders. In: Pathy, S.J. (ed.): *Principles and Practice of Geriatric Medicine*, 2nd edn. Wiley, Chichester, 1991, pp. 253–264.

Spiegel, R., Devos, J.E.: Central effects of guanfacine and clonidine during wakefulness and sleep in healthy subjects. *Br. J. Clin. Pharmacol.* **10**, 165S–168S, 1980.

Spiegel, R., Dixon, K.: Psychotropic drug experiments in normal subjects: Their relation to animal studies and clinical trials. In: Spiegelstein, M.Y., Levy, A. (eds): *Behavioral Models and the Analysis of Drug Action.* Proc. 27th OHOLO Conf., Elsevier, Amsterdam, 1982, pp. 39–55.

Spiegelstein, M.Y., Levy, A. (eds): *Behavioral Models and the Analysis of Drug Action.* Proc. 27th OHOLO Conf., Elsevier, Amsterdam, 1982.

Spitzer, R.L.: Discussion of paper by Weissman *et al.* (1976). In: Spitzer, R.L., Klein, D.F. (eds): *Evaluation of Psychological Therapies.* Johns Hopkins University Press, Baltimore/London, 1976, pp. 178f.

Spitzer, R.L., Robins, E., Endicott, J.: Research diagnostic criteria: rationale and reliability. *Arch. Gen. Psychiatry* **35**, 773–782, 1978.

Squire, L.R.: Mechanisms of memory. *Science* **232**, 1612–1619, 1986.

Staehelin, J.E., Kielholz, P.: Largactil, ein neues vegetatives Dämpfungsmittel bei psychischen Störungen. *Schweiz. Med. Wschr.* **83**, 581–586, 1953.

Steardo, L., Barone, P., Monteleone, P., Iovino, M., Cardone, G.: Is the dexamethasone suppression test predictive of response to specific antidepressant treatment in major depression? *Acta Psychiatr. Scand.* **76**, 129–133, 1987.

Steimer, J.-L., Ebelin, M.-E., van Bree, J.: Pharmacokinetic and pharmacodynamic data and models in clinical trials. *Eur. J. Drug Metab. Pharmaco-Kinet.* **18**, 61–76, 1993.

Steinhausen, H.C., Kreuzer, E.M.: Learning in hyperactive children: are there stimulant-related and state-dependent effects? *Psychopharmacology* **74**, 389–390, 1981.

Sternbach, H.: The serotonin syndrome. *Am. J. Psychiatry* **148**, 705–713, 1991.

Sternbach, L.: The benzodiazepine story. In: Jucker, E. (ed.): *Progr. Drug Res.* Vol. 22. Birkhäuser, Basel, 1978, pp. 229–266.

Sternberg, D.E., Jarvik, M.: Memory functions in depression. *Arch. Gen. Psychiatry* **33**, 219–224, 1976.

Sternberg, D.E., Van Kammen, D.P., Lerner, D., Bunney, W.E.: Schizophrenia: dopamine-beta-hydroxylase activity and treatment response. *Science* **216**, 1423–1425, 1982.

Stoll, W.A.: Lysergsäure-Diäthylamid, ein Phantasticum aus der Mutterkorn-Gruppe. *Schweiz. Arch. Neurol. Psychiatr.* **60**, 279–323, 1947.

Subhan, Z., Harrison, C., Hindmarch, I.: Alprazolam and lorazepam single and multiple-dose effects on psychomotor skills and sleep. *Eur. J. Clin. Pharmacol.* **29**, 709–712, 1986.

Sulser, F., Vetulani, J., Mobley, Ph.L.: Mode of action of antidepressant drugs. *Biochem. Pharmacol.* **27**, 257–261, 1978.

Summers, W.K., Majovski, L.V., Marsh, G.M., Tachiki, K., Kling, A.: Oral tetrahydroaminoacridine in long-term treatment of senile dementia, Alzheimer type. *N. Engl. J. Med.* **315**, 1241–1245, 1986.

Sunderland, T., Tariot, P.N., Cohen, R.M. *et al.*: Anticholinergic sensitivity in patients with dementia of the Alzheimer type and age-matched controls. *Arch. Gen. Psychiatry* **44**, 418–426, 1987.

Suzman, M.M.: Use of ß-adrenergic receptor blocking agents in psychiatry. In: Palmer, G.C. (ed.): *Neuropharmacology of Central Nervous System and Behavioral Disorders*. Academic Press, New York, 1981, pp. 339–391.

Swanson, J.M., Kinsbourne, M.: Stimulant-related state-dependent learning in hyperactive children. *Science* **192**, 1354–1357, 1976.

Swazey, J.P.: *Chlorpromazine in Psychiatry*. MIT Press. Cambridge, MA, 1974.

Swire, F.M.M., Marsden, C.A., Barber, C., Birmingham, A.T.: Effects of a sedative and of a non-sedative H1-antihistamine on the event-related potential (ERP) in normal volunteers. *Psychopharmacology* **98**, 425–429, 1989.

Szasz, I.: Some observations on the use of tranquilizing drugs. *Arch. Neurol. Psychiatry* **77**, 86–92, 1957.

Szelies, B.,: Brain mapping zur Darstellung altersabhängiger Veränderungen in Abgrenzung von Demenz. *Nervenarzt* **63**, 609–618, 1992.

Tanimukai, H., Ginther, R., Spaide, J., Bueno, J.R., Hinwich, H.E.: Detection of psychotomimetic *N*, *N*-dimethylated indoleamines in the urine of four schizophrenic patients. *Brit. J. Psychiat.* **117**, 421–430, 1970.

Taylor, J.L., Tinklenberg, J.R.: Cognitive impairment and benzodiazepines. In: Meltzer, H.Y. (ed.): *Psychopharmacology: The Third Generation of Progress*. Raven, New York, 1987, pp. 1449–1454.

Tecce, J.J., Savignano-Bowman, J., Cole, J.O.: Drug effects on contingent negative variation and eyeblinks: The distraction–arousal hypothesis. In: Lipton, M.A., DiMascio, A., Killam, K.F. (eds): *Psychopharmacology: A Generation of Progress*. Raven, New York, 1978, pp. 745–758.

Thompson, C.: The use of high-dose antipsychotic medication. *Br. J. Psychiatry* **164**, 448–458, 1994.

Thompson, P.J.: Antidepressants and memory: A review. *Hum. Psychopharmacol.* **6**, 79–90, 1991.

Thompson, R.F.: The neurobiology of learning and memory. *Science* **233**, 941–947, 1986.

Tiller, J.W.G.: Antidepressants, alcohol and psychomotor performance. *Acta Psychiatr. Scand.* Suppl. 360: 13–17, 1990.

Tölle, R.: *Psychiatrie.* Springer, Berlin/Heidelberg/New York, 1985.

Tulving, E.: How many memory systems are there? *Am. Psychol.* **40**, 385–398, 1985.

Turner, P.: Drugs and the special senses. *Semin. Drug Treatm.* **1**, 335–353, 1971.

Uhlenhuth, E.H.: Depressives, doctors, and antidepressants. *JAMA* **248**, 1879–1880, 1982.

Uhlenhuth, E.H., DeWitt, H., Balter, M.B., Johanson, Ch.E., Mellinger, G.D.: Risks and benefits of long-term benzodiazepine use. *J. Clin. Psychopharmacol.* **8**, 161–167, 1988.

Uhr, L., Miller, J.C.: *Drugs and Behavior.* Wiley, New York, 1964.

Ulrich, G., Kriebitzsch, R.: Ein rechnergestütztes visuomotorisches Tracking-Verfahren zur trennscharfen Objektivierung zentralnervöser Pharmakaeffekte. *Arzneimittelforschung* **37**, 472–475, 1987.

Varga, E., Sugerman, A.A., Varga, V. *et al.*: Prevalence of spontaneous oral dyskinesia in the elderly. *Am. J. Psychiatry* **139**, 329–331, 1982.

Vestergaard, P., Poulstrup, I., Schou, M.: Prospective studies on a lithium cohort. *Acta Psychiatr. Scand.* **78**, 434–441, 1988.

Vogel, G.W., Buffenstein, A., Minter, K., Hennessey, A.: Drug effects on REM sleep and on endogenous depression. *Neurosci. Biobehavioral Rev.* **14**, 49–63, 1990.

Wardle, J.: Behaviour therapy and benzodiazepines: Allies or antagonists? *Br. J. Psychiatry* **156**, 163–168, 1990.

Ware, J.C., Pittard, J.T.: Increased deep sleep after trazodone use: a double-blind placebo-controlled study in healthy young adults. *J. Clin. Psychiatry* **51**, (Suppl.): 18–22, 1990.

Warner, K.E., Luce, B.R.: *Cost–benefit and cost-effectiveness analysis in health care: Principles, practice and potential.* Health Administration Press, Ann Arbor, MI, 1982.

Warot, D., Danjou, P., Lacomblez, L., Diquet, B., Puech, A.J.: Effets de trois doses de maprotiline (25, 50 et 75 mg) sur la vigilance et la mémoire chez le volontaire sain. *Thérapie* **44**: 257–261, 1989a.

Warot, D., Molinier, P., Lacomblez, L. *et al.*: Dose related effects of trimipramine on psychomotor function, memory, and autonomic nervous system activity in healthy volunteers. *Hum. Psychopharmacol.* **4**, 121–127, 1989b.

Warrington, S.J.: Clinical implications of the pharmacology of serotonin reuptake inhibitors. *Int. Clin. Psychopharmacol.* **7**, Suppl. 2, 13–19, 1992.

Weingartner, H.: Human state dependent learning. In: Ho, B.T., Richards, D.N., Chute, D.L. (eds): *Drug Discrimination and State Dependent Learning.* Academic Press, New York, 1978, pp. 361–382.

Weingartner, H.: Models of memory dysfunction. *Ann. NY Acad. Sci.* **444**, 359–369, 1985.

Weingartner, H., Silberman, E.: Models of cognitive impairment: Cognitive changes in depression. *Psychopharmacol. Bull.* **18**, 27–42, 1982.

Weingartner, H.J., Hommer, D., Lister, R.G., Thompson, K., Wolkowitz, O.: Selective effects of triazolam on memory. *Psychopharmacology* **106**, 341–345, 1992.

Weintraub, S., Mesulam, M.M.: Mental state assessment of young and elderly adults in behavioral neurology. In: Mesulam, M.-M. (ed.): *Principles of Behavioral Neurology, second edition.* Davis, Philadelphia, 1986, pp. 71–123.

Weiss, B., Laties, V.C.: Enhancement of human performance by caffeine and the amphetamines. *Pharmacol. Rev.* **14**, 1–36, 1962.

Weiss, G., Hechtman, L.T.: *Hyperactive Children Grown Up: Empirical Findings and Theoretical Considerations*. Guilford Press, New York, 1986.

Weissman, M.M.: Psychotherapy and its relevance to the pharmacotherapy of affective disorders: From ideology to evidence. In: Lipton, M.A., DiMascio, A., Killam, K.F. (eds): *Psychopharmacology: A Generation of Progress*. Raven, New York, 1978, pp. 1313–1321.

Weissman, M.M., Klerman, G.L., Paykel, E.S., Prusoff, B., Hanson, B.: Treatment effects on the social adjustment of depressed patients. *Arch. Gen. Psychiatry* **30**, 771–778, 1974.

Weissman, M.M., Prusoff, B.A., Di Mascio, A. *et al.*: The efficacy of drugs and psychotherapy in the treatment of acute depressive episodes. *Am. J. Psychiatry* **136**, 555–558, 1979.

Weissman, M.M., Jarrett, R.B., Rush, J.A.: Psychotherapy and its relevance to the pharmacotherapy of major depression: A decade later (1976–1985). In: Meltzer, H.Y. (ed.): *Psychopharmacology: The Third Generation of Progress*. Raven, New York, 1987, pp. 1059–1069.

Welkowitz, L.A., Papp, L.A., Cloitre, M. *et al.*: Cognitive-behavior therapy for panic disorder delivered by psychopharmacologically oriented clinicians. *J. Nerv. Ment. Dis.* **179**, 473–477, 1991.

Welner, A., Welner, Z., Robins, E.: Effect of tricyclic antidepressants on individual symptoms. *J. Clin. Psychiatry* **41**, 306–309, 1980.

Whalen, C.K., Henker, B., Collins B.E., Finck, D., Dotemoto, S.: A social ecology of hyperactive boys: Medication effects in structured classroom environments. *J. Appl. Behav. Anal.* **12**, 65–81, 1979.

WHO Guidelines: *Guidelines for the Clinical Investigation of Anxiolytic (Hypnotic, Antidepressant, Neuroleptic) Drugs*. World Health Organization, Regional Office for Europe, Copenhagen, 1985.

WHO: *The ICD-10 Classification of Mental and Behavioral Disorders. Clinical descriptions and diagnostic guidelines*. World Health Organization, Geneva, 1992.

Wiggins, J.G.: Would you want your child to be a psychologist? *Am. Psychol.* **49**, 485–492, 1994.

Wilens, T.E., Biederman, J.: The stimulants. *Psychiatr. Clin. North Am.* **15**, 191–222, 1992.

Wilson, W.W., Ban, T., Coleman, B., Vause, B., Papadatos, J.: The effects of clovoxamine on sleep in normal volunteers. *Drug Dev. Res.* **9**, 293–298, 1986.

Wirshing, W.C., Marder, S.R., van Putten, T., Ames, D.: Acute treatment of schizophrenia. In: Bloom, F.E., Kupfer, D.J. (eds): *Psychopharmacology: The Fourth Generation of Progress*. Raven Press, New York, 1995, pp. 1259–1266.

Wistedt, B., Jorgensen, A., Wiles, D.: A depot neuroleptic withdrawal study. *Psychopharmacology* **78**, 301–304, 1982.

Wittenborn, J.R.: Reliability, validity, and objectivity of symptom-rating scales. *J. Nerv. Ment. Dis.* **154**, 79–87, 1972.

Wittenborn, J.R.: Behavioral toxicity in normal humans as a model for assessing behavioral toxicity in patients. In: Lipton, M.A., DiMascio, A., Killam, K.F. (eds): *Psychopharmacology: A Generation of Progress*. Raven, New York, 1978, pp. 791–796.

Wittenborn, J.R.: Effects of benzodiazepines on psychomotor performance. *Br. J. Clin. Pharmacol.* **7**, 61–67, 1979.

Wittenborn, J.R.: Pharmacotherapy for age-related behavioral difficulties. *J. Nerv. Ment. Dis.* **169**, 139–156, 1981.

Wittern, R.: Die Geschichte psychotroper Drogen vor der Aera der modernen Psychopharmaka. In: Langer, G., Heimann, H. (eds): *Psychopharmaka: Grundlagen und Therapie*. Springer, Wien/New York, 1983, S. 3–19.

Woggon, B.: Neuroleptika-Absetzversuche bei chronisch schizophrenen Patienten. *Int. Pharmacopsychiatry* **14**, 34–56, 1979.

Woggon, B.: Prädiktoren für das Ansprechen bei Psychopharmaka. In: Riederer, P., Laux, G., Pöldinger, W. (HRSG): *Neuropsychopharmaka, Bd.I.* Springer, Wien, 1992, pp. 475–484.

Woggon, B.: Gibt es Antidepressiva, die bei bestimmten Depressionen speziell indiziert sind? *Schweiz. Med. Wochenschr.* **123**, 1312–1319, 1993.

Wolkowitz, O.M., Pickar, D.: Benzodiazepines in the treatment of schizophrenia: a review and reappraisal. *Am. J. Psychiatry* **148**, 714–726, 1991.

Wooley, D.W., Shaw, E.: A biochemical and pharmacological suggestion about certain mental disorders. *Proc. Nat. Acad. Sci. USA* **40**, 228–231, 1954.

Yesavage, J.A., Tinklenberg, J.R., Hollister, L.E., Berger, P.A.: Vasodilators in senile dementia. A review of the literature. *Arch. Gen. Psychiatry* **36**, 220–223, 1979.

Zametkin, A.J., Rapoport, J.L.: Noradrenergic hypothesis of attention deficit disorder with hyperactivity: A review. In: Meltzer, H.Y. (ed.): *Psychopharmacology: The Third Generation of Progress.* Raven Press, New York, 1987, pp. 837–842.

Zarkin, G.A., Grabowski, H.G., Mauskopf, J., Bannerman, H.A., Weisler, R.H.: Economic evaluation of drug treatment for psychiatric disorders: The new clinical trial protocol. In: Bloom, F.E., Kupfer, D.J. (eds): *Psychopharmacology: The Fourth Generation of Progress.* Raven Press, New York, 1995, pp. 1897–1905.

Zerssen, D. von: Beschwerden-Liste. In: *Internationale Skalen für Psychiatrie.* CIPS – Collegium internationale psychiatriae scalarum, Berlin, 1986a.

Zerssen, D. von: Bf-S (Befindlichkeits-Skala) In: *Internationale Skalen für Psychiatrie.* CIPS – Collegium internationale psychiatriae scalarum, Berlin, 1986b.

Zerssen, D. von, Koeller, D.-M., Rey, E.-R.: Die Befindlichkeits-Skala (B-S)-ein einfaches Instrument zur Objektivierung von Befindlichkeitsstörungen, insbesondere im Rahmen von Langsschnitt-Untersuchungen. *Arzneimittel-Forschung.* **20**, 915–918, 1970.

Zimmermann Tansella, Ch.: The long-term treatment with benzodiazepines: Suggestions for further research. *Int. Pharmacopsychiatry* **15**, 99–104, 1980.

Zung, W.W.K.: A self-rating depression scale. *Arch. Gen. Psychiatry* **12**, 63–70, 1965.

Index

Index compiled by C. Purton